3 P's:

Pathophysiology, Pharmacology, and Physical Assessment

Edited By:

Cathleen Crowley-Koschnitzki, DNP, CNM, WHNP-BC, FNP-C, PMHNP-BC

Cara Wallace, PhD, RN

Katie Kay, DNP, RN, PCCN-CMC

Kevin Letz, DNP, MBA, APRN, CNE, FNP-BC, ANP-BC, PNP-BC, FAANP

ACNPF.org

ISBN: 978-0-9714762-4-0

Contributions and Acknowledgements

Gulenia "GK" Rikabi, DNP, FNP-BC

Susan Sanner, PhD, APRN, FNP-BC

Kristina Martinez, DNP, RN-BC, ANP-BC, CRNP

Kelly Holben, DNP, APRN, FNP-BC, PMHNP-BC

Rhoda Murray, Ph.D, NP-C

Nancy Winters, PhD, RN, ANP-C

Shanna Chapman, DNP, APRN, FNP-C, FAANP

Omotolu Aje-Omokore, DNP, FNP, PMHNP

Katie Kay, DNP, RN, PCCN-CMC

Mindy Thompson, DNP, APRN, FNP-C, CNE

Pamela Porter, DNP, APRN, FNP-BC, CNS, PA-S

Patty Roof, EdD/CI, APRN, FNP-C, MSN/ED

Adrienne Small, DNP, FNP-C, CNE, CHSE

Michelle Krawczyk, DNP, ARNP-BC, CNE

Yvette T. Wilson, DNP, APRN, FNP-BC

Vannessa Davis, DNP, APRN, FNP-C, CNN

Cameron Duncan DNP, MS, APRN, FNP-C, PMHNP-BC

Shay A. Schroetter, DNP, APRN, ANP-BC

Cara Wallace, PhD, RN

Nicole Sinkler, DNP, MS, APRN, FNP-C

Mary Sizemore, DNP, APRN-FNP

Joel Regalado, DNP, ACNP-BC, CCRN-CMC, PCCN

Tracy Stogner, DNP, APRN, PMHCNS-BC

Susan A. Simmons, DNP, FNP-C

Alex Bahadori, DNP, MS, FNP-C

Dana Y. Preston, DNP, APRN, FNP-BC

Sherri Richardson, DNP, APRN-CNP

LaTonya Carroll, DNP, FNP-C, CPNP-PC

Nathalie Grant, EdD, APRN, ADM-BC

Tiney Ray, PhD, DNP, FNP-BC

Candice Phillips, PhD, RN, APRN, CNM, CNE

Diana Meeks PhD, RN, MSN, CS, CNE, NE-BC, FNP

Amanda Marshall, DNP, APRN, WHNP-BC

Cathleen Crowley-Koschnitzki, DNP, CNM, WHNP-BC, FNP-C, PMHNP-BC

Patricia D Bailey, PhD, MSN, CNP, CNE, CME

Angela Golden, DNP, FNP-C, FAANP

Kevin Letz, DNP, MBA, APRN, CNE, FNP-BC, ANP-BC, PNP-BC, FAANP

Claudia Griffin, DNP, MSN, CPNP, RN

Linda Wilson, DNP, FNP-C

Table of Contents

Chapter 1: HEENT

Conjunctivitis

Otitis

Rhinitis

Sinusitis

Pharyngitis

Diagnosis: Conjunctivitis

ICD-10 H10: Conjunctivitis

Claudia Griffin, DNP, CPNP

Pathophysiology

Conjunctivitis, known also as “pink eye”, is the inflammation of the thin membrane that covers the inside of the eyelids. There are three main types of conjunctivitis: allergic, viral, and bacteria.

Assessment

Subjective and Objective Data

The signs and symptoms of conjunctivitis depend on their type. For the allergic type, patients may have redness, itching, watery eyes (bilaterally). Viral symptoms include pinkness, swelling, watery eyes, which are sensitive to light (may occur in one or both eyes). The bacterial type includes red or pink eyes, pain, itching, green or yellow discharge, crusted eyes (occurs in mostly one eye).

Laboratory/Diagnostics

Conjunctivitis is diagnosed with presenting signs/symptoms and history.

Pharmacological Management

Eye drops may help with itching. Additionally, oral antihistamines may be used. Contagious conjunctivitis is often self-limiting so no treatment is needed. Contagious forms may need antibiotic eye drops; polymyxin B or erythromycin are common first line treatments.

Non-pharmacologic treatment includes limiting exposure to allergic triggers. Cool, wet compresses may also be beneficial. Patients should avoid using eye makeup and wearing contacts.

Special Considerations

Neonatal conjunctivitis occurs when an infant is exposed to bacteria in the birth canal or may have a blocked tear duct. Chlamydia trachomatis and Gonococcal conjunctivitis are the most common causes of neonatal conjunctivitis, which can result in blindness and could indicate an underlying systemic infection in the bloodstream, lining of the brain, or the spinal cord. Conjunctivitis is treated with oral antibiotics. Newborns are treated with erythromycin eye drops after they are born to help prevent conjunctivitis.

Chemical conjunctivitis can occur when a substance gets in the eye and could lead to redness or burning. The eyes can be flushed with water to remove the substance; however, depending on the substance, a referral to and ophthalmology may be required.

Referrals

Referral should be made to an ophthalmologist if conjunctivitis is not clearing up, the patient reports vision problems, or the pain intensifies.

Diagnosis: Acute Otitis Media (AOM)

Acute Infection of the Middle Ear

ICD-10 H65.0: Acute serous otitis media

Kevin Letz, DNP, MBA, APRN, CNE, FNP-BC, ANP-BC, PNP-BC, FAANP

Pathophysiology

AOM presents itself often after an upper respiratory infection or with forms of rhinitis whereas there is an increased amount of nasal draining and nasal congestion. This then leads to middle ear effusion making for a breeding ground for infections. Remember the eustachian tubes drain within the nasal cavity and the middle ear is closed off to the outer ear by the tympanic membrane. Infections can be both viral and bacterial and the more frequent bacterial infectious agents include *H. influenzae*, *S. pneumoniae*, and *S. aureus*.

Physical Assessment

Subjective Data

Ear pain is the most common complaint. This may manifest in children as ear tugging or rubbing. Other symptoms include hearing loss, draining if the drum is perforated, and fever in about a third of those with AOM. Younger children may present with only general fussiness or other nonspecific symptoms.

Objective Data

The assessment for AOM includes an otoscopic examination to visualize the tympanic membrane (TM). A normal TM is translucent, mobile, and intact; therefore, no aeration to the outer ear occurs. In AOM the TM can be erythematous (red), yellow, white, or opaque. The color alone, such as redness, does not necessarily indicate AOM as bulging can be seen, as well as immobility. Bulging of the drum is a better hallmark than redness. Decreased immobility, in and of itself, is not diagnostic without a constellation of findings.

Pharmacologic Management

The approach to treatment can be watchful observation or the use of oral antibiotics. Amoxicillin is typically the first line bacterial therapy in those without a penicillin allergy and those without recent beta-lactam treatment. Amoxicillin with clavulanate is used in cases of increased risk of resistance or for those who are unresponsive to amoxicillin. Algorithms and guidelines exist on unresolved cases along with those with penicillin allergy.

Pharmacologic pain management can include systemic agents such as acetaminophen and ibuprofen and/or topical agents including benzocaine and lidocaine which can be used in children older than two years old. Topical agents are not commonly used.

Complications

The most common complication is a ruptured TM. A more rare and severe complication would be an extension of the infection, which can occur with mastoiditis and meningitis.

Referrals

Recurrent or chronic AOM is typically referred to an otolaryngology (Ear, Nose, and Throat Specialist) or to an allergy specialist. Surgical intervention with TM tubes, treatment of chronic rhinitis, and prolonged antibiotics can be the next steps.

Diagnosis: Rhinitis

ICD-10 J30.9: Allergic rhinitis, unspecified

Claudia Griffin, DNP, CPNP

Pathophysiology

Rhinitis is an inflammation and swelling in the mucous membranes of the nose caused by an allergic reaction to allergen triggers; or it may be viral in nature. Rhinitis causes rhinorrhea, congested sounding speech, and mouth breathing due to nasal congestion and edema. The pathophysiology, assessment findings, and treatment for allergic and viral rhinitis are found in Table 1 below.

Table 1.1: Allergic and Viral Rhinitis

	Allergic Rhinitis	Viral Rhinitis
Pathophysiology	IgE Mediated in response to seasonal allergic triggers such as grass, pollens, and mold Persistent triggers include dust mites and animal dander	Most commonly caused by the adenovirus
Assessment	*Subjective symptoms*: • Rhinorrhea • Stuffiness • Sneezing • Itchy, watery eyes *Objective findings*: • Edematous Nasal turbinates	*Subjective symptoms*: • Headache • Occasional mild fever • Sneezing • Coughing • Sore throat *Objective findings*: • Edematous nasal turbinates and tonsillar edematous • Postnasal drip
Pharmacologic Treatment	Nasal corticosteroids, OTC antihistamines including oral and nasal sprays	OTC acetaminophen or ibuprofen to treat fever and pain Nasal decongestants for rhinorrhea
Non-Pharmacologic Treatment	Avoiding allergic triggers Nasal saline flushes	Nasal saline flushes Salt-water gurgle for sore throat

Diagnosis: Sinusitis

ICD-10 J01.90: Acute sinusitis, unspecified

Claudia Griffin, DNP, CPNP

Pathophysiology

Sinusitis is the inflammation of the tissues lining the sinuses. The sinuses produce more mucus when a viral infection starts in the lining of the sinuses. The body responds by producing more mucous and the sinuses are unable to drain the fluid due to the inflammation. The back up of fluid leads to an ideal environment for bacteria to grow.

Physical Assessment

Subjective Data

- Reports of a gradual onset, recurrent or chronic dull, constant pain over the affected sinuses.
- Can report retro orbital pain or tooth pain.
- Pain described as throbbing and worsens with coughing or sudden head movements, especially bending forward.
- Complaints can include nasal congestion, mucopurulent rhinorrhea, cough, pharyngitis and fatigue.
- May report cough due to pharyngeal drainage.

Objective Data

- Tenderness elicited over affected sinus
- Highly erythematous nasal mucosa

- Purulent nasal secretions noted on exam

Viral sinusitis: With viral sinusitis, symptoms last less than 7 days with consistent improvement.

***Bacteria sinusitis*:** Symptoms last greater than ten days or symptoms become worse after three to four days. Symptoms will be more severe and can include a fever above 102°F.

Pharmacologic Management

Viral Sinusitis

- OTC medications for symptom relief.
- Acetaminophen for patients with a fever
- Nasal decongestants for rhinorrhea.

Bacterial Sinusitis

Check for the most up-to-date clinical guidelines, which typically advise against the early use of antibiotics with symptoms less than 10-14 days.

First Line Treatment: Amoxicillin-clavulanate

Second Line/Penicillin Allergy: Doxycycline

Diagnosis: Acute Pharyngitis

ICD-10 J02.9: Acute pharyngitis, unspecified

Claudia Griffin, DNP, CPNP

Pathophysiology

Acute pharyngitis is one of the most common conditions found in outpatient clinical practices. Most cases are caused by respiratory viruses and are self-limited. Treatable disease does exist in a smaller percentage of patients in the form of group *A. streptococcus* (GAS), which is important for the practitioner to identify and treat appropriately given the associated complications.

Pathophysiology, Physical Assessment and Pharmacological Treatment

Table 2 below provides an overview of the pathophysiology, physical assessment and pharmacological treatment associated with allergic, viral, and bacterial pharyngitis.

Table 1.2: Pathophysiology, Physical Assessment and Pharmacological Treatment

	Pathophysiology	Physical Assessment	Pharmacological Treatment
Allergic	IgE mediated diseases in response to triggers Common triggers can be seasonal such as grass, pollens, and mold Persistent allergic triggers include dust mites and animal dander	*Subjective symptoms*: • Postnasal drip • Sneezing • Itchy, watery eyes • Sore throat *Objective findings*: • Bilateral injected conjunctiva, clear discharge • Pharynx: edema with minimal redness, clear	OTC antihistamines can be used including diphenhydramine, loratadine, cetirizine, and fexofenadine For throat pain, throat lozenges, acetaminophen, or ibuprofen can

		exudate	be used as needed
Viral	Common agents include human rhinovirus and adenovirus	*Subjective symptoms*: • Conjunctivitis • Cough • Hoarseness • Rhinorrhea • Occasional fever • Headache • Sore throat *Objective findings*: • Possible fever • Unilateral or bilateral injected conjunctiva • Pharynx; edematous, pale, boggy, slightly injected, no exudate	OTC antihistamines can be used including diphenhydramine, loratadine, cetirizine, and fexofenadine For fever and headaches, acetaminophen or ibuprofen can be used as needed For throat pain, throat lozenges, acetaminophen, or ibuprofen can be used as needed
Bacterial (AKA Strep Throat)	Group A beta-hemolytic streptococcus is caused by *S. pyogenes* *S. pyogenes* is transmitted primarily via saliva and droplets, making it highly contagious	*Subjective symptoms*: • Severe sudden onset sore throat • Headache • Nausea, vomiting *Objective findings*: • Fever > 101° F • Pharyngeal erythema and edema • Patchy pharyngeal exudate • Tonsil inflammation • Tender anterior cervical lymphadenopathy • Possible scarlatiniform rash • Positive rapid antigen detection test and/or	*Antibiotics*: • Penicillin V • For patients with a penicillin allergy, use Cephalexin OTC antihistamines can be used such as diphenhydramine, loratadine, cetirizine,

		culture of a throat swab	fexofenadine as needed For fever and headache, acetaminophen or ibuprofen can be used as needed For throat pain, throat lozenges, acetaminophen, or ibuprofen can be used as needed

Physical Assessment

Center criteria can help guide the decision to test for GAS; however, it should not replace testing nor be used to determine the need to treat patients with antibiotics.

Complications

A number of complications exist for GAS including acute rheumatic fever (ARF), poststreptococcal reactive arthritis (PSRA), scarlet fever, streptococcal toxic shock syndrome, acute glomerulonephritis, and pediatric autoimmune neuropsychiatric disorder associated with group *A. streptococci* (PANDAS).

Referrals

Chronic pharyngitis can be referred to otolaryngology or to allergy/immunology specialists.

Chapter 2: Musculoskeletal

Low Back Pain

Fractures

Osteoporosis

Rheumatoid Arthritis

Diagnosis: Low Back Pain

ICD 10 M54.5 Low back pain

Gulenia "GK" Rikabi, DNP, FNP-BC

Cathleen Crowley-Koschnitzki, DNP, CNM, FNP-C, PMHNP-BC

Pathophysiology

Low back pain (LBP) can occur due to changes or damages to the muscles, the ligaments, the spine, or the nerves. Most common low back pain involves the lumbar spine. Changes within any structure in the lumbar spine leads to secretion of cytokine that increases numbers of neutrophils forcing nerve fibers to grow into the injured area. The nerves fibers cause spinal nerve sensitivity and back pain. Changes in the lumbar area might be due to deterioration of the spine cartilage such as osteoarthritis, forced movement causing ligaments sprain or tear, muscles strain, or nerves compression by a spinal disc. Other possible changes are due to tumors such as hemangiomas, cancer, post-surgery infection, or an autoimmune disease such as ankylosing spondylitis.

Physical Assessment

Subjective Data

LBP can present differently in every patient. The assessment of back pain includes a focused history. A focused history on lower back pain includes onset of pain to establish an acute or chronic compliant. Location questions include whether pain is noted in the mid, right, or left side of the lumbar area. Duration of pain will establish constant or intermittent symptoms which characteristics will establish the type of pain and include any radiation. Ask about weakness in the lower extremities or referred pain to one or both legs. LBP can affect activities of daily living, inquire about barriers to bending, going up the stairs, sitting or standing for a long time.

Previous medical history should include any history of bone deformity such as scoliosis, osteoarthritis, herniated disk, sciatica or trauma from sports activities or falls. Assess for a history of long-term corticosteroid use, this can weaken ligaments causing a sprain or tear. Assess for family history of spinal degenerative disease.

Objective Data

Lumbar pain assessment includes:

- patient's weight- obesity can contribute to LBP.
- Inspection of the lower back with particular attention to the painful area. Assess for kyphosis and scoliosis.
- Assess skin for brusing, or rashes which can indicate shingles or contact dermatitis.
- Palpate skin temperature and assess pain, tenderness, or bruising.
- A positive straight leg test indicates sciatica

- A neuro exam for L1- L5: check for lower extremities strength, sensitivity to touch and reflexes. Any abnormalities can further differentiate a diagnosis.
- A positive costovertebral angle tenderness (CVAT) requires further assessment for nephrolithiasis and pyelonephritis.
- Loss of anal sphincter tone and significant motor deficits is indicative of cauda aquina.

Laboratory/Diagnostics

Imaging is not recommended in the first 6 weeks, only with specific indications such as severe or progressive neurological deficits or osteomyelitis.

- X-ray imaging-changes in spine such as arthritis, degenerative disease, fracture, scoliosis, or kyphosis.
- Magnetic Resonance Imaging (MRI)- most used to show any abnormalities such as sprain or strain, infection, tumors, disc disease or compression, or spine misalignment.
- Labs are not required unless the patient pain is unbearable, suspected vitamin D deficiency or swelling post-surgery to rule out infection. Labs include CBC and CRP to check for any sign of infection. Inflammation biomarkers such as cytokines which are elevated in spinal stenosis and herniated disc.

Pharmacological Management

First Line Treatment

National Institute of Neurological Disorders & Stroke (2020) recommends Tylenol as a first line of pain treatment. Nonsteroidal anti-inflammatory drug (NSAID) medications, and muscle relaxants.

- Acetaminophen (Tylenol)- an analgesic, excreted through urine. Half-life 2-4 hours. (Epocrates, 2021).
- Ibuprofen (Motrin)- a nonsteroidal antinflammatory, NSAIDS inhibits cyclooxygenase decreasing prostaglandin synthesis (Epocrates, 2021).
- Cyclobenzaprine (Flexeril)- a muscle relaxant, potentiates norepinephrine to bind to serotonin receptors decreasing muscle spasms. Excreted through urine. (Epocrates, 2021).

Do not prescribe opiates for acute back pain prior to a trial of first line treatment to prevent misuse, abuse and dependence.

Special Considerations

Elderly

The most common cause of low back pain in older adults might be due to degenerative disease, spinal stenosis, or spondylolisthesis. Acetaminophen (Tylenol) is the first line rcommendation for pain in the elderly. To avoid gastrointestinal bleeding and ulcer, aplastic or hemorrhagic anemia, hypertension or myocardial infarction caused by oral NSAIDS, Diclofenac sodium 1% gel

(Voltatren) is preferred. Ali et al. (2018) recommends serotonin-norepinephrine reuptake inhibitors such as venlafaxine for neuropathic or chronic pain in the elderly.

Pregnant women

Hormones during pregnancy cause the ligaments to soften, affecting spinal support. Additionally, the center of gravity moves forward where the baby weight is. The extra weight added during the pregnancy second and third trimester can stress the softened ligaments and muscles of the spine. Acetaminophen is safe to prescribe in pregnancy. Muscle relaxants can be prescribed for moderate to severe pain.

Pediatrics

Most common causes of back pain in pediatrics are scoliosis, muscle strain, trauma, kyphosis, and herniated disc. Back pain treatment in pediatric patients includes rest and minimal use of NSAIDs. If pain persists imaging is recommended.

Complications

Complications of LBP can include the following:

Cauda Equina Syndrome occurs due lumbar disc herniation that impairs nerve function. The syndrome causes sciatica, urinary retention, or incontinence. Inquire about patient's bowel or bladder dysfunction.

Referrals

Neurosurgeon if there's loss of function, numbness, weakness in any lower extremity, or nerve injury. Pain management if the pain is uncontrollable.

Diagnosis Fractures

ICD 10 S52 Fracture, the ICD 10 code varies based on fracture site.

Gulenia Rikabi, DNP, FNP-BC

Pathophysiology

A fracture is a break or a crack in the bone and may be direct or indirect. Direct injury to the bone may be due to physical abuse, a fall, trauma, or sports activities. Indirect injury may be caused by osteoporosis or the use of medications such as corticosteroids. Bone fractures range from a small crack in the bone called a stress fracture to a complete bone fracture, displacement or malalignment. With open fractures there are skin lacerations or abrasions. Closed fractures occur where the skin is intact.

Physical Assessment

Subjective Data

Patients might present with pain, weakness of the affected limb, swelling or deformity, or a history of numbness in the affected limb after the fracture occurred. . Patients may report the pain to be dull, intermittent, or constant; pain may be increased with severe edema of the affected limb. Patients might report an injury from a fall or sporting activity. Past medical history may include osteoporosis, knee instability, or an unsafe home environment (often for elderly patients). Family history includes low vitamin D_3 or osteoporosis.

Objective Data

Upon examination, identify the fracture location, assessing for tenderness, bruising, deformity, pain, warmth, or cold skin over the affected area.

Laboratory/Diagnostics

X-ray imaging can assist in ruling out a fracture, as well as identifying the type of fracture. The imaging might show displacement, fragmentation, misalignment, a hairline fracture, or edema. Labs are not required unless the pain is unbearable and severe swelling exists to rule out an infection and compartment syndrome. A CBC and CRP are used to check for signs of infection. An MRI might be needed if tendons or ligaments are affected.

Pharmacological Management

Pharmacological management depends on the severity, extent, and location of the fracture. Non-pharmacological management may include RICE (rest, ice, compression, elevation), splint, cast, surgery or a traction.

Acetaminophen (Tylenol) or Ibuprofen are most commonly used for mild to moderate pain. Tylenol is an analgesic, the mechanism of action for Tylenol is unknown; however, it has analgesic and antipyretic effects.

Narcotics such as hydrocodone can also be prescribed if the patient has severe pain as a result of an extended injury with an open fracture, fragmented bone; if the patient is postoperative surgery or if the bone is misaligned.

Hydrocodone/Acetaminophen (Vicodin), an opioid, binds to opioid receptors causing sedation and analgesia.

Special Considerations

Elderly patients may easily suffer a bone fracture due a deficiency in vitamin D3. Additionally, the elderly are at risk for falls or injury due to weakness, falls, osteoporosis, or decreased vision in the evening while going to the restroom.

Healthy pregnant women pain control should be determined based on severity of fracture. Tylenol is considered safe in pregnancy. Ibuprofen should be avoided within the third trimester of pregnancy.

Pediatric patients present with fractures of the digital forearm, tibia, ankle, clavicles, hand, and foot phalanges. Causes of pediatric fractures may be due to falls, physical abuse, or sports in high school.

Complications of Fractures

1. Loss of function
2. Compartment syndrome, swelling or an injury that blocks the blood supply to muscles and nerves
3. Deep vein thrombosis (DVT)
4. Bleeding that leads to joint edema and loss of function
5. Casting might lead to bone immobility, as well as foul smelling skin
6. Bone healing issues due to a deficiency of vitamin D3
7. Infection due to an open fracture or skin laceration

Referrals

Patients are referred to Orthopedics to evaluate and manage the extent of the fracture. A neurology consult might be need if the patient demonstrates loss of function, numbness or has nerve injury.

Diagnosis: Osteoporosis

ICD-10 M81.0: Age-related Osteoporosis without current pathological fracture

Susan Sanner, PhD, APRN, FNP-BC

Pathophysiology

Osteoporosis is a disorder of bone thinning in which bone absorption exceeds bone formation to the degree that bone density is insufficient to meet skeletal needs. In measureable terms, it is defined as bone density more than 2.5 standard deviations below the average bone mass for a healthy young adult. Bone is a dynamic tissue that is remodeled constantly throughout life. The arrangement of compact and cancellous bone provides strength and density that promotes mobility and protection. In adults, bone remodeling is the major metabolic skeletal process.

The two primary functions of bone remodeling in adults is to repair microdamage within the skeleton to maintain skeletal strength and to supply calcium when needed from the skeleton to maintain serum calcium. Remodeling can be activated by excessive stress put on the bone. Bone remodeling is also regulated by multiple hormones (estrogens, androgens, vitamin D and parathyroid hormone (PTH) and other locally produced growth factors. These factors control the rate at which new remodeling sites are activated. This process results initially in bone resorption by osteoclasts, followed by a period where new bone tissue is synthesized by osteoblasts. Estrogen deficiency is a major risk factor for the development of osteoporosis and is most common in postmenopausal women. This produces an imbalance between bone resorption and bone formation. The result is the thinning of the bone.

Physical Assessment

Subjective Data

Patients with osteoporosis are often asymptomatic until a fracture occurs. Back pain, with varying degrees of severity, might be reported. Patients might also experience a loss of height.

Objective Data

Patients may present with thoracic kyphosis, which is a rounding of the back. Height loss can be commonly found:

- Historical height loss >1.5 cm (difference between current height and peak height at age 20)
- Prospective height loss >2 cm (difference between current height and previously documented height)

Laboratory/Diagnostics

To diagnose osteoporosis, a dual-energy x-ray absorptiometry (DXA or DEXA) of the lumbar spine/hip is the gold standard.

Pharmacologic Management

Alendronate (Fosamax), a Bisphosphonate derivative, is the first line treatment for patients with osteoporosis. Alendronate inhibits bone resorption via actions on osteoclasts or on osteoclast precursors. It also decreases the rate of bone resorption, leading to an indirect increase in bone mineral density.

Special Considerations

Avoid alendronate in women with reproductive potential until more data is available regarding fetal safety.

Complications

Complications of osteoporosis include the following:

- Bone fractures
- Bone, joint, muscle pain
- Gastrointestinal mucosa irritation
- Hypocalcemia
- Ocular effects: conjunctivitis, uveitis, episcleritis
- Osteonecrosis of the jaw

Referrals

Patients with osteoporosis may be referred to orthopedics for follow-up.

Diagnosis: Rheumatoid Arthritis

ICD-10 M06.9: Rheumatoid Arthritis, unspecified

Susan Sanner, PhD, APRN, FNP-BC

Pathophysiology

Rheumatoid Arthritis (RA) is an autoimmune, systemic musculoskeletal disease that causes chronic inflammation in the synovial membranes and underlying cartilage, as well as the bone of multiple joints. Joints of the hands and feet are typically affected first. Larger joints can be involved anytime.

The synovial membrane is a thin layer of connective tissue that normally covers most articular surfaces, tendon sheaths and bursae and consists of two types of cells. Type A synoviocytes are derived from macrophages and Type B synoviocytes are derived from fibroblasts. The synovial fibroblasts are the most abundant and produce the structural components of joints (collagen, fibronectin, and laminin). Chronic inflammation causes structural damage to cartilage and bone by osteoclasts. They appear at the pannus-bone interface where they eventually form localized lesions where the synovial membrane inserts into the periosteal surface at the edges of bones close to the rim of articular cartilage and at the attachment sites of ligaments and tendon sheaths. Another form of bone loss is periarticular osteopenia that occurs in joints with active inflammation.

Physical Assessment

Subjective Data

RA patients may present with symmetrical joint stiffness, lasting approximately one hour, which worsens upon wakening, as well as joint pain and joint swelling. Patients may report symptoms such as malaise, anorexia, weight loss, and low-grade fevers.

Objective Data

Proximal Interphalangeal Joints:

- Fusiform swelling, pain, tenderness on palpation
- Swan neck deformities
- Boutonniere deformities
- Ligament instability
- Rheumatoid nodules

Metacarpophalangeal Joints:

- Swelling, pain and tenderness on palpation
- Flexion deformities
- Ulnar drift and subluxation

Wrists

- Dorsal swelling, pain, and tenderness
- Radial deviation
- Flexor tendon thickening with nodules

Laboratory/Diagnostics

Non-Specific Inflammatory Markers

- Erythrocyte Sedimentation Rate (ESR) – elevated
- C-Reactive Protein (CRP) - elevated
- Rheumatoid Factor (RF)
- Anti-cyclic citrullinated peptide (anti-CCP)
- IgM – found in 75-80% of patients with RA

Synovial Fluid Analysis

- WBC count in the range between 5000-50,000 WBC/μL
- Neutrophils

Joint Imaging

- Plain radiography can be used for diagnosis
- MRI and Ultrasound may be used in certain cases to guide clinical decision making

Pharmacologic Management

Methotrexate, a Disease Modifying Anti-Rheumatic Drug (DMARD), is the first line treatment for RA. Methotrexate inhibits DNA synthesis, repair, and cellular replication. Additionally, it irreversibly binds to and inhibits dihydrofolate reductase, inhibiting the formation of reduced folates, and thymidylate synthetase. This results in inhibition of purine and thymidylic acid synthesis which interferes with DNA synthesis repair and cellular replication.

Special Considerations

Methotrexate is contraindicated in pregnancy, may cause embryo-fetal toxicity and fetal death. Methotrexate is also contraindicated in alcoholism, alcoholic liver or other chronic liver disease and immunodeficiency syndromes. Methotrexate complications include acute renal failure, bone marrow suppression and neurotoxicity.

Referrals

Patients with RA may be referred to a rheumatologist for follow-up.

Chapter 3: Endocrine

Diabetes (Type 1, Type 2)

Hyperthyroidism

Hypothyroidism

Goiter

Cushing's Syndrome

Addison's Disease

Diagnosis: Diabetes Type 1 and Diabetes Type 2

ICD-10 E10.9: Diabetes Type 1 without complications

ICD-10 E11.9: Diabetes Type 2 without complications

Susan Sanner, PhD, APRN, FNP-BC

Pathophysiology

Diabetes Mellitus (DM) is a disorder of the endocrine pancreas and is defined by the presence of hyperglycemia due to a functional deficiency of insulin action. Deficient insulin action can result from 1) a decrease in insulin secretion by the beta cells of the pancreas, 2) a decreased response to insulin by target tissues (insulin resistance) and/or 3) an increase in the counter-regulatory hormones that oppose the effects of insulin. These three factors form the basis for the classification of diabetes into either Type 1 or Type 2.

Type 1 DM is characterized by the autoimmune destruction of pancreatic beta cells leading to a severe insulin deficiency. It is caused by the selective destruction of pancreatic beta cells by T- lymphocytes that results in islet cell inflammation and destruction. This occurs over time and therefore, beta cell destruction may not be recognized quickly. Islet cell antibodies (ICAs) appear early in the course of the disease and are thought to serve as markers of beta cell destruction.

Type 2 DM accounts for the majority of cases of DM and has a stronger genetic component than Type 1 DM. Insulin resistance is the hallmark of Type 2 DM. In the majority of cases, two metabolic defects are responsible for hyperglycemia: 1) target tissue resistance to the effects of insulin and 2) inadequate pancreatic beta cell insulin secretion in the setting of insulin resistance. Hyperglycemia will appear after a long, progressive decline in beta-cell function. Because individuals have varying amounts of residual insulin secretion that prevents severe hyperglycemia or ketosis early on, they may be asymptomatic and not diagnosed for several years after its onset when a fasting glucose is elevated on a routine screening test. Obesity is a major factor in the development of Type 2 DM with insulin resistance being the key factor that links obesity and Type 2 DM. Excess eating leads to increased free fatty acid storage as triglyceride in adipose tissue which is resistant to insulin.

Physical Assessment

Subjective Data

Depending upon the type of DM, patients will report different types of symptoms, as demonstrated in Table 3.

Table 3.1: Type 1 and Type 2 Diabetes Subjective Symptoms

Symptoms	**Type 1 DM**	**Type 2 DM**
Polyuria and thirst	Yes	Yes
Weakness or fatigue	Yes	Yes
Polyphagia with weight loss	Yes	No
Recurrent blurred vision	Yes	Yes
Vulvovaginitis or pruritis	Yes	Yes
Peripheral neuropathy	Yes	Yes
Often asymptomatic	No	Yes

Objective Data

Upon examination, objective data varies for patients with Type 1 or Type 2 DM. Type 1 DM objective findings include weight loss, blurred vision, loss of subcutaneous fat and muscle wasting, and postural hypotension. In contrast, Type 2 DM objective findings include overweight/obesity, local fat deposits on upper segment of the body (abdomen, chest, face, and neck), high weight circumference (men >40 inches; women >35 inches), acanthosis nigricans (dark discoloration of body folds and creases), and hypertension.

Laboratory/Diagnostics

The following laboratory and/or diagnostic tests may be ordered for patients with actual or suspected Type 1 or Type 2 DM:

- Urine glucose
- Urine ketones
- Fasting plasma or serum glucose (126 mg/dL or more) documented on more than one occasion
- Oral glucose tolerance test if fasting plasma glucose is less than 126 mg/dL)
- Glycated hemoglobin (HbA1C) measurements
- Serum Fructosamine
- Self-monitoring blood glucose

Pharmacologic Management

Insulins used in the treatment of Type 1 DM are classified as either short-acting, rapid onset of action, short-acting regular, intermediate-acting, and long-acting. The table below (see Table 4) depicts the variety of insulins available within these categories along with their onset, peak and duration. The nurse practitioner will consider the overall status of the patient as well as cost when determining the type of insulin prescribed.

Table 3.2: Type 1 DM Insulin

Insulin Type	Onset	Peak	Duration
Short-acting, rapid onset of action (lispro insulin solution Humalog)	15–30 min, give within 15 min or right after meals	30 min–2.5 hr.	3–6.5 hr.
Short-acting, rapid onset of action (aspart insulin solution NovoLog)	10–20 min, give 5–10 min before meals	1–3 hr.	3–5 hr.
Short-acting, rapid onset of action (insulin glulisine Apidra)	10–15 min, give within 15 min or right after meals	1–1.5 hr.	3–5 hr.
Rapid-acting inhaled (insulin human Afrezza)	15–30 min, administer at the beginning of a meal	~53 min	2.5–3 hr.
Short-acting regular Humulin R, Novolin R	30 min–1 hr.	2–3 hr.	4–6 hr.
Intermediate-acting (NPH Novolin N, Humulin N)	1–2 hr.	6–14 hr.	16–24 hr.
Long-acting (insulin glargine solution ,Lantus, Toujeo)	Clinical effect about 1 hr. after injection	None	≥24 hr.

Long-acting (insulin detemir solution Levemir)	Approximately 1–2 hr.	6–8 hr. (minimal peak)	Dose dependent; 12 hr. for 0.2 units/kg, 20 hr. for 0.4 units/kg Albumin bound
Long-acting (insulin degludec Tresiba)	Unknown, not stated in product information	~12 hr.	At least 42 hr. (after the last dose of a series of 8 once-daily doses)

When treating patients with Type 2 DM, there are a variety of drug classifications available (see Table 3.3).

Table 3.3: Type 2 DM Drugs

Drug Classification	Mechanism of Action	Daily Dose	Duration of Action
Sulfonylureas Glipizide	Stimulates insulin release from the pancreatic beta cells; reduces glucose output from the liver; insulin sensitivity is increased at peripheral target sites	2.5–40 mg as a single dose or in two divided doses 30 minutes before meals	6–12 hours
Meglitinide Analogs Repaglinide (Prandin)	Blocks ATP-dependent potassium channels, depolarizing the membrane and facilitating calcium entry through calcium channels. Increased intracellular calcium stimulates insulin release from the pancreatic beta cells.	0.5 to 4 mg three times a day before meals	3 hours
Biguanides Metformin (Glucophage)	Decreases hepatic glucose production, decreases intestinal absorption of glucose and improves insulin sensitivity by increasing peripheral glucose uptake and utilization	1–2.5 g; 1 tablet with meals two or three times daily	4 hours
Thiazolidinediones Pioglitazone (Actos)	Improves target cell response to insulin, without increasing pancreatic insulin secretion.	15–45 mg daily	Up to 24 hours

GLP-1 Receptor Agonists Dulaglutide (Trulicity)	Is an agonist of human glucagon-like peptide-1 (GLP-1) receptor and augments glucose dependent insulin secretion and slows gastric emptying.	0.75 mg subcutaneously once weekly. Dose can be increased to 1.5 mg if necessary.	1 week
DPP-4 Inhibitors Saxagliptin (Onglyza)	Inhibits dipeptidyl peptidase IV (DPP-IV) enzyme resulting in prolonged active incretin levels. Incretin hormones regulate glucose homeostasis by increasing insulin synthesis and release from pancreatic beta cells and decreasing glucagon secretion from pancreatic alpha cells.	2.5 mg or 5 mg once daily. CrCl ≤ 50 mL/min or if also taking drugs that are strong CYP3A4/5 inhibitors such as ketoconazole: 2.5 mg daily.	24 hours
SGLT2 Inhibitors Empagliflozin (Jardiance)	Inhibits sodium-glucose cotransporter 2 (SGLT2) in the proximal renal tubules which reduces reabsorption of filtered glucose from the tubular lumen. The result is a lowered renal threshold for glucose which results in increased urinary excretion of glucose leading to reduced plasma glucose concentrations.	10 mg daily. 25-mg dose can be used if necessary.	24 hours

Special Considerations

The incidence of diabetes in pregnancy is increasing. Preconceptual counseling should include the need for maintaining normal glucose levels in pregnancy. Risks of diabetes (hyperglycemia) in pregnancy include spontaneous abortion, fetal anomalies, fetal demise, and macrosomia. Infants born to diabetic mothers have risk for neonatal hypoglycemia, respiratory distress, and hyperbilirubinemia. Women are at higher risk of death from cardiovascular disease and are more likely to die following a myocardial infarction; therefore, they must be treated aggressively to achieve glycemic targets. In the elderly, co-morbid conditions in addition to diabetes must be adequately managed to avoid compounding the effects of diabetes on other body systems.

Complications of DM

Patients with Type 1 or Type 2 DM may experience some of the following complications as the result of their disease process.

Ocular Complications

- Diabetic cataracts
- Diabetic retinopathy
- Glaucoma
- Diabetic nephropathy
- Diabetic neuropathy
- Peripheral neuropathy

Autonomic Neuropathy

- Nausea, vomiting, dysphagia
- Gastric reflux
- Constipation, diarrhea
- Delayed gastric emptying
- Incomplete emptying of the bladder
- Erectile dysfunction

Cardiovascular Complications

- Hypertension
- Peripheral vascular disease

Skin and Mucous Membrane Complications

- Gangrene
- Diabetic ulcers

Bone and Joint Complications

- Progressive joint stiffness
- Carpal tunnel syndrome
- Gout
- Bursitis

Referrals

Patients with Type 1 or Type 2 DM should be referred to an endocrinologist for consultation and initial management. Nurse practitioners can continue treatment in consultation with the endocrinologist.

Diagnosis: Hyperthyroidism

ICD-10 E05.00: Thyrotoxicosis (hyperthyroidism)

Susan Sanner, PhD, APRN, FNP-BC

Pathophysiology

Hyperthyroidism (thyrotoxicosis) is an autoimmune disorder that affects the thyroid gland. It is characterized by an increase in the synthesis and release of thyroid hormones. The autoantibodies involved are thyroid-stimulating immunoglobulins (TSI) or thyroid-stimulating hormone (TSH) receptor antibodies. These receptor antibodies bind to the TSH receptor in thyroid cell membranes and stimulate the gland into a hyperfunction state. Major etiologies of thyrotoxicosis are hyperthyroidism caused by Graves' disease, toxic multinodular goiter, and toxic adenomas.

Physical Assessment

Subjective Data

Patients with hyperthyroidism may experience various signs and symptoms such, including:

- Hyperactivity, irritability, dysphoria
- Heat intolerance and sweating
- Palpitations
- Fatigue and weakness
- Weight loss and increased appetite
- Diarrhea
- Polyuria
- Oligomenorrhea, loss of libido

Objective Data

Upon examination, patients with hyperthyroidism may demonstrate:

- Tachycardia; atrial fibrillation in the elderly
- Tremor
- Goiter
- Warm, moist skin
- Muscle weakness, proximal myopathy
- Lid retraction or lag
- Gynecomastia

Laboratory/Diagnostics

The following laboratory and/or diagnostic testing may be useful in the diagnosis of hyperthyroidism:

- TSH (suppressed)
- Free T4 (FT4) (elevated)
- Free T3 (FT3) (elevated)
- T4 (elevated)
- Thyroid-stimulating immunoglobulins (TSHrAb) detectable
- Antithyroperoxidase or antithyroglobulin antibodies elevated by non-specific
- Serum antinuclear antibodies elevated
- Hypercalcemia, hypokalemia, hypophosphatemia

- Increased liver enzymes
- Increased alkaline phosphatase
- Anemia
- Radioisotope Uptake and imaging
- Thyroid ultrasound
- MRI or CT scanning

Pharmacologic Management

An antithyroid agent, methimazole, is the first line treatment for patients with hyperthyroidism. Methimazole inhibits the synthesis of thyroid hormones by blocking the oxidation of iodine in the thyroid gland; blocks synthesis of thyroxine and triiodothyronine (T_3); does not inactivate circulating T_4 and T_3.

There are special considerations when prescribing methimazole, as it crosses the placenta. Birth defects have been observed in neonates exposed to maternal methimazole in the first trimester of pregnancy and include anomalies of the upper gastrointestinal tract (esophageal atresia or tracheoesophageal fistula), respiratory tract (choanal atresia), skin (aplasia cutis), and facial dysmorphism.

Complications

Complications of hyperthyroidism include:

- Bleeding
- Bone marrow suppression
- Dermatologic reactions

- Fever
- Hepatic effects
- Hypothyroidism
- Lupus-like syndrome
- Vasculitis

Referral

Patients with hyperthyroidism may be referred to an endocrinologist for follow up.

Diagnosis: Hypothyroidism

ICD-10 E03.9: Hypothyroidism

Susan Sanner, PhD, APRN, FNP-BC

Pathophysiology

Hashimoto thyroiditis is the most common cause of hypothyroidism. It is characterized by marked lymphocytic infiltration of the thyroid that leads to atrophy of the thyroid follicles accompanied by oxyphil metaplasia, absence of colloid and mild to moderate fibrosis. Thyroid cell destruction is primarily mediated by the CD8+ cytotoxic T cells. Local production of cytokines such as tumor necrosis factor (TNF), interleukin-1 (IL-1) and interferon y (IFN-y), renders the thyroid cells more susceptible to apoptosis. Cytokines (HLA class I and class II molecules) also impair thyroid cell function directly. Antibodies to TPO and thyroglobulin (Tg) are clinical markers of thyroid autoimmunity.

Physical Assessment

Subjective Data

Patients with hypothyroidism may experience a variety of symptoms, including:

- Weight gain
- Fatigue, lethargy
- Depression
- Weakness
- Dyspnea on exertion

- Arthralgias or myalgias
- Muscle cramps
- Menorrhagia
- Constipation
- Dry skin
- Headache
- Paresthesias
- Cold intolerance
- Carpal tunnel syndrome
- Raynaud's phenomenon

Objective Data

Upon physical examination, patients with hypothyroidism may exhibit:

- Bradycardia
- Diastolic hypertension
- Thin, brittle nails
- Thinning of hair
- Peripheral edema
- Puffy face and eyelids
- Skin pallor or yellowing
- Delayed relaxation of deep tendon reflexes
- Palpable thyroid goiter

Laboratory/Diagnostics

A thyroid-stimulation hormone (TSH) may be elevated; however, note that reference ranges may vary. FT4 The amount of free thyroxine, or FT4, in the blood may be low or normal. Diagnostic imaging is usually not indicated but can reveal a retrosternal goiter.

Pharmacologic Management

Levothyroxine (T_4), a thyroid product, is the first line treatment for patients with hypothyroidism. Levothyroxine is a synthetic form of thyroxine, an endogenous hormone secreted by the thyroid gland. T_4 is converted to its active metabolite, L-triiodothyronine (T_3). Thyroid hormones (T_4 and T_3) then bind to thyroid receptor proteins in the cell nucleus and exert metabolic effects through control of DNA transcription and protein synthesis; involved in normal metabolism, growth, and development; promotes gluconeogenesis, increases utilization and mobilization of glycogen stores, and stimulates protein synthesis, and increases basal metabolic rate.

Special Considerations

Levothyroxine has not been shown to increase the risk of congenital abnormalities or miscarriage. Maternal hypothyroidism, however, can be associated with adverse effects in the mother and fetus, including spontaneous abortion, stillbirth, premature birth, low birth weight, impaired neurocognitive development in the offspring, abruptio placentae, gestational hypertension, and preeclampsia. Due to alterations of endogenous maternal thyroid hormones, hypothyroid patients treated with levothyroxine prior to pregnancy require a dose increase as soon as pregnancy is confirmed. Levothyroxine is to be avoided in postmenopausal women, elderly patients, patients with cardiovascular disease, osteoporosis, large thyroid nodules, or long-standing goiters, or low-normal TSH levels

Complications

Complications associated with hypothyroidism include:

- Adrenal insufficiency
- Benign thyroid nodules
- Cardiovascular disease
- Diabetes
- Osteoporosis
- Sub-acute thyroiditis

Referral

Patients with hypothyroidism may be referred to an endocrinologist for follow up.

Diagnosis: Goiter

ICD-10 E04.9 Nontoxic goiter, unspecified

Kristina Martinez, DNP, RN-BC, ANP-BC, CRNP

Pathophysiology

An abnormal growth in the thyroid gland is referred as goiter. However, the presence of a goiter does not always mean there is a malfunction of the thyroid gland. A goiter can occur in euthyroidism, hyperthyroidism or hypothyroidism.

Common Causes

Hashimoto's thyroiditis (chronic autoimmune thyroiditis) is the predominant cause of a goiter in United States. This results in an increase in thyroid stimulating hormone (TSH) secretion from thyroid failure.

Grave's disease is an autoimmune disorder where thyrotropin receptor immunoglobulins (thyroid-stimulating antibodies [TSab]) activate the TSH receptors on the surface of thyroid cells and trigger synthesis of excess thyroid hormone and growth (causing a diffuse goiter).

Multinodular goiters are common in older adults. Multiple nodules are either toxic or nontoxic. Toxic Multinodular Goiter (Plummer Disease) are prevalent among middle aged and elderly persons. It is often associated with a long-standing simple goiter which results from diffuse hyperplasia of thyroid follicular cells whose activity is independent of TSH regulation.

Nontoxic multinodular goiter refers to a nodular goiter not associated with increased thyroid hormone production. The nodules are composed of a great deal of fibrous tissue and often do not shrink much.

Physical Assessment

Subjective Data

- If due to Hashimoto's thyroiditis or severe iodine deficiency, symptoms of hypothyroidism such as cold intolerance, fatigue, constipation may be present
- If due to a multinodular goiter or Grave's disease, symptoms of hyperthyroidism such as palpitations, dyspnea on exertion and unexplained weight loss may be present
- Exertional dyspnea is common in patients with obstructive cervical or substernal goiter

Objective Data

- Thyroid may become nodular and very large
- Tracheal deviation may be visible or palpable if the goiter is symmetric

Laboratory/Diagnostics

- Thyroid function test: TSH. When TSH value is decreased, it should be followed by free thyroxine (FT4) and free triiodothyronine (FT3)
- Thyroid ultrasound
- Thyroid Peroxidase (TPO) antibodies if TSH values are increased

- Fine-needle aspiration biopsy is indicated if there is a history of rapid growth, pain or tenderness

Management

For a nontoxic nodular goiter, use observation with monitoring, thyroidectomy, radioiodine (option for patients who have nontoxic benign goiters that continue to grow or prefer to avoid surgery). With benign nodules, levothyroxine (LT4) is not recommended. Levothyroxine should be considered in Hashimoto's thyroiditis patients with elevated serum TSH levels. Treatment with thyroid hormone may reduce the size of the goiter. Levothyroxine is a synthetic thyroxine (T4) which is converted to an active metabolite, L-triiodothyronine (T_3). Thyroid hormones (T_4 and T_3) then bind to thyroid receptor proteins in the cell nucleus and exert metabolic effects through control of DNA transcription and protein synthesis. Grave's Disease is treated with antithyroid drugs, radioiodine, or surgery.

Surgery (total or subtotal thyroidectomy) is primarily indicated in patients who have an obstructive goiter or a very large goiter; in patients with moderate to severe, active orbitopathy who desire definitive therapy for their hyperthyroidism; in pregnant women who are allergic to antithyroid drugs; and in patients who have allergies or poor compliance on antithyroid drugs but refuse radioiodine. Surgery would also be indicated if there was a coexisting suspicious or malignant thyroid nodule or primary hyperparathyroidism.

Pharmacological management

Antithyroid drugs (thionamides) such as Methimazole 15-60mg/d can be used depending on the severity. Methimazole inhibits the synthesis of thyroid hormones by blocking the oxidation of iodine in the thyroid gland; Methimazole has better compliance rate due to once-daily dosing and is less toxic.

Radioiodine (RAI), a thyrotoxic isotope of iodine that emits radiation) is administered as a capsule or, less commonly, an oral solution of sodium iodine-131 (I-131), which is rapidly absorbed from the GI tract and concentrated in thyroid tissue. Radioiodine induces extensive tissue damage, resulting in ablation of the thyroid within 6 to 18 weeks. RAI should not be used during pregnancy.

Special Considerations

Thyroid problems during pregnancy can lead to miscarriage, preterm delivery, low birth weight and intellectual problems in the newborn. Clients who ingest RAI must follow radiation precautions to limit radiation exposure to other people.

Complications

Large goiters may cause compression of the trachea, with tracheomalacia and asphyxiation. Autoimmune goiters may develop lymphoma. Nodular goiters may cause pain, intramodular necrosis, and hemorrhage.

Referrals

If a solitary nodule is detected in a clinically euthyroid patient, a referral to perform fine needle biopsy should be made. Referral to an endocrinologist can be made for hyperthyroidism, enlarging goiter, suspicious nodules

Diagnosis: Cushing's Syndrome

ICD-10 E24.9: Cushing's syndrome, unspecified

Kristina Martinez, DNP, RN-BC, ANP-BC, CRNP

Pathophysiology

Cushing's syndrome refers to manifestations of excessive corticosteroids as a result of corticosteroid drugs. Cushing's disease is caused by pituitary corticotropin (ACTH)-secreting tumors.

Physical Assessment

Subjective Data:

- Fatigue and reduced endurance
- Muscle atrophy causes weakness, with difficulty standing up from a seated position or climbing stairs
- Oligomenorrhea or amenorrhea in women, erectile dysfunction in men
- Backache, headache

Objective Data:

- Truncal obesity with reddish purple cutaneous striae over the abdomen and other parts
- Dryness and pigmentation of the skin and fragility of skin vessels
- Excessive facial hair and baldness
- Cyanosis and mottling of the skin of the extremities
- Osteoporosis

- Thoracic kyphosis
- Proximal muscular weakness
- Hypertension
- glycosuria

Laboratory/Diagnostics

- Late night salivary cortisol (two measurements)
- 24-hour urinary free cortisol excretion (two measurements)
- Overnight 1 mg dexamethasone suppression test (DST)
- MRI with and without contrast for suspicion of brain tumor

Pharmacologic Management

Adrenal Enzyme Inhibitors

Ketoconazole

Ketoconazole inhibits the first step in cortisol biosynthesis. It also inhibits ACTH secretion. Dosing is 200 to 400mg two to three times a day. Ketoconazole is not the treatment of choice during pregnancy.

Metyrapone

Metyraprone is a 11-beta-hydroxylase (P450c11) inhibitor that blocks the final step in cortisol biosynthesis. A dose of 500 to 750 mg three or four times a day is usually required in these patients. Metyrapone has also been used in pregnancy but its efficacy is unclear.

Adrenolytic Agent

Mitotane

Mitotane is an adrenocorticolytic drug that is used primarily for the treatment of adrenal carcinoma. It has a direct cytotoxic action on the adrenal cortex. Dosing is 1 to 3 g per day. Mitotane should not be prescribed to pregnant women.

Dopamine Agonist

Cabergoline

Caberogline is a dopamine agonist with a high affinity for the dopamine receptor type 2, which is expressed by most corticotroph adenomas and is prescribed to treat hyperprolactinemia.

Glucocorticoid Receptor-Directed Treatment

Mifepristone

Can be used therapeutically as an antiprogestin (i.e., for the treatment of endometriosis and uterine myomas). Dosage is 300-1200 mg per day. Mifepristone, at much higher doses, can be used as a glucocorticoid receptor antagonist.

Pasireotide

Pasireotide is a somatostatin receptor (SST) agonist that binds to 4 of the 5 SST subtypes with substantially higher affinity for SST1 and SST5 than octreotide or lanreotide. Corticotroph tumors have a high expression of SST4, and pasireotide decreases ACTH secretion and cell proliferation in cultured human corticotroph tumors.

Additional Management

Management of Cushing's can also include transsphenoidal microadenomectomy and pituitary irradiation. Management for Cushing's syndrome due to exogenous therapy is stopping the use of glucocorticoids.

Complications

Complications associated with Cushing's syndrome includes osteoporosis, infection, pulmonary thromboembolism, cardiovascular complications, mood, and cognitive impairment.

Referrals

Patients with Cushing's syndrome should be referred to an endocrinologist for follow-up and management.

Diagnosis: Addison's Disease

ICD-10 E27.1: Primary adrenocortical insufficiency

Kelly Holben, DNP, APRN, FNP-BC, PMHNP-BC

Introduction

Addison's disease is considered rare, affecting 1 in 100,000 people in the United States and effects men and women equally (New, 2018). Prevalence is an estimate, since the disease tends be under and undiagnosed (New, 2018). 75% of Addison's disease cases are from an autoimmune reaction, which damages the adrenal glands. Addison's disease was first discovered by Dr. Thomas Addison in 1855 after describing the symptoms and on autopsy found that the "suprarenal capsules are diseased" (Bishop, 1950).

Pathophysiology

There are primary, secondary, and tertiary causes of adrenal insufficiency. Initially, there is adrenal failure that results in decreased cortisol production then a decrease of aldosterone. This econdition will cause an increase in adrenocorticotropic hormone (ACTH) and a rise in plasma renin levels due to the loss of the negative feedback loop (Munir & Wassem, 2020). If caused by autoimmunity, the wasting of the adrenals is a progressive asymptomatic process, the subclinical prodromal stage can last years (Nieman, 2019). Antibodies, lymphatic and endocrine deficiencies are usually present (Nieman, 2019).

There are four stages for adrenal insufficiency which are:

1. High plasma renin activity and normal to low aldosterone

2. Impaired serum cortisol response to cosyntropin stimulation
3. Increased morning ACTH and normal serum cortisol
4. Low morning cortisol (Nieman, 2019).

The autoantibodies associated with autoimmune adrenal insufficiency attack the CYP21A2 gene , which results in a high concentration of autoantibodies in the blood stream and has a strong association to the magnitude of renal insufficiency. Clinical symptoms will not be noticed until at least 90% of the adrenal cortex is destroyed. This is the damage to the zona fasciculata, which secretes cortisol and zona glomerulosa which secrete aldosterone and are the outermost layers of the adrenal gland. Primary adrenal insufficiency occurs when the production of cortisol and aldosterone are no longer produced by the adrenal cortex. 75% of the cases of primary adrenal insufficiency is caused by an autoimmune reaction that is idiopathic (Neiman, 2018; Barthel, Willenberg, Gruber, Bornstein, 2019; New, 2019; Munir & Wassem, 2020),

In secondary adrenal insufficiency there is dysfunction of the hypothalamus and pituitary gland. This is characterized by a decrease in cortisone, low to normal ACTH concentration, and normal aldosterone. This is due to the adrenal gland not being affected, but the pituitary gland. Aldosterone is regulated the renin-angiotensin system that works independently of the hypothalamus and pituitary (Barthel, Willenberg, Gruber, Bornstein, 2019). There are other causes of secondary adrenal insufficiency and depending on if there is pituitary involvement or interruption ACTH. Drugs that can cause secondary adrenal insufficiency are high dose progestins (megestrol acetate, medroxyprogesterone, and opioids) (Neiman, 2018; Barthel, Willenberg, Gruber, Bornstein, 2019).

In tertiary adrenal insufficiency there are causes that are due to hypothalamic abnormalities which decrease the corticotropin-releasing hormone (CRH) which suppresses ACTH. Those on chronic high-dose glucocorticoid therapy, however, normal doses can also suppress CRH synthesis and secretion when there is drug-drug interaction with medications such as fluticasone or ritonavir (Neiman, 2018).

Physical Assessment

Subjective Data:

- Fatigue is noted in 84-95% of the patients most non-specific complaint along with GI complaints.
- Weight loss 66-76% can be from anorexia mainly, however, dehydration can also be a cause, major weight loss may not be seen until advance adrenal failure
- Salt craving 38-64% such as drinking pickle juice
- GI complaints: such as nausea, vomiting, abdominal pain 49-62%
- Reproductive issues: decreased axillary and pubic hair along with loss of libido with 25% with amenorrhea and autoimmune-mediated primary ovarian insufficiency; men less so since androgen production is mainly in the testes.

- Musculoskeletal issues: muscle and joint pain 35-40%; myalgia and arthralgia, which will correct with glucocorticoid and mineralocorticoid replacement, and some with contracture which will require orthopedic measures to correct
- Psychiatric issues: Depression noted in 20-40% with amotivation and anhedonia; psychosis in 20-40% noted as social isolation, negativism irritability, agitation, poor judgement, 40% hallucinate, and about 85 with catatonia, paranoid and bizarre behavior. Anxiety is noted in about 24%; Mania is noted in about 12%; disorientation in about 20%. Organic brain syndrome is seen in about 5-20% and can range from mild to moderate as well as changes in memory that precede confusion, delirium, and stupor. Psychiatric symptoms are noted early in Addison's and before other symptoms which makes this difficult to diagnose. Improvement is not noted with correction of medical interventions such as correcting hyponatremia. Psychosis can last for months and many symptoms will resolve with steroid use.
- Hypotension: seen as postural dizziness and hypotension and syncope. The aldosterone deficiency will contribute to volume depletion. Glucocorticoids are needed for epinephrine that is derived from the adrenal medullary cortex. Hypertension is a rule out for adrenal insufficiency.

- Hyperpigmentation: The most characteristic finding in all those with adrenal insufficiency and is noted in all patients with primary adrenal insufficiency not seen in secondary. The hyperpigmentation is most noted in areas exposed to the sun and to continual friction. There is an increase in melanin syntheses causing the hyperpigmentation. Hair and nails become darker and nails have longitudinal lines noted. Freckles that are present may become darker and freckles may increase in number. Hyperpigmentation begins to fade with treatment
- Auricular-cartilage calcification: This only seen in men and is the calcification of auricular cartilage from chronic adrenal insufficiency and doesn't resolve with treatment.
- Vitiligo: Is seen in 10-20% of those with autoimmune adrenal insufficiency, however, not in other causes. Vitiligo is patches of depigmented skin mainly on the trunk (Neiman, 2018).

Objective Data

Hypotension systolic BP of < 110 and postural hypotension can be found upon assessment. Weight loss is noted in all patients with Addison's. Hyperpigmentation, an increase in freckles, as well as vitiligo on the trunk may be seen.

Laboratory/Diagnostics

The gold standard diagnostic lab is a short corticotropin test of 25 mcg to establish the diagnosis for primary adrenal insufficiency (Bornstein et al.,2016). Serum electrolytes can demonstrate low sodium, elevated potassium (not seen in secondary adrenal insufficiency), rarely elevated calcium, BUN possibly elevated. Blood sugar can be decreased and patients will present with hypoglycemia. The CBC can demonstrate anemia both normocytic and pernicious, eosinophilia; however, other allergic or infectious reactions need to be ruled out. Cortisol levels might show morning serum levels (drawn between 8-9:00am) less than 3mcg/dL. An ACTH stimulation test is done when the morning cortisol is inconclusive; serum ACTH can be used for differentiating between primary, secondary, and tertiary adrenal insufficiency, plasma renin activity, plasma aldosterone, plasma DHEA and DHEAS, adrenal antibodies, insulin hypoglycemic test, overnight single dose metyrapone test. Adrenal CT and MRI may also be ordered.

Pharmacologic Management

Glucocorticoid therapy is the first line treatment and is used in all patients with primary adrenal insufficiency.

Hydrocortisone is a CYP3A4 (minor) short-acting corticosteroid. There is minimal sodium retaining potential and reduces inflammation by suppression of polymorphonuclear leukocytes and reversal of increased capillary permeability (Lexicomp, 2020). In adults, hydrocortisone 15-25mg or cortisone acetate 20-35 mg is prescribed twice a day (bid) or three times a day (tid) with the highest dose taken upon waking; the next dose is to be taken two hours after lunch for bid or at awakening, lunch, and afternoon for patients taking tid (Bornstein et al., 2016). Adjust dosing for stressors and illness.

Special Considerations

In pregnant women without adrenal insufficiency there have been some studies showing first trimester teratogenic effects with systemic corticosteroids such as oral clefts; there are some reports of low birth weights and hypoadrenalism in newborns with maternal use (Lexicomp, 2020). For pregnant women with primary adrenal insufficiency, hydrocortisone is preferred with adjustments to dosing as pregnancy continues with stress dosing during labor with monitoring at minimum once each trimester (Bornstein et al., 2016; Lexicomp, 2020). It is important to monitor women breastfeeding, as corticosteroids are present in the breast milk.

Pediatric dosing with hydrocortisone is accomplished tid or qid with a total daily dose of 8mg/m2 body surface area; avoid synthetic long-acting glucocorticoids such as prednisolone or dexamethasone (Bornstein et al., 2016). Children should be monitored via clinical assessment such as height, weight, blood pressure and energy levels (Bornstein, et al., 2016).

Complications

Patients in adrenal crisis need to be provided an immediate dose of 100mg (50mg/m2 for pediatrics) hydrocortisone followed by fluid resuscitation and 200 mg (50-100mg/m2 pediatric) of hydrocortisone continual IV drip (Bronstein et al., 2016).

Referrals

Referral to an endocrinologist is recommended at least annually for adults and pediatric patients with primary adrenal insufficiency; for infants follow up is recommended every three to four months (Bornstein et al., 2016).

Chapter 4: Neurology

Headache (Migraine)

Headache (Tension)

Cerebral Vascular Accident

Transient Ischemic Attack

Dementia (Alzheimer's, Vascular)

Multiple Sclerosis

Seizure Disorder

Diagnosis: Migraine Headache

ICD-10 G43.9: Migraine, unspecified

G43.11 Migraine with aura

G43.7 Chronic migraine without aura

G43.839 Menstrual migraine

Kristina Martinez, DNP, RN-BC, ANP-BC, CRNP

Pathophysiology

Migraine is a leading cause of disability worldwide but is often underdiagnosed and undertreated. Migraine pathogenesis is uncertain, although it is thought to be related to neurologic dysfunction in the trigeminal system which results to the release of vasoactive neuropeptides such as calcitonin gene-related peptide (CGRP) leading to neurogenic inflammation, sensitization, and headache. Migraine Headache is classified into episodic and chronic migraine.

Physical Assessment

Subjective Data

Migraines are a heritable disorder and are more common in women than men. For women, there is often an association with the menstrual cycle. Patients may exhibit the following symptomology:

- Headache that is characteristically unilateral, with pulsating quality, moderate or severe intensity, aggravated with physical activity
- Headache attacks lasting 4 to 72 hours (treated unsuccessfully or untreated)

- May have an aura of transient neurological symptom (most commonly visual)
- Commonly, head pain does not have an aura
- Nausea and/or vomiting
- Photophobia and phonophobia
- Exacerbated by exercise

Patient reports of a sudden-onset headache that reaches maximal and severe intensity within seconds or a few minutes ("thunderclap" headache) is an emergency and requires workup for subarachnoid hemorrhage.

Objective Data

Upon examination, vital signs and neurological exams are normal. Exam findings may include vomiting, photophobia, phonophobia.

Laboratory/Diagnostics

Neuroimaging is not necessary among patients diagnosed with migraine headache who have a normal neurologic examination. However, a head CT (Computed Tomography) scan (with and without contrast) may be indicated in the following clinical situations:

- First or worst migraine
- New or unexplained neurologic symptoms
- New onset headaches in patients with cancer or HIV infection
- Episodic headache with hypertension, palpitations, and diaphoresis

- Associated symptoms: fever, stiff neck, papilledema, cognitive impairment, personality change
- New onset headache after 50 years of age

Magnetic Resonance Imaging (MRI) can be used when there is a suspicion of posterior fossa lesions or cerebrospinal fluid (CSF) leak is suspected. Magnetic Resonance Angiography (MRA) and Magnetic Resonance Venography (MRV) are indicated when arterial or venous lesions are suspected.

Pharmacologic Management

Pharmacologic management of acute migraines depends upon the severity of onset. For mild to moderate attacks, the following agents are recommended:

- NSAIDS (including aspirin, diclofenac, ibuprofen, Naproxen)
- Acetaminophen
- Caffeinated analgesic combinations (e.g. aspirin+acetaminophen + caffeine)

The following are recommended for management of moderate to severe migraine attacks:

- Dihydroergotamine (DHE)- alpha adrenergic blocker that has a weaker arterial vasoconstrictor. It is also a potent 5-HT 1b/1d receptor agonist.
- Triptans – Serotonin 1b/1d agonist. Inhibit the release of vasoactive peptides promote vasoconstriction and block pain pathways in the brainstem.

- Sumatriptan (3, 4 or 6 mg SC and intranasal and inhaled powder formulations) Almotriptan, Eletriptan, Naratriptan, Rizatriptan, Zolmitriptan
- Ubropegant (Ubrelvy) and erenumab-aooe (Aimovig), both CGRP receptor antagonists have been proven effective for acute treatment of migraine in adults. Ubropegant (Ubrelvy) has been approved for migraine treatment in children.
- Lasmiditan, a selective serotonin (5-HT 1F) receptor agonist, is thought to block the release of CGRP and glutamate. This blockade is thought to prevent or reverse central sensitization.

Nonpharmacological treatments for acute migraines include single pulse transcranial magnetic stimulation (sTMS) and Noninvasive vagus nerve stimulator (nVNS). Migraine prevention is managed by various pharmacological means, as described in Table 6 below.

Table 4.1: Migraine Prevention

Type	Mechanism of Action
Antiepileptic Drugs: • Divalproex sodium, • Valproate sodium (titration to therapeutic level from 250 mg 3x daily),	Causes increased availability of gamma-aminobutyric acid (GABA), an inhibitory neurotransmitter, to brain neurons or may enhance the action of GABA or mimic its action

• Topiramate (25-100 mg twice daily)	at postsynaptic receptor sites.
Beta Blockers: • Metoprolol (50 to 200 mg/d • Propranolol (40-320 mg/d) • Timolol (10-30 mg/d)	Blood pressure treatment reduces the prevalence of a headache. Blockade of beta-adrenergic receptors result in the inhibition of arterial dilatation. Vasodilation is associated with migraines.
5-$HT_{1B,1D}$ Receptor Agonist: • Frovatriptan for short term preventive treatment of menstrual migraine	Interacts with serotonin 5-HT_{1B} and 5-HT_{1D} receptors, which interrupts the cycle of neurotransmitter-mediated inflammation and pain.
Antidepressants: • Amitriptyline (TCA) (10-150 mg/d) • Venlafaxine (SNRI) (starting at 37.5 mg, dose range is 75-150 mg/d)	TCA increases the synaptic concentration of serotonin and/or norepinephrine in the central nervous system by inhibition of their reuptake by the presynaptic neuronal membrane pump. SNRI potent inhibitors of neuronal serotonin and norepinephrine reuptake and weak inhibitors of

	dopamine reuptake/
Onabutolinumtoxin (Botox)	Neurotoxin produced by *Clostridium botulinim* affects the presynaptic membrane of the neuromuscular junctions in humans. This blocks neurotransmitters that carry pain signals form the brain.
Calcitonin Gene-Related Peptide (CGRP) Antagonists: • Erenumab (70-, 140 mg once monthly, subcutaneous injection) • Fremanezumab (225 mg or 675 mg once monthly, subcutaneous injection) • Galcanezumab (loading dose of 240 mg followed by 120mg, once monthly, subcutaneous injection)	Human monoclonal antibody that binds to and inhibits the CGRP receptor.

Special Considerations

Due to birth defects, Topamax must not be prescribed to pregnant women or women with childbearing potential who are not using a reliable contraceptive method. NSAIDS can cause serious gastrointestinal and cardiovascular side effects.

Triptans and ergotamine derivatives should be avoided or used with caution in patients with coronary artery disease, peripheral vascular disease, uncontrolled hypertension, and other vascular risk factors and disorders.

Coadministration of triptans with other serotonergic medications can increase the risk of serotonin syndrome

Patient reports of a sudden-onset headache that reaches maximal and severe intensity within seconds or a few minutes ("thunderclap" headache) is an emergency and requires workup for subarachnoid hemorrhage.

Complications

Complications associated with migraines include:

- Status migranosus
- Migrainous infarction
- Persistent aura without infarction
- Migraine aura-triggered seizure

Referrals

A neurology consult may be warranted if the patient has episodes of transient neurologic dysfunction, unilateral headache increasing in frequency and severity, a change in personality, or if there is suspicion of a mass lesion. A vision examination with an ophthalmologist may be warranted for patients who have prolonged close work resulting in a headache. Finally, patients with chronic, intractable tension type-headaches may be referred to a psychiatrist for follow up.

Diagnosis: Tension Headache

ICD-10 G44.209: Tension-type headache, unspecified

Rhoda Murray, Ph.D., NP-C

Pathophysiology

The exact pathophysiologic cause of tension headaches is unclear. Tension headaches are thought to be multifactorial. A tension headache may be caused by a central nervous system disorder, muscular issues, or by psychogenic factors.

Physical Assessment

Subjective Data

A tension headache is the most common type of primary headache. Tension headaches mainly affect adults. Although tension headaches can occur in both sexes, it is more commonly found in women. Patients may complain of a generalized headache described as a tight band squeezing the head or as holocranial pain and pressure. The headache is often nonthrobbing with a gradual onset.

Additional features may include:

- Episodic, may be chronic
- Pain is bilateral, mild to moderate in intensity and does not worsen with activity
- No associated nausea or vomiting.
- May have associated photophobia or phonophobia

- Triggers can include stress, fatigue, loud noises, bright light, anxiety, or depression.

Objective Data

Tenison headaches are diagnosed based on upon patient symptoms. Patients may present with normal vital signs neurological examinations. It may be challenging to distinguish tension-type headaches from migraines without aura. Encourage patients to keep a headache diary to better identify causative factors associated with the headaches being experienced.

Laboratory/Diagnostics

There are no current laboratory or diagnostic tests suggested for tension-like headaches. If there is a suspected secondary cause associated with the headache, the practitioner may perform diagnostic and further workup.

Pharmacologic Management

Medications used for treatment of tension headaches are similar to those used to treat migraines with the exception of triptans and ergotamines. The first line treatment is NSAIDS (including ibuprofen, aspirin, Naproxen, and Tylenol).
If anxiety and depression are triggers, headaches may need treatment with antianxiety and antidepressant medications.

Nonpharmacological management focuses upon identifying and avoiding triggers, minimizing stress, as well as encouraging relaxation techniques.

Special Considerations

The use of NSAIDs may lead to gastrointestinal and cardiovascular complications, especially in the elderly. Some migraine medications are contraindicated in pregnancy or in women of childbearing age who are not on birth control.

Complications

An overuse of medication can lead to rebound headaches. Additionally, gastrointestinal bleeding may result from chronic NSAID use.

Referrals

For patients who do not respond to treatment, a neurology consult may be warranted. If appropriate, patients may be referred to a pertinent specialist to identify secondary causes.

Diagnosis: Cerebrovascular Accident (CVA) and Transient Ischemic Attack (TIA)

ICD-10 CM163: Cerebral infarction due to unspecified occlusion or stenosis of unspecified cerebral artery

ICD-10 G45.9: Transient cerebral ischemic attack, unspecified

Nancy Winters, PhD, RN, ANP-C

Pathophysiology

There are two major types of strokes, ischemic and hemorrhagic. The pathophysiology of these types of strokes varies. Regardless of type, a CVA (Cerebrovascular Accident) occurs when a portion of the brain is deprived of oxygen rich circulatory blood.

Ischemic Stroke

In ischemic stroke, oxygen deprivation causes a hypoxic state. Cellular function deficits result from impaired neurons resulting in the eventual death of brain cells. Causes of occlusion include atherosclerotic and/or arteriosclerotic changes, drugs that cause vasoconstriction (i.e., nicotine), or by a blood clot (thrombus or embolus), which blocks the circulatory pathway.

Hemorrhagic Stroke

Hemorrhagic stroke is typically caused by hypertension but may also be caused by other factors such as aneurysms and arteriovenous malformations. There is a weakening of the walls of blood vessels, causing eventual rupture. A cascade of events occurs following the rupture; the most significant of which is an increase in intracranial pressure and the risk of cerebral herniation. Remember that the skull is a hard, closed box which has no space for expanding size.

Transient Ischemic Attack

A transient ischemic attack (TIA) is a brief episode of a neurologic deficit that often comes and goes quickly. Symptoms are identical to the two major stroke types, but do not last as long, as they usually disappear in less than an hour and involve complete neurologic recovery. TIAs are typically reoccurring, and their occurrence signify an increased risk of a future cerebral infarct.

Physical Assessment

Subjective and Objective Data

The acuity, appropriate treatment, and potential patient outcomes can be assessed utilizing valid and reliable measures such as the National Institutes of Health Stroke Scale (NIHSS). Subjective and Objective findings associated with ischemic and hemorrhagic strokes are explained in Table 7 below.

Table 4.2: Subjective and Objective Data of Strokes

	Ischemic	**Hemorrhagic**
Subjective Data	• Unilateral numbness • Difficulty talking/understanding • Confusion • Sudden onset of visual deficit	• Unilateral numbness • Difficulty talking/understanding • Difficulty understanding • Confusion

	• Sudden weakness, typically unilateral • Sudden loss of balance or coordination • Sudden onset of severe headache	• Sudden onset of visual deficit • Sudden weakness, typically unilateral • Sudden loss of balance or coordination • Sudden onset of severe headache
Objective Data	• Change in level of consciousness • Difficulty following commands • Unilateral weakness • Asymmetrical smile • Arm drift • Lack of coordination/sensation • Aphasia • Dysarthria • Hypertension	• Change in level of consciousness • Difficulty following commands • Unilateral weakness • Asymmetrical smile • Arm drift • Lack of coordination/sensation • Aphasia • Dysarthria • Hypertension

Laboratory/Diagnostics

When suspecting a stroke, differentiation between the two types is essential, as treatment for varies. Providing the wrong treatment can cause death. To differentiate between the two, a non-contrast CT (Computed Tomography) scan or an MRI (Magnetic Resonance Imaging) may be ordered. Both diagnostic tests have similar sensitivity and specificities for the hemorrhagic stroke type; however, for the ischemic stroke, the CT scan is more sensitive. Laboratory analysis includes coagulation studies, CBC w/platelets, and a complete metabolic panel.

Pharmacological Management

First line treatment depends upon the type of stroke involved, as demonstrated in Table 8 below.

Table 4.3: Stroke First Line Treatment

Ischemic	Hemorrhagic	TIA
Tissue plasminogen activator – r-tPA (alteplase) is the gold standard in treating ischemic stroke. **Drug class**: Thrombolytic (fibrinolytic) **Mechanism of action** converts	Treatment is focused on: • Stopping the bleeding (Vitamin K, dabigatran, rivaroxaban, apixaban, or edoxaban). • Managing hypertension	Treatment is aimed at preventing another TIA (Transient Ischemic Attack). First line prevention treatment is clopidogrel (Plavix). **Drug class**: antiplatelet agent **Mechanism of**

plasminogen to plasmin, which then degrades fibrin in clots (dissolves the clot).	(labetalol, hydralazine, or nicardipine). • And, decreasing intracranial pressure (mannitol).	**action** inhibits platelet aggregation by irreversibly inhibiting the binding of ATP (Adenosine triphosphate) to platelet receptors.

Special Considerations

Endovascular removal of clots is strongly recommended in eligible patients. However, this should be done within six hours of the start of stroke symptoms. tPA is never given to those having a hemorrhagic stroke, as this will lead to increased bleeding and cause death.

Complications

Complications of stroke include bleeding, hemiparesis, hemiplegia, aphasia, dysphagia, and death.

Referrals

Stroke patients should be referred to neurologists and/or neurosurgeons.

Diagnosis: Dementia and Alzheimer's Disease

ICD-10 F03.90: Unspecified dementia without behavioral disturbance

ICD-10 G30.9: Alzheimer's disease without behavioral disturbance

Nancy Winters, PhD, RN, ANP-C

Pathophysiology

Dementia occurs when cells in certain areas of the brain are damaged, affecting the brain cells ability to send messages from one area of the brain to another. Typically, the cells of the hippocampus are damaged first. The hippocampus is responsible for memory; therefore, this damage causes memory difficulties. The damage is permanent and gradual. The three most common types of dementia are vascular dementia, Lewy body dementia, and Alzheimer's disease.

Vascular Dementia

In vascular dementia, brain cells are damaged due to a reduction of oxygenated blood flow. This can be due to multiple embolic infarcts, anoxic brain damage, atherosclerosis, hypotension, and hypertensive vessel damage. The more brain tissue damaged; the more dementia is recognized.

Lewy-Body Dementia

Lewy-body dementia is a progressive form of dementia in which brain cells are damaged due to a buildup of a protein called alpha-synuclein. Additionally, a loss of dopamine-producing neurons and acetylcholine is evident.

Alzheimer's Disease

Alzheimer's disease is progressive, degenerative, and associated with microscopic changes in the brain long before memory loss is evident. Brain cells are damaged due to beta-amyloid protein fragment buildup (plaques) between nerve cells and tau protein build up (tangles) within cells. Over time, these plaques and tangles spread throughout the cortex interfering with brain cell communication causing memory and language difficulty. Alzheimer's disease is more prevalent in women.

Physical Assessment

Individuals may exhibit dementia-like symptoms in the absence of a disease pathology. A urinary tract infection can lead to a reversible form of dementia. The first step of assessment is to determine what is causing the dementia. A comprehensive medical history, physical exam, neuropsychological testing, and laboratory assessment should be completed. History includes a timeline and speed of progression of symptoms. Practitioners should thoroughly review medications including any over the counter and herbal supplements using Beers Criteria to assess for polypharmacy. Additionally, it is important to assess for alcohol and substance abuse. Client or another informant such as family members will endorse memory loss, impairment of activities of daily living (ADLs) and other symptoms, which vary on the type of dementia.

Subjective and Objective Data

Table 9 provides an overview of the various subjective and objective data findings associated with vascular dementia, Lewy-body dementia, as well Alzheimer's disease.

Table 4.4: Subjective and Objective Data Findings

	Vascular dementia	**Lewy-body dementia**	**Alzheimer's disease**
Subjective	• Abrupt onset • Fluctuating symptoms • Psychosis • Depression	• Fluctuating cognition mimicking delirium • Recurrent well-formed visual hallucinations • Spontaneous features of Parkinsonism • Sleep disturbances	• Slow, insidious onset • Short-term memory loss (early) • Anxiety/depression (early) • Poor judgment (middle) • Hallucinations (middle)
Objective	• Focal neurological symptoms (gait change)	• Tremor • Motor impairment • Postural instability • Increased sensitivity	• Difficulty word finding (early middle) • Disorientation

	• Hypertension	to neuroleptics	(middle) • Paranoia/Delusions (middle) • Incontinence (middle) • Motor rigidity (late) • Apraxia/agnosia (late) • Severe cognitive and language impairment (late) • Brain atrophy on MRI (Magnetic Resonance Imaging).

Laboratory/Diagnostics

Screenings tests include Mini-Cog, Memory Impairment Screen, and General Practitioner Assessment of Cognition, Geriatric Depression Scale. All clients with cognitive impairment require depression screening. To rule out reversible causes of dementia the following laboratory and diagnostic tests should be ordered:

- Thyroid studies to rule out hypothyroidism
- CBC & folate to assess for anemia and infection
- Vitamin B12 to assess for deficiency
- LFTs, metabolic panel, drug and alcohol levels
- Urinalysis to assess for infection
- Medications levels (e.g. carbamazepine and divalproex)
- Sleep study to rule out obstructive sleep apnea
- MRI without contrast- preferred imaging for assessment of atrophy.
- Amyloid Positron Emission Tomography (PET) visualizes beta-amyloid plaques to attempt to diagnose Alzheimer's disease.
- Cerebrospinal fluid analysis can assess for presence of CSF 14-3-3 (Creutzfeldt-Jakob disease)

APOE-e4, the strongest risk gene for Alzheimer's disease, is controversial and still under research. This gene mutation indicates greater risk but does not indicate that an individual has or will develop this condition.

Pharmacologic Management

While there is no cure for Alzheimer's disease and other pathologic forms of dementia, there are treatment options to slow progression regardless of type. Treatment for Alzheimer's is focused on treating symptoms such as memory loss, confusion, thinking, language, judgment, and reasoning. Pharmacologic management for Alzheimer's disease and other forms of dementia are provided in Table 4.5.

Table 4.5: Pharmacologic Management for Dementia

N-methyl-D-asparate (NMDA)	Cholinesterase Inhibitors
Drug: Memantine (Namenda) This may be combined with a cholinesterase inhibitor for moderate-severe dementia. Mechanism of action: Selectively blocks the effects of abnormal glutamate release.	Drugs: Donepezil (Aricept), Rivastigmine (Exelon), and Galantamine (Razadyne) These are for mild-moderate dementia. Mechanism of action: Inhibits acetylcholinesterase which leads to an increase in circulating acetylcholine in the brain.

Special Considerations

Patients with forms of dementia require safety considerations including assessment for driving competency and self-care. Patients and families should be consulted on securing a healthcare proxy, durable power of attorney, as well as a living will.

Complications

Due to memory loss, the following complications may occur in patients:

- Driving impairment and accidents
- Getting lost
- Contractures
- Pressure ulcers
- Frequent urinary tract infections

- Pneumonia
- Immobility.
- Nutritional deficits
- Apraxia
- Aphasia
- Death

Referrals

Patients with Alzheimer's or other forms of dementia may require referral to the following specialists:

- Neurology
- Neurosurgery
- Physical therapy
- Speech therapy
- Nutrition therapy
- Neuropsychologist

Diagnosis: Multiple Sclerosis

ICD-10 G35: Multiple Sclerosis

Shanna Chapman, DNP, APRN, FNP-C, FAANP

Pathophysiology

Multiple Sclerosis (MS) is a debilitating, inflammatory disease that attacks the myelin sheath of nerve fibers, which interrupts the communication pathway. While the exact etiology for MS is unknown, it is immune mediated destruction of CNS components. The destruction of the sheath causes a space that is devoid of nerve impulses or a "lesion". These lesions, also known as plaques, are the characteristic hallmark sign of MS. Symptoms experienced indicate the plaque locations. Lesions may form in areas of the white matter of the brain and the spinal cord.

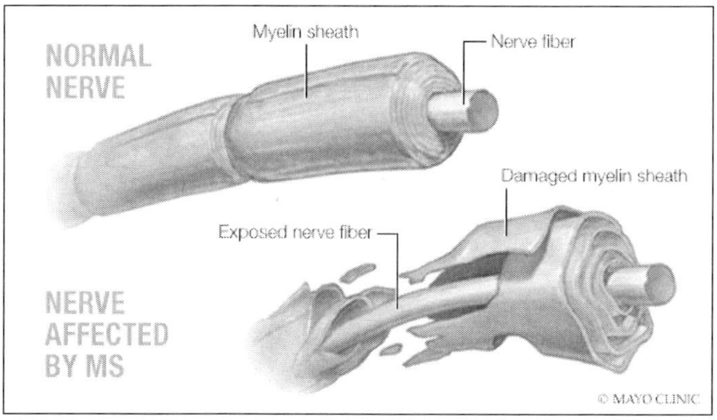

Physical Assessment

Children, adolescents, and adults often experience similar symptoms. Symptoms usually correlate with plaque location (lesion) within the brain or spinal cord. Symptoms may arise gradually or suddenly. Patients may have one symptom, or they may have several symptoms depending on plaque severity or the location within the brain or spinal cord.

Subjective Data

Patients will often experience optic neuritis or visual changes as their first symptom. Patients can also experience muscle cramps/spasticity, vertigo, disequilibrium, fatigue, malaise, memory loss, weakness, paralysis, incoordination, tremor, slurred speech, and/or incontinence.

Objective Data

A comprehensive physical examination including a complete neurological exam is necessary. The provider should note any signs of weakness, spasticity, or unequal muscle tone. All cranial nerves should be tested, as well as tandem walking, DTRs (Deep Tendon Reflexes) in both upper and lower extremities and bulbar function testing. An eye exam should be completed. Assessment for any signs of infection is also particularly important.

Laboratory/Diagnostics

Laboratory and diagnostic data may include the following:

- CBC to rule out infection
- Vitamin B12 & D to rule out abnormalities

- Copper level should be drawn to rule out Wilson's Disease
- TSH to rule out thyroid disease
- ANA, ESR, CCP to rule out autoimmune factors.
- MRI Brain and/or Spinal Cord (depending on symptoms/assessment) with contrast
- lumbar puncture per neurologist as well as definitive diagnosis.

Pharmacologic Management

Medications in primary care settings often seek to reduce the symptoms until the patient can be seen by the neurologist. Once the diagnosis is confirmed, disease modifying drugs (DMDs) are prescribed which include immunomodulating (recepting modulator) or immunosuppressives.

First line treatment is prednisone, a corticosteroid, which suppresses immune response and inflammation. The goal is to stop the inflammatory response of an active plaque by inhibiting leukocyte infiltration. Immunomodulators can slow disability and decrease exacerbations in relapsing MS. Immunosuppressants can delay disease progression by suppressing the immune reaction.

Complications

Complications of MS include cognitive dysfunction, fatigue, spasticity, bowel and bladder problems, and pain.

Referrals

Patients with MS should be referred to ophthalmology to check for optic lesions. Additionally, a neurology referral is necessary to start DMDs and monitor the patient. A lumbar puncture (LP) may also be necessary.

Diagnosis: Seizure Disorders (Convulsion and Epilepsy)

ICD-10 R56.9: Unspecified convulsions

ICD-10 G40.909: Epilepsy, unspecified, not retractable, without status epilepticus

Omotolu Aje-Omokore DNP, FNP, PMHNP

Pathophysiology

A seizure occurs when there is disruption of the normal balance between excitation and inhibition due to genetic or acquired causes.

This imbalance results from an alteration of brain function - from genes and subcellular signaling cascades to widespread neural circuitry. Genetic pathologies of epilepsy can occur anywhere from the circuit level (i.e., abnormal synaptic connectivity in cortical dysplasia) to the receptor level (i.e., abnormal γ-aminobutyric acid [GABA] receptor subunits in Angelman syndrome) to abnormal ionic channel function. Acquired cerebral insults can result from structural changes in hippocampal circuitry after prolonged febrile seizures or head trauma.

Seizures are divided into three categories: focal, generalized, and epileptic spasms. Focal seizures originate in neuronal networks limited to part of one cerebral hemisphere. Generalized seizures occur in the bilateral distributed neuronal networks. Epileptic spasms can begin focally and later generalize. Seizures can originate in the cortex or in subcortical structures.

The main subtypes of generalized seizures are:

- Atypical absence seizure: staring spell characterized by partial impairment of consciousness

- Generalized Tonic–Clonic (GTC)/(Grand-mal): consist of bilateral symmetric convulsive movements (stiffening followed by jerking) of all limbs with impairment of consciousness.
- Myoclonic: consist of sudden, brief ("lightning-fast") movements that are not associated with any obvious disturbance of consciousness. These brief involuntary muscle contractions may affect one or several muscles; therefore, myoclonic seizures can be generalized or focal.
- Atonic: involves the loss of body tone, often resulting in a head drop or fall.
- Absence (formerly called petit mal): involve staring with unresponsiveness to external verbal stimuli, sometimes with eye blinking or head nodding.

Physical Assessment

Subjective Data

Taking a thorough history is essential. The most important subjective data usually includes information from observers as well as the patient.

Previous medical and social history includes:

- History of seizures and description of the most current seizure
- Stroke or other epilepsy risk factors
- Other medical conditions
- Current medications, noting predispose to seizures via either intoxication (e.g., stimulants, many other drugs) or withdrawal (e.g., benzodiazepines, sedatives)
- Substance use including alcohol

Objective Data

The neurologic examination reflects the location and severity of seizure foci. A physical examination performed shortly after a seizure usually shows a more severe deficit. If a large stroke or other structural lesion is present, a postictal or Todd's paralysis may persist for hours or days.

Laboratory/Diagnostics

The following laboratory and diagnostic testing may be used for patients with seizure disorders:

- Complete Metabolic panel: evaluation is aimed at ruling out metabolic factors that could predispose to seizures such as: glucose, electrolyte, BUN, ammonia, and renal indices
- Toxicology screens: to check for presence of drugs or alcohol
- Complete Blood Count: to check for elevated WBC as related to infection
- Anticonvulsant levels: to check if anticonvulsant medications are within therapeutic window
- MRI or CT of brain: MRI is a preferred over CT because it has superior sensitivity for detecting a variety of acute and remote causes of seizure and epilepsy, however either image is still beneficial per guidelines from the American Academy of Neurology (AAN), and the American College of Emergency Physicians

- Lumbar Puncture: if clinical presentation is suggestive of an acute infectious process that involves the central nervous system.
- Electroencephalogram (EEG): the fundamental diagnostic exam for patients with seizures and is indicated in all children with the first nonfebrile seizure. The main EEG manifestation after stroke is focal slowing. The development of a seizure focus may be accompanied by the appearance of epileptiform discharges such as sharp waves, spikes, or periodic lateralized epileptiform discharges (PLEDs).

Pharmacologic Management

Pharmacologic management depends on the type of seizure (see Table 11).

Table 4.6: Pharmacologic Management of Seizures

Types of Seizures	**First-Line Agents**	**Alternative agents**
Focal/Partial:	• Carbamazepine	• Levetiracetam
• Simple partial	• Phenytoin	• Topiramate
• Complex Partial	• Oxcarbazepine	• Tiagabine
• Secondarily generalized	• Valproic acid	• Zonisamide
		• Gabapentin
		• Phenobarbital
		• Primidone
		• Felbamate
		• Eslicarbazepine

		• Vigabatrin • Lacosamide • Pregabalin • Rufinamide
Primary Generalized: • Atypical absence • Myoclonic • Tonic-clonic (grand-mal) • Status epileptic	• Valproic acid • Lamotrigine • Topiramate	• Zonisamide • Felbamate • Phenytoin • Carbamazepine • Oxcarbazepine • Phenobarbital • Primidone
Unknown Onset: • Absence (petit mal)	• Valproic acid • Ethosuximide	• Lamotrigine • Clonazepam

Special Considerations

Extra care should be taken when prescribing to pediatric patients for accuracy and efficacy. Pregnant patients on anticonvulsants should be monitored closely for safety reasons. Studies show that there is an increased risk of congenital malformations in infants born to mothers on anticonvulsant medications. Breastfeeding is not a contraindication for mothers on anticonvulsant medications if the infant is closely monitored for blood levels and safety limits.

Optimal treatment outcome of seizure control with minimal dosage of medication is key in managing the elderly population with seizures –to avoid toxicity, imbalanced absorption, polypharmacy, and weight gain.

Complications

Complications of seizures include:

- Anticonvulsant toxicity
- Metabolic acidosis
- Autoimmune reaction
- Psychosis
- Hyponatremia
- Hypoxia
- Death

Referrals

It is suggested to refer all patients with first-time seizures to a neurologist, as well as uncontrolled/recurrent seizure episodes in established patients

Chapter 5: Respiratory

Asthma

Chronic Obstructive Pulmonary Disease

Pneumonia

Pulmonary Embolism

Obstructive Sleep Apnea

Diagnosis: Asthma

ICD-10 J45.90: Unspecified asthma

Katie Kay DNP, RN, PCCN-CMC

Introduction

Asthma is a chronic lung disease that involves the airways in the lungs. It is a common disease impacting 8-10% of the patient population resulting in nearly ten million office visits and 1.8 million emergency room visits. A person with the diagnosis of asthma is impacted by airways that are inflamed resulting in tightening and constricting that triggers symptoms of coughing, shortness of breath, chest tightness, and wheezing.

Patients can present with multiple types of asthma, the most common being exercise-induced bronchoconstriction or EIA for exercise-induced asthma. Additionally, allergic asthma, occupational asthma, or childhood asthma may all be seen in the primary care setting. While there is no cure, proper diagnosis, treatment, and management will improve the quality of life for this patient population. When asthma is well controlled, evidence demonstrates that patients have reduced morbidity rates, improved quality of life, and overall improved health outcomes.

Pathophysiology

Bronchoconstriction is the main physiological event resulting in patients presenting with clinical symptoms. This is further defined as the narrowing of the airway which results in airflow interference. In an acute asthma exascerbation, the bronchial smooth muscle rapidly contracts in response to a trigger or irritant.

As the disease becomes more persistent and inflammation more progressive, other factors further limit airflow. These include edema, inflammation, mucus hypersecretion and the formation of mucus plugs, as well as structural changes to the airway smooth muscle including hypertrophy and hyperplasia. These latter changes may not respond to traditional treatment.

In some patients who have asthma, airflow limitation may be only partially reversible. Permanent structural changes can occur to the airway. Airway remodeling involves permanent changes to the respiratory system which increases airflow obstruction and airway responsiveness and reduces the patient's responsiveness to therapy. These structural changes can include airway smooth muscle hypertrophy and hyperplasia, blood vessel proliferation and dilation, as well as mucous gland hyperplasia and hypersecretion.

Physical Assessment

Subjective Data

Patients with asthma often report symptoms or flare-ups with exercise, exposure to allergens including dust, pollen, or pet dander or even non-allergic triggers which might include elements such as pollution or changes in the weather. Patients might report flare-ups even in times of increased stress. Obtain a full medication history to determine if any new medications might have triggered an asthmatic event.

Objective Data

During a physical exam for asthma a full assessment of the ears, nose, throat, eyes, skin, chest, and lungs should be performed. Auscultate lungs for any wheezing that could indicate inflammation while also assessing the nose and throat for any swelling or drainage. Clinical diagnosis can be based on the presence of symptoms such as cough, wheeze, breathlessness and chest tightness. Providers need to assess if the symptoms are intermittent and what provokes those symptoms as gained from the subjective data. Additional physical assessment findings that increase the probability of asthma include nasal mucosal swelling, increased secretions, and eczema, atopic dermatitis or other allergic skin disorders may also be present.

Laboratory/Diagnostics

Pulmonary function tests including spirometry which measures forced vital capacity before and after the administration of a short-acting bronchodilator help determine airflow obstruction and determine reversibility. Peak flow expiratory flow monitoring help quantify asthma severity ad further help base treatment decisions for the provider. An arterial blood gas measurement may indicate respiratory alkalosis in a mild asthma exacerbation.

Pharmacologic Management

The goal of treatment is to minimize chronic symptoms and to prevent recurrent exascerbations. Asthma medications are categorized as being a reliever medication to relax the bronchial smooth muscles and stop acute obstruction and the second category is to medicate for long-term control to reduce the need for reliever medications (see Tables 5.1and 5.2).

Table 5.1: Common Asthma Controller Medications

Class	Generic Names	Mode of Action	Common S/E	Considerations
Inhaled Steroids	fluticasone proprionate, budesonide, ciclesonide, beclomethasone dipropionate, mometasone	Anti-inflammatory, inhibits multiple inflammatory mediators	Oral thrush, hoarseness	Typically, 1st line therapy, should be used daily
Long Acting Broncho Dilators-Beta-2 Agonists	salmeterol, formoterol, vilanterol, tiotroprium, olodaterol	Selectively stimulates beta-2 adrenergic receptors which relaxes airway smooth muscle	Tremor, nervousness, tachycardia	Should be used in conjunction with inhaled steroid as a controller due to increased risk of death when used alone
Leukotriene Inhibitors	montelukast, zileuton, zafirlukast	Inhibit leukotrienes	Headache, influenza like Sx, neuropsychiatric symptoms	Caution and monitoring with liver disease particularly zafirlukast, monitor for behavioral changes, can be first line therapy although not as effective as inhaled steroids
Mast cell stabilizers	cromolyn	Stabilize mast cell decreasing mediator release	Few, throat irritation, dry throat	Relatively weak controller albeit low S/E profile
Systemic	omalizumab	Inhibits IgE binding to	Hypersensitivity	Injectable, high cost

non-steroidal Anti-IgE		mast cells decreasing mediator release	reactions, injection site reactions	
Systemic non-steroidal Interleukin antagonists	duplimab, resilizumab, benralizumab, mepolizumab	Binds to and inhibits interleukin	Hypersensitivity, fever, injection site reactions	Injectable, high cost

Table 5.2: Bronchodilators

Short Acting Bronchodilator Beta 2 Agonists	albuterol, levalbuterol, pirbuterol	Selectively stimulates beta-2 adrenergic receptors which relaxes airway smooth muscle	Tremor, nervousness, tachycardia	All asthmatics should have available
Short Acting Bronchodilator Muscarinic Antagonists	ipratropium bromide	Antagonizes acetylcholine receptors, producing broncho dilators	Nervousness, cough, oral irritation	Not as effective as beta-2 agonists in most, can be used adjunctively, can be more effective in those w/ COPD and Asthma

Special Considerations

Patients with a diagnosis of asthma should receive annual influenza and Pneumovax.

Complications

A severe exacerbation of asthma can be life-threatening, all treatment should be started immediately including the administration of oxygen, a high dose inhaled SABA, and a systemic corticosteroid.

Referrals

Asthma can be treated successfully in primary care in the majority of cases. Referral to an Allergist or Immunologist might also be indicated depending on the patient's severity of symptoms. A primary care provider should refer with atypical presentation or uncertain diagnosis of asthma, in cases of complicated comorbidities, uncontrolled symptom management, any life-threatening asthma exacerbations in the past twelve months or with more than two courses of oral prednisone therapy in the past twelve months.

ICD-10 J44.9: Chronic obstructive pulmonary disease, unspecified

Katie Kay DNP, RN, PCCN-CMC

Introduction

Chronic obstructive pulmonary disease (COPD) is a chronic inflammatory lung disease that causes obstructed airflow from the lungs. Emphysema and chronic bronchitis are the two most common conditions that contribute to COPD. Often the conditions can overlap with one being more predominant in clinical presentation. Cigarette smoking and other forms of chronic inhalation exposure often precipitate a diagnosis of COPD.

While there is no cure for COPD, it is treatable. With appropriate management, most people with COPD can achieve symptom control, report a higher quality of life, and have a reduced risk of complications.

Pathophysiology

Chronic bronchitis is inflammation of the lining of the bronchial tubes, which carry air to and from the air sacs (alveoli) of the lungs. It's characterized by daily cough and mucus (sputum) production.

Emphysema is a condition in which the alveoli at the end of the smallest air passages (bronchioles) of the lungs are destroyed as a result of damaging exposure to cigarette smoke and other irritating gases and particulate matter.

Physical Assessment

Subjective Data

Patients will report excessive cough, sputum production, and shortness of breath. Loss of appetite and loss of weight may also be reported. Additional complaints of increasing dyspnea or shortness of breath occurring more frequently are often reported. A full medication history should be obtained when a patient presents with a potential diagnosis of COPD.

Objective Data

Clinical presentation may vary based on if the underlying cause is related to emphysema or bronchitis. With emphysema, cough and mucous is rarer, patients will often present thin with recent weight loss, chest sounds might be quiet and often there is a lack of peripheral edema. A patient presenting with bronchitis would have a very productive cough, peripheral edema, rhonchi, and wheezes are common on auscultation.

Laboratory/Diagnostics

A diagnosis of COPD can often be made through imaging, lab findings, and clinical presentation. In Emphysema, hyperinflation and a flat diaphragm will be seen on chest xray. A barrel chest may be noted on lateral view. In chronic bronchitis, bronchial wall thickening and enlarged vessels may be noted as well as cardiomegaly. Spirometry can assess pulmonary function as well as evaluate response to therapy. An arterial blood gas should be obtained in acute situations.

Pharmacologic Management

The treatment of COPD is guided by the severity of the symptoms. Always refer to the most up-to-date guidelines for treatment of COPD. Supplemental oxygen therapy has demonstrated improvement in COPD patient lifespan. Patients also may be prescribed inhaled bronchodilators and corticosteroids. Antibiotics are commonly given to treat acute bronchitis as well as administered prophylactically to prevent chronic bronchitis (Papadakis & McPhee, 2020).

First line daily treatment consists of a long-acting bronchodilator typically in the form of a LAMA or alternatively a LABA. More severe cases can consist of dual therapy (LABA/LAMA) or even triple therapy (adding inhaled steroid). All COPD patients should have a short acting bronchodilator (see Table 5.3).

Table 5.3: Common Bronchodilators

Class	Generic Names	Mode of Action	Common Side Effects	Considerations
Inhaled Steroids	fluticasone proprionate, budesonide, ciclesonide, beclomethasone dipropionate, mometasone	Anti-inflammatory, inhibits multiple inflammatory mediators	Oral thrush, hoarseness	Can be used in combination w/ long acting bronchodilators in those with component of asthma or eosinophil count >300
Long Acting Broncho Dilators (LABA) Beta-2	salmeterol, formoterol, vilanterol, tiotroprium, olodaterol	Selectively stimulates beta-2 adrenergic receptors which relaxes	Tremor, nervousness tachycardia	1st line therapy, LAMA's are superior to LABA's

Agonists		airway smooth muscle		with regard to number of exacerbations
Long Acting Muscarinic Antagonists (LAMAs)	Umeclidinium, aclidinium, glycopyrrolate, tiotroprium, revefenacin	Antagonizes acetylcholine receptors, producing bronchodilators	Nervousness, cough, oral irritation	1st line therapy preferred. Can be used in combination with LABAs in more severe cases
Short Acting Bronchodilator Beta 2 Agonists	albuterol, levalbuterol, pirbuterol	Selectively stimulates beta-2 adrenergic receptors which relaxes airway smooth muscle	Tremor, nervousness tachycardia	All COPD patients should have available or a muscarinic antagonist
Short Acting Bronchodilator Muscarinic Antagonists	ipratropium bromide	Antagonizes acetylcholine receptors, producing bronchodilator	Nervousness, cough, oral irritation	Can be more effective in those w/ COPD and Asthma

Special Considerations

In general, COPD is largely preventable; as such, the primary care provider should focus preventative care promoting smoking cessation as well as decreased exposure to other inhaled toxins. Patients with a diagnosis of COPD should obtain an annual influenza vaccine as well as regular pneumococcal vaccinations to help prevent the frequency of community-acquired pneumonia.

Complications

Patients with worsening symptoms that do not respond to treatment may need inpatient care. Additionally, patients presenting with worsening hypoxemia, peripheral edema and altered mental status need transferred to an acute care setting and should not be managed in an outpatient clinic.

Referrals

The patient should be referred to a pulmonologist if they have a diagnosis of COPD before the age of 40; have more than two exacerbations per year; experience rapidly progressing symptoms; or have comorbidities impacting the progression of the disease.

Diagnosis: Pneumonia

ICD-10 J18.9: Pneumonia, unspecified organism

Katie Kay DNP, RN, PCCN-CMC

Introduction

Pneumonia is an infection that inflames the air sacs in one or both lungs. Community-Acquired Pneumonia (CAP) is a common disorder that results in over 4 million patients diagnosed each year. Those patients that are of advanced age, have a history of alcohol or tobacco use or other comorbidities are at greater risk for pneumonia. While pneumonia can have bacterial, viral, or fungal etiologies, bacterial is the most common.

Pneumonia can range in seriousness from mild to life-threatening and is one of the leading causes of death in the United States. Pneumonia demonstrates higher mortality rates on those older than age 65 or those with other health problems resulting in weakened immune systems.

Pathophysiology

The most common cause of pneumonia is the inhalation of a bacteria or virus triggering alveolar inflammation and edema. When this occurs, the capillaries become enlarged with blood resulting in the breakdown of the alveolocapillary membrane. The alveoli fill with blood and inflammatory exudates which then results in atelectasis. Most common bacterial pathogens consist of streptococcus pneumoniae, haemophilus influenzae, mycoplasma pneumoniae legionella pneumophila, and chlamydia pneumoniae.

Physical Assessment

Subjective Data

Patients will have symptoms of feeling feverish, generally unwell, with complaints of shortness of breath, loss of appetite, chest discomfort and sweats or chills. A full medication history should be obtained when a provider suspects pneumonia.

Objective Data

Patients will often present with tachypnea, cough, dyspnea, and may either have a fever or be hypothermic. Bronchial breath sounds, as well as crackles on inspiration, are often present.

Laboratory/Diagnostics

In most outpatient cases, clinical presentation and evaluation are sufficient for the diagnosis of pneumonia. . Chest imaging can be helpful to display effusions and consolidation but does not guide antibiotic selection. The patient will often have an elevated white blood cell count on a complete blood count (Papadakis & McPhee, 2020). In some instances and to help guide antibiotic therapy additional diagnostics might be required. Two separate sets of blood cultures drawn prior to antibiotic administration should be obtained if inpatient treatment is required. Sputum analysis for pathogens can also be obtained.

Pharmacologic Management

Prompt initiation of antibiotic therapy is indicated to ensure improved outcomes and is considered the first line treatment for pneumonia. Outpatient therapy is directed at covering the most common bacterial causes as noted above and expanded for those with comorbidities. Initial therapy without complications often consists of a beta-lactam in the form of high dose amoxicillin or amoxicillin/clavulanate as these medications cover most strains of the most common pathogen S. Pneumoniae. A macrolide or doxycycline can be added to target additional pathogens or added to a cephalosporin for those with penicillin hypersensitivity. Lastly, for more complicated cases a quinolone can be used with broad coverage but should be reserved for the complicated cases related to side effects along with avoiding resistance.

Special Considerations

Pneumococcal vaccinations should be encouraged to prevent or lessen the severity of pneumonia. Those in long-term care settings are particularly vulnerable to pneumonia. The absence of fever in older adults does not indicate the absence of infection. Often, a slight alteration in mental status might be the first clinical indicator of infection.

Complications

Pneumonia can be a very serious condition if left untreated or if the patient is unresponsive to treatment. Respiratory failure and septic shock can result. Earlier initiation of antibiotic therapy is associated with improved patient outcomes.

Referrals

If it is safe to treat the patient at home the patient will not need further referrals unless there is a failure to respond to treatment, symptoms worsen, or the pneumonia could impact an underlying disease process, such as heart failure.

Diagnosis: Pulmonary Embolism

ICD-10 I26: Pulmonary embolism

Katie Kay DNP, RN, PCCN-CMC

Pathophysiology

A pulmonary embolism (PE) is a life-threatening emergency that occurs when a blood clot/thrombus, from another part of the body, enters the pulmonary circulation and obstructs a pulmonary vessel/artery. The majority of PEs are caused by thrombi from the legs, arm, or pelvis. The pulmonary occlusion results in impaired gas exchange, circulation, ventilation-perfusion mismatch, and increased pulmonary vascular resistance.

Physical Assessment

Patients may present with no symptoms, nonspecific dyspnea, or symptoms related to a cardiac insult. Due to the life-threatening nature of pulmonary emboli, early recognition and treatment are critical to prevent death.

Subjective Data

Patients may report a history of DVT, immobility, long car/plane rides, major general surgery, pregnancy, major trauma, or recent fracture. Nonspecific classic symptoms include:

- Sudden onset of severe dyspnea
- Chest pain
- Hypoxia
- Productive cough (maybe frothy phlegm)
- Hemoptysis

- Anxiety

Objective Data

Upon examination, patients with a PE may display the following symptomology:

- Cyanosis
- Hypoxemia
- Hypotension
- Tachycardia
- Tachypnea
- S3 gallop
- Distended neck veins
- Unilateral lower extremity edema

Laboratory/Diagnostics

A CT scan of the lungs with contrast is the diagnostic test used to confirm a PE diagnosis, a CT has high specificity for PE. The Ventilation Perfusion scan is another conclusive diagnostic test that should be used in patients who have contraindications for IV contrast. The VQ scan will more than likely reveal a perfusion defect. Additional diagnostics include an ECG, chest X-ray, ultrasound of the legs to look for a DVT, pulmonary angiogram, and a variety of labs to assess clotting factors/abnormalities.

Pharmacological Management

Anticoagulants or thrombolytics are the first-line drugs for PE and should be started as soon as possible to improve mortality.These drugs help to break up the clot and prevent it from getting bigger.

For the hemodynamically unstable patient, thrombolytic therapy should be given via IV.

For hemodynamically stable patients, low molecular weight or unfractionated heparin can be started:

- Heparin-Unfractionated and low molecular weight
- Dalteparin
- Enoxaparin
- Rivaroxaban, Apixaban, Dabigatran

Special Considerations

Assessment in pregnant patients is difficult due to similarity of many of the presenting signs and symptoms being common in pregnancy. Low molecular weight heparin is recommended for use in hemodynamically stable pregnant patients. Coumadin is contraindicated in the beginning stages of pregnancy, as it can lead to fetal defects. Monitor for bleeding in all patients.

Complications

Complications of PD include hemorrhage and death.

Referrals

Patients with a PE should be referred to a pulmonologist and/or hematologist.

Diagnosis: Obstructive Sleep Apnea

ICD-10 G47.33: Sleep apnea, unspecified

Rhoda Murray, Ph.D., NP-C

Pathophysiology

The cause of obstructive sleep apnea (OSA) is multifactorial. OSA varies between patients due to different anatomical and neuromuscular anatomy. In OSA, anatomical and neuromuscular abnormalities lead to nasopharyngeal and oropharynx collapse and upper airway obstruction during inspiration when sleeping.

Physical Assessment

Subjective Data

Patients with sleep apnea may report the following signs/symptoms:

- Patient or spouse reports snoring
- Frequent awakening at night/disturbed sleep
- Morning drowsiness
- Excessive daytime sleepiness
- Reports of waking up tired or fatigued
- Morning headaches
- Reports of sore or dry throat

During the exam, assess medication, sleep, respiratory, neurological, and mental health history.

Objective Data

The physical exam findings can be normal. The patient with OSA may present as hypertensive, obese, with a short neck, narrow oropharynx, tonsillar hypertrophy, large uvula, poor nasal airflow, or a deviated septum. Hypertension secondary to OSA is due to the drop in blood oxygen levels resulting in cardiovascular strain and an increase in blood pressure.

Assess for the following risk factors:

- Age, OSA is more common in patients over 40.
- Male
- Obesity
- Smoking
- Alcohol/Sedative use at bedtime
- Tonsillar hypertrophy
- Nasal obstruction

Laboratory/Diagnostics

An overnight sleep study (polysomnogram) is the gold standard for diagnosing OSA.

Pharmacological Treatments

There are no pharmacological treatments for OSA; practitioners may need to treat secondary hypertension or other identified comorbidities.

Nonpharmacological treatments include:

- Lifestyle modifications, such as encouraging weight loss or decreasing alcohol intake, optimize sleep schedule, etc.
- CPAP (continuous positive airway pressure) is the gold standard treatment for OSA.
- CBC to evaluate for polycythemia, which is caused by chronic hypoxemia.

Complications

Patients with OSA may have underlying cardiovascular disorders such as myocardial infarction, hypertension, and cardiovascular disease; as well as neurological disorders such as stroke.

Referrals

Patients may be referred to a sleep lab/sleep specialist for a sleep study. Additionally, referral may include an ENT or surgery for upper airway abnormalities/deviated septum repair.

Chapter 6: Cardiovascular

Angina

Myocardial Infarction

Atherosclerosis

Arrhythmias

Heart Failure

Hypertension

Peripheral Vascular Disease

Varicose Veins

Diagnosis: Angina

ICD-10 I20.9: Angina pectoris, unspecified

Katie Kay DNP, RN, PCCN-CMC

Introduction

Angina, or angina pectoris, is often described as chest pain usually precipitated by stress or exertion and relieved rapidly with rest or nitrates. Those with angina report varying symptoms including chest pain categorized as squeezing while others describe the pain like a heavy weight being placed on the chest. Angina is relatively common, and usually due to atherosclerotic heart disease.

Pathophysiology

Angina is chest pain that is associated with decreased blood flow or ischemia to the myocardial tissue. The decreased blood flow may be the result of atherosclerosis or coronary artery spasm. Neural pain receptors are stimulated by accelerated cellular metabolism, chemical changes, and imbalances.

Physical Assessment

Subjective Data

Patients may have complaints of chest heaviness, chest pressure, squeezing or fullness. Sometimes this pain radiates to the left shoulder and arm while others report pain in the jaw. Generally, the attack length can range anywhere between three minutes to twenty minutes. Attacks reported at greater than thirty minutes are concerning and could indicate the development of acute coronary syndrome.

A full medical history should be obtained for those patients being evaluated for a potential diagnosis of angina, including the circumstances that precipitate and relive the chest pain. Additionally, providers should determine the level of discomfort, location, any radiation of pain as well as the effect of nitroglycerin.

Objective Data

If the client is not experiencing angina at the time of exam, the exam will be normal. Evaluation during an episode of angina often will demonstrate an elevation of blood pressure. In some cases, a gallop rhythm and apical murmur may be present with pain.

Laboratory/Diagnostics

Laboratory tests are drawn to assess for the cause of angina. A troponin and CK-MB should be drawn to evaluate for acute coronary symptoms as well as for anemia which might be contributing to ischemic chest pain. An ECG should also be obtained to rule out acute coronary syndrome.

Pharmacologic Management

Nitroglycerin, a nitrate, is the medication of choice for acute management of an anginal episode. Nitroglycerin relaxes and widens the blood vessel promoting easier blood flow to the heart muscle._Dosing of nitroglycerin is 0.3-0.6 mg by translingual spray or sublingual tablet every five minutes, as indicated with a max of 3 doses in 15 minutes.

There is a wide range of pharmacological agents that patients with angina might need for longstanding management. Beta-Blockers should be considered, as they have demonstrated to prolong life in patients with coronary artery disease post-myocardial infarction (Papadakis & McPhee, 2020). ACE inhibitors are also effective as they reduce afterload resulting in the heart to work against less resistance.

Special Considerations

Women often present with vague symptoms that could be dismissed without full work-up. Additionally, those with comorbidities are at additional risk and providers should encourage approaches to relieve underlying additional risk factors for further complications including smoking cessation, weight control, and management of hypertension as well as cholesterol. Adolescents and younger adults should be investigated for potential drug use or abuse as vasospasm or constriction can result in angina.

Complications

While the prognosis of angina pectoris has improved with new therapies, mortality rates are largely related to the number of diseased vessels as well as those patients with accelerating symptoms. Risks include further complications and potential acute coronary syndrome.

Referrals

Patients with angina should be referred to a specialist with new and worsening symptoms of angina. Further procedures that can promote revascularization may be indicated. Cardiology, Interventional Cardiology, or Cardiothoracic Surgery may be indicated depending on the further workup of the patient.

Diagnosis: Myocardial Infarction

ICD-10 121.9: Acute myocardial infarction, unspecified

Katie Kay DNP, RN, PCCN-CMC

Introduction

A myocardial infarction (MI) occurs when blood flow to the heart is minimized. The blockage is most often caused by a buildup of cholesterol, which forms a plaque in the arteries that circulate oxygenated blood flow to the myocardium. When the plaque breaks away it can form a clot, interrupting or completely blocking blood flow and destroying a part of the heart muscle.

Pathophysiology

During a myocardial infarction there is an imbalance between myocardial oxygen supply and demand. Prolonged ischemia (>30 minutes) from the lack of circulating blood flow to the myocardium results in cellular death, further impacting the heart's ability to function. Depending on the extent of the cell death, the heart might have decreased contractility resulting in wall function abnormalities further placing the patient at risk for decompensation.

Physical Assessment

Subjective Data

Unlike with an episode of angina, those experiencing a myocardial infarction often report symptoms of pain at rest. The pain is often reported as more severe and likely will not be relieved with nitroglycerin. Patients might also report being light-headed or have increased feelings of anxiety or impending doom. Additional symptoms of nausea may be reported, which is more common in right coronary artery occlusion.

Objective Data

On assessment, the patient may exhibit diaphoresis, syncope, dyspnea, orthopnea, wheezing, or vomiting.

Laboratory/Diagnostics

Troponins are the most indicative lab test and are more sensitive than CK-MB. Circulating troponins often stay elevated for one week after infarction however in those patients with chronic kidney disease low levels of troponin may remain and do not indicate or relate to acute coronary disease.

An ECG will often demonstrate ST-segment elevation or new left bundle branch block. The extent of the ECG changes is often indicative of the extent of the damage.

Management

Patients presenting with acute myocardial infarction will need reperfusion therapy or fibrinolytic therapy. To decrease mortality rates, reperfusion through PCI needs to be completed within 90 minutes of presentation to the emergency room.

Special Considerations

It is important to note that over 30% of patients with an acute myocardial infarction do not report chest pain. Often this is seen in women as well as elderly adults or patients with diabetes. Post myocardial treatment should also focus on health and wellness including the administration of annual influenza and pneumonia vaccination.

Complications

Without treatment, those with acute myocardial infarction can develop severe life-threatening cardiac arrhythmias, acute left ventricular failure, hypotension, shock, myocardial rupture and other life-threatening complications. Mortality rates increase without fibrolytic therapy within the first 30 minutes of hospitalization or revascularization of the coronary artery or arteries through PCI within the first 90 minutes of hospitalization. Immediate intervention for acute myocardial infarction is indicated to improve survival rates.

Referrals

All patients with an acute myocardial infarction need immediate reperfusion therapy and activation of the emergency response team is indicated. Immediate consult to cardiology is warranted.

Diagnosis: Atherosclerosis

ICD-10 170.90: Unspecified atherosclerosis

Katie Kay DNP, RN, PCCN-CMC

Introduction

Atherosclerosis occurs when the blood vessels that carry oxygen to organs and tissues is restricted. This is the result of the hardening of the vessels from buildup of fats, cholesterol, and other substances in and on the artery walls. This process usually occurs very gradually, over several years. The formed plaque can burst, triggering a blood clot.

Pathophysiology

Atherosclerosis is an inflammatory process that begins with damage to the endothelium often the result of hypertension, smoking, high cholesterol or other risk factors. The endothelium develops a fatty streak which further develops into a fibrous plaque and then complicated lesion.

Physical Assessment

Subjective Data

Family medical history and personal medical history should be reviewed for risk factors, including level of physical activity, tobacco, use, and dietary habits. A review of symptoms including recent and increasing fatigue, as well as fluid retention should be completed. A medication history should be obtained to determine risk factors including high cholesterol, hypertension, or diabetes.

Objective Data

While a full physical assessment should be performed, particular attention to pulse deficits, neck vein distention, edema, and calf pain can further contribute to the diagnosis.

Laboratory/Diagnostics

Stress tests (either exercise or pharmacological), chest x-ray, and 12-lead ECG should all be performed. An Ankle-Brachial index might also be performed to assess blood pressure in the extremities.

Pharmacologic Management

The first line treatment includes antiplatelet medications, statins, and angiotensin-converting enzyme (ACE) inhibitors. Aspirin, a commonly used antiplatelet, inhibits platelet function through irreversible inhibition. Statins can help reduce inflammation, modify the composition of plaque and promote vessel stabilization. ACE inhibitors are also effective, as they relax blood pressure and reduce the work and pressure the heart must overcome to circulate oxygenated blood to the body.

Special Considerations

Atherosclerosis can be effectively managed with lifestyle management modifications in addition to medical management. Lifestyle modifications include smoking cessation and a healthy diet in combination with regular exercise.

Complications

Without effective follow-up and therapy, a patient with atherosclerosis is at risk for the development of aneurysms, angina, coronary artery disease, acute myocardial infarction, heart failure, peripheral artery disease, stroke, and chronic kidney disease.

Referrals

Referral to cardiology is indicated. Patients with worsening or progressive symptoms as well as pain with rest need to be referred to a vascular specialist.

Diagnosis: Arrhythmias

ICD-10 149.9: Cardiac arrhythmia, unspecified

Mindy Thompson DNP, APRN, FNP-C, CNE

Pathophysiology

Contraction of the heart is dependent on several factors. The first, and perhaps most important factor, is the ability of the heart to complete the electrical signaling of muscle tissue. This is achieved through specialized cardiac muscle fibers also knows as myocardial fibers. Cardiac muscle is smooth muscle that include the intercalated discs that contain desmosomes.

Desmosomes prevent myocardial muscle cells from coming apart during contraction. Additionally, gap junctions allow ions to move from cell to cell allowing the transmission of impulses to happen very rapidly. All of this happens in a way that assures the two atria contract together followed by contraction of the two ventricles. While all myocardial cells are capable of initiating impulses, normal conduction begins at the sinoatrial (SA) node within the wall of the right atrium. This signal then travels to the atrioventricular (AV) node and then up through the bundle of His that innervates the septum and the Purkinje fibers that innervate the ventricles.

There are several arrhythmias that can occur depending on where the conduction error occurs. Rate and rhythm both help to illustrate where the issue in the conduction system is occurring while an electrocardiogram helps to illustrate the issue. The presence of a P wave indicates a signal from the SA node. The QRS wave on the electrocardiogram is the image of the electrical movement through the ventricles and the T wave shows the repolarization of the ventricles. Repolarization is an electrical description meaning the tissue is losing its electrical change and preparing to receive the next signal. A delay or blockage of the signal in any part of this system can then result in various different arrhythmias. There are four types of arrhythmias, as described below:

Bradyarrhythmia

This is a sinus rhythm originating from the SA node; it is just slower than 50-60 beats per minute (bpm). Depending on the source, some define bradycardia as less than 50 bpm and some reference it as less than 60 bpm. However, there is also a need to consider someone's athleticism as someone with a strong cardiovascular stroke volume may naturally have a slower heart rate and no further work up is needed.

Premature or Extra Beats

This is another type of arrhythmia group which is exactly how it sounds. Either the SA node or the VA node will initiate a beat prematurely or just a random extra beat. Depending on which node initiates the extra beat will determine how this is seen on electrocardiogram in its respective wave.

Supraventricular Arrhythmias

These arrhythmias begin in the right atrium of the heart and this is why they are called supra for above and ventricular for the ventricles. Supraventricular arrhythmias are identifiable by heart rates over 100 bpm (tachycardia) at rest. The rhythm can be regular or irregular. Types of supraventricular arrhythmias are:

- Atrial fibrillation, one of the most common types of arrythmias seen around the world, can produced extremely fast heart rates.
- Atrial flutter differs from atrial fibrillation in that the signal does not make it all the way through both atria to achieve a full contraction thus also resulting in a slower rate than seen in atrial fibrillation. The signal usually encounters some type of damaged myocardial tissue and the signal get stuck in a loop that causes the atria to attempt contraction repetitively. Because of this, the atria and ventricles beat at different rates.
- Paroxysmal supraventricular tachycardia (PSVT) occurs during vigorous activity and tends to occur in young people. Like the other supraventricular arrhythmias, this one too begins in the SA Node. However, in PSVT, the electrical signal makes it to the AV node to trigger the ventricles so the tachycardic rate is successful in both the upper and lower chambers of the heart. While these rates can be very high and concerning, this is usually short in duration.

Ventricular Arrhythmias

Ventricular arrhythmias originate in the ventricles and also create tachycardia. However, ventricular arrhythmias can be perilous and often require expedited medical attention. Types of ventricular arrhythmias include:

- Ventricular tachycardia can be dangerous when it lasts for any considerable length of time. Furthermore, this rhythm can advance into more serious rhythms such as ventricular fibrillation.
- Ventricular fibrillation is the result of unorganized electrical impulses that result in the ventricles quivering instead of creating a full contraction to pump the blood out of the heart. In this scenario, sudden cardiac arrest and death is possible within just a few minutes.

Physical Assessment

Subjective Data

Patients with arrhythmias may report a variety of symptoms or none at all. Some patients report having palpitation or the feeling of a skipped beat or their heart racing. Other symptoms of arrhythmias that can be more serious include anxiety, vision changes, chest pain, dyspnea, syncope, fatigue, diaphoresis, or dizziness.

Additional subjective information providers should solicit include information around the timing of symptoms and how symptoms relate to rest and activity. As noted above, some arrhythmias occur during rest and some during exertion so this piece of information can help narrow potential diagnoses in some cases.

Objective Data

Physical assessment findings that may be seen with an arrhythmia include dependent edema, irregular pulses, and a heart murmur. Thyroid abnormalities may coincide with arrhythmias if there is alteration in thyroid hormones.

Laboratory/Diagnostics

Electrocardiogram is the first and most valuable diagnostic tool when an arrhythmia is suspected. A chest x-ray can also be done to ascertain myocardial size and the potential impact on cardiac rhythm and function . Once confirmed, lab values to consider ordering include thyroid stimulating hormone and electrolytes such as potassium, magnesium, calcium, and sodium. A cardiologist may order additional tests such as an echocardiogram, cardiac CT scan, cardiac monitor, loop recorder, sleep study, or a stress test.

Pharmacologic Management

There is not a singular first line treatment for arrhythmia. There are several medications that can be used on their own or in combination with other drugs to achieve rate and/or rhythm control.

Special Considerations

Cardiac arrhythmias can be precipitated by pregnancy with the risk of arrhythmia being slightly higher during labor and delivery. With pregnancy related changes such as hormones, hemodynamic alterations, and electrolyte imbalances, arrhythmias can occur at any time throughout gestation. Management of arrhythmias in a pregnant patient is like that of a non-pregnant patient. The special consideration arises in relation to the pharmacological management selected should avoid negative effects to the fetus.

Arrhythmias in the older population can carry additional risks due to hemodynamic sensitivity. While treatments remain the same, the pharmacokinetics and distribution need to be evaluated carefully in the older population. Additionally, older patients experience symptoms of hemodynamic instability faster than other patient populations and rebound slower. Symptoms are often vague in this population and easily mistaken for other problems. A careful and thorough assessment and history is paramount followed by a mindful and considerate treatment plan.

Complications

Complications of arrhythmias include blood clots, stroke, heart failure, or cardiac death. Additionally, vascular dementia is a potential long-term complication (Dunphy, 2015).

Referrals

A cardiologist should be consulted to establish a plan of care and determine the extent of additional testing needed.

Diagnosis: Heart Failure

ICD-10 150.9 Heart failure, unspecified

Pamela Porter DNP, APRN, FNP-BC, CNS, PA-S

Pathophysiology

Heart failure is a complex clinical syndrome that results from structural or functional impairment of ventricular filling or ejection of blood, which in turn leads to the cardinal clinical symptoms of dyspnea and fatigue, edema, and rales. Because many patients present without signs or symptoms of volume overload, the term heart failure is preferred over the older term Congestive heart failure.

Classification of Heart Failure

The New York Heart Association (2021) developed the following functional classification system for heart failure diagnoses:

Table 6.1: New York Heart Association Heart Failure Classifications

Classification	Objective Assessment of clients with cardiac disease	
Class I	No physical activity limitation	Ordinary physical activity does not cause fatigue, palpitations, dyspnea, or anginal pain.
Class II	Slight physical activity limitation. *comfortable at rest	Ordinary physical activity results in fatigue, palpitation, dyspnea, or anginal pain.
Class III	Marked physical activity limitation. *comfortable at rest.	Less than ordinary activity causes fatigue, palpitation, dyspnea, or anginal pain.
Class IV	inability to carry on any physical activity without discomfort. *Symptoms of heart failure or angina may be present at rest.	discomfort is increased with any physical activity.

Stages of Heart Failure

The following table presents the four stages of heart failure, as defined by the American Heart Association and American College of Cardiology:

Table 6.2: Stages of Heart Failure

Stage	Criteria
A	Heart disease risk, no structural changes
B	Structural disease no symptoms of heart failure present
C	Structural disease with current or past heart failure symptoms
D	End stage disease, nonresponsive to treatment

Physical Assessment

Subjective Data

The following subjective data may be found in patients with heart failure:

- Pre-existing conditions such as diabetes, liver failure, renal disease, anemia.
- Dyspnea on exertion, orthopnea, paroxysmal nocturnal dyspnea (PND), nocturnal angina, Cheyne-Stokes respirations (ask families or caretaker)
- Fatigue, lethargy, decreased functional capacity
- Patient takes medications as directed, observing, and adhering to dietary requirements
- Alcohol or tobacco use
- History of rheumatic heart disease or Chaga's disease

Objective Data

Upon examination, patients with heart failure may present with the following:

- discomfort when laying down; feels better when sitting upright
- Inability to complete sentences when talking
- Hypertension, systolic BP > 160
- Fine pulmonary crackles, rales, expiratory wheezes, tachypnea, and hypoxia
- Bilateral pleural effusions can occur, but when they present as unilateral it is more frequently in the right pleural space
- Tachycardia, and narrowed pulse pressure due to increased sympathetic tone
- S3 gallop, paradoxical splitting of the S2, jugular venous distention (JCD), hepatojugular reflux, congestive hepatomegaly, ascites, and peripheral edema seen in dependent tissues and extremities
- Point of maximal impulse (PMI0 is displaced below the fifth intercostal space or lateral to the midclavicular line and palpable over two intercostal spaces
- Murmurs of mitral and tricuspid regurgitation present in advanced disease
- Peripheral vasoconstriction, peri-oral and peripheral cyanosis, decreased capillary refill, pulsus alternans, cool extremities from the decreased cardiac output
- Skeletal muscle abnormalities

- With severe, chronic heart failure, may present with cardiac cachexia and marked weight loss

Laboratory/Diagnostics

To diagnose heart failure, laboratory tests include:

- CBC, electrolytes, BUN, serum creatinine, hepatic enzymes, and a urinalysis to screen for diabetes mellitus
- Fasting lipid panel and TSH
- B-type natriuretic peptide (BNP) and N-Terminal pro-BNP (NT-proBNP) are released from a failing heart and a sensitive marker for the presence of HF
- Newer markers, soluble ST-2, and galectin-3 are used to determine the prognosis of HF patients (Yancy et al., 2017).

The following diagnostic testing may also be considered:

- Chest Xray to show the size and shape of the heart, as well as pulmonary vasculature
- Electrocardiogram 12-lead; assess for cardiac rhythm, and if LV hypertrophy is present, prior MI, QRS width. A normal ECG can exclude any LV systolic dysfunction.
- Echocardiogram two-dimensional (2-D) assessment of LV size and function, as well as valvular function or dysfunction and wall motion

abnormalities (indicative of prior MI damage). With Doppler can also assess RV size and pulmonary pressures for evaluation and management of cor-pulmonale.

- MRI is the gold standard for assessing LV mass and volume

Pharmacological Management

First line pharmacological management of heart failure is as follows:

Asymptomatic Treatment

Ace Inhibitor – Venous/Arterial vasodilation

- Drug/Dosing: Enalapril 2.5mg three times a day

Angiotensin II Receptor Blocker – Venous/Arterial vasodilation

- Drug/Dosing: Losartan 25-40mg per day

Symptomatic Treatment

Beta Blockers – Blocks receptors of adrenergic nervous system

- Drug/Dosing: Coreg 6.25-25mg twice a day

HCN Channel Blockers – Blocks Hyperpolarization-Activated Cyclic Nucleotide-Gated Channel (HCN) in SA node to decrease heart rate

- Drug/Dosing: Corlanor 5mg twice a day for two weeks, then 5mg per day

Diuretics – Inhibits sodium chloride reabsorption

- Drug/Dosing: HCTZ 12.5-50mg per day
- Drug/Dosing: Lasix 20-80mg per day

Antiarrhythmics – Inhibits sodium-potassium ATPase

- Drug/Dosing: Digitalis 3.4-5.1mcg/kg per day

Non-Pharmacological Management

Non-pharmacological management focuses on correcting precipitating factors such as increased sodium load, medication non-compliance, ischemia, infections, and anemia. Providing education and support associated with the patient's diet, salt restriction (2 gm /day), and lifestyle modifications (i.e., exercise) is essential. Patients should avoid NSAID's, antiarrhythmic drugs, calcium channel blockers, thiazolidinediones. Fluid intake should be restricted to two liters per day in a patient who has hyponatremia. Caloric supplementation may be provided to patients to maintain weight, prevent muscle wasting and further weight loss. Use of a CPAP may be beneficial if the patient has sleep apnea. Pneumococcal and annual influenza vaccinations are also suggested in patients with heart failure.

Referrals

Heart failure is a complex clinical syndrome with many variables. Therefore, patients should be referred to a cardiologist for initial treatment and follow up as their condition changes/progresses.

Diagnosis: Hypertension

ICD-10 I10: Essential (primary) hypertension

I15:Secodary hypertension

Gulenia "GK" Rikabi, DNP, FNP-BC

Pathophysiology

Hypertension, or elevated blood pressure (BP) is a result of pressure of increased resistance to arterial blood flow. Primary or essential hypertension is caused by sedentary life, familial or genetic in nature, high intake of salt, unhealthy diet, or obesity. Secondary hypertension is linked to medical conditions that affect the kidneys, aortic or renal artery, excess cortisol, heart disease, hyperparathyroidism, obesity, Cushing syndrome, or aldosteronism.

Physical Assessment

Subjective Data

Patients with hypertension usually have no symptoms unless BP is significantly elevated. Patients can report occipital or generalized headaches, dizziness, blurred vision, or extreme fatigue. To determine if the hypertension is primary or secondary, a thorough health history includes past and present medical history of nicotine dependency, obesity, thyroid issues, cardiovascular disease, and dietary habits. Family history should be assessed for hypertension, stroke, heart disease, diabetes, or hyperlipidemia.

Objective Data

Hypertension is diagnosed after two consecutive clinic visits with high BP readings $\geq$ 130/80. Assessment of patients with hypertension includes:

- Body Mass Index -often elevated
- carotid bruits may be auscultated
- lower extremities edema may be present in heart failure
- full assessment of other systems based upon presenting symptoms or history

Laboratory/Diagnosis

Laboratory tests include

potassium- Low potassium can increase BP

Sodium- high sodium levels can elevate BP

Blood glucose and HgA1C to assess for hyperglycemia and diabetes

Lipid panel to assess for hyperlipidemia or metabolic syndrome

Creatinine and blood urea nitrogen and ultrasound of kidneys to assess for secondary hypertension.

TSH and T4 to assess for secondary hypertension due to abnormal thyroid function.

Pharmacologic management

Nonpharmacological Treatment

Lifestyle modification include actions which promote weight loss. These include increased physical activity, a low sodium diet with decreased intake of processed and canned food, cheese, pickles and alcohol. Smoking cessation if the patient is nicotine dependent.

First Line Treatment

- Thiazides -Hydrochlorothiazide- diuretic. Thiazide diuretics inhibits sodium absorption.
- ACE inhibitor (ACEI) Accupril: Angiotensin-converting enzyme (ACE) inhibitors, inhibits conversion of Angiotensin I to Angiotensin II.
- Angiotensin receptor blocker (ARB) Valsartan- blocks Angiotensin II that constricts blood vessels.
- Calcium channel blockers (CCBs)- Amlodipine. Calcium channel blockers relax smooth muscles of the blood vessels and the myocardium

Ethnic considerations when prescribing:

Thiazides or Calcium channel blockers (CCBs) are first line for African Americans.

Angiotensin-converting enzyme (ACE I) for patients with coronary artery disease, heart failure or kidney failure.

Angiotensin II receptor blockers (ARB), ACEI, Thiazides, or CCBs for Whites/Caucasian.

ACEI or ARB for patients with chronic kidney disease with or without diabetes for all races and ages.

ACEI, ARB, or CCBs for diabetes in non-Blacks.

Special Considerations

Comorbidities

Hypertension is often accompanied by comorbidities such as diabetes and hyperlipidemia known as metabolic syndrome. Accurate and timely diagnosis and treatment of comorbid conditions is essential for successful hypertension management.

Pregnancy

Up to 1.5 pregnant women have chronic hypertension prior to pregnancy. First line medication in pregnancy is Labetalol. Extended release Nifedipine, hydrochlorothiazide, and Methyldopa are also considered safe in pregnancy. Pregnant women with chronic hypertension or preeclampsia must be on low dose Aspirin between week 12 and week 28 of gestation.

Pediatrics

Hypertension in pediatrics is considered when BP is ≥130/80. Hypertensive pediatric patients are screened for diabetes, hyperlipidemia, and cardiac diseases. Treatment includes lifestyle changes. Obese children and adolescents should be encouraged to increase physical activities and enroll in sports. Healthy meals and snacks are enforced. Kids pharmacological treatment includes Thiazides, ACE1, CCB, and ARB.

Elderly

Hypertension treatment guidelines for adults ≥ 60 years:

65-79 years old initiate antihypertensive medications if BP ≥140/90 mmHg.

For the very old > 80 years old initiate medications if BP $\geq$ 160/90 mmHg.

For elderly persons with cardiac diseases or stroke- treatment is individualized.

Complications

Uncontrolled primary hypertension may lead to chronic kidney disease, stroke, and heart diseases. Uncontrolled secondary hypertension may cause aneurysm, kidney disease, metabolic syndrome, atherosclerosis, and stroke.

Referrals

Referrals includes cardiology if patient has history of cardiac diseases or has heart failure, nutritionist to help the patient learn low sodium healthy eating habits, and nephrology to prevent or treat kidney diseases or failure, polycystic kidney disease or glomerulonephritis.

Diagnosis: Peripheral Vascular Disease

ICD-10 173.9: Peripheral vascular disease, unspecified

Patty Roof, EdD/CI, APRN, FNP-C, MSN/ED

Pathophysiology

Atherosclerosis is the most common cause of peripheral artery disease (PVD). Atherosclerosis is characterized by changes in the vascular wall and occurs in either arteries or veins causing wall vessel inflammation and changes in circulation. Patients are often asymptomatic and should have their risk factors controlled, as there is a high incidence for death from cardiac-associated causes relating to PVD.

Physical Assessment

Subjective Data

Risk factors including a history of smoking, obesity, diabetes, hyperlipidemia, hypertension, and increased age (>65 and >50 with risk factors of atherosclerosis). A family history of PVD, heart disease or stroke can also increase the risk for patients. The following are symptoms of PVD, which patients may report:

- cramp like muscle pain in one or both legs; pain with rest; pain with walking which does not improve with rest.
- Skin color changes, edema, or tenderness in arms/legs
- Color changes in fingers or toes
- Coldness, numbness, and weakness in one leg compared to the other

- For males, changes in sexual function, erectile dysfunction

Objective Data

Exam findings in PVD can vary based on severity. Skin may be cool to touch and pale, red, or blue in color. Pedal pulses may be diminished or absent. A femoral artery bruit may be noted.

Laboratory/Diagnostics

Measurement of ABI (Ankle-Brachial Index) may be needed, as well as a duplex ultrasound. An ABI <0.9 is indicative of PVD. A lipid profile may be ordered; dependent upon the underlying problem associated with PVD, the patient may need additional laboratory testing (refer to the specific problem for recommended laboratory testing).

Pharmacologic Management

Medications are dependent on the underlying problem associated with PVD; medications focus on reducing the risk factor for cardiovascular mortality and morbidity. If appropriate, the provider may prescribe statins, ACE Inhibitors, anti-platelet therapy, as well as beta-blockers.

Non-Pharmacologic Management

Non-pharmacological management primarily focuses on lifestyle modifications including exercise, smoking cessation, and diabetes control through a healthy diet.

Special Considerations

Patients with PVD should avoid the use of pseudoephedrine found in over-the-counter medications, which can constrict the blood vessels.

Pregnant women with PVD may have edema of their lower extremities and develop varicose veins in the third trimester. The dorsalis pedis (DP) and posterior tibial (PT) pulses may be more difficult to palpitate in elderly patients.

Complications

Patients may experience arteriosclerosis obliterans, acute arterial occlusion, Raynaud's disease, Raynaud's phenomenon, superficial thrombophlebitis, deep venous thrombosis (DVT), chronic venous insufficiency, thromboangiitis obliterans, compartment syndrome, acute lymphangitis, leg/foot ulcers, stroke, and heart attack.

Referrals

Dependent upon the physical assessment, and the severity of the condition, patients may be referred to Cardiovascular Medicine/Surgery or Vascular and Endovascular Surgery.

Diagnosis: Varicose Veins

ICD-10 183.813: Varicose veins of bilateral lower extremities with pain

Patty Roof, EdD/CI, APRN, FNP-C, MSN/ED

Pathophysiology

Varicosities occur with vein dilatation, which is often associated with factors that leads to increase pressure and distention of veins as well as tortuous vein appearance. Pooling of blood is an associated factor as well as venous value incompetence which allows for retrograde blood flow. While superficial varicose veins may often be benign; venous stasis can be the result of a much more severe case of varicose veins.

Physical Assessment

Subjective Data

Patients with varicose veins may report pain, cramping, itching, or burning/throbbing of the legs. It is important to determine when these symptoms occur, as well as what relieves any pain, feelings of heaviness, burning, swelling, and itching. Risk factors for the development of varicose veins include advanced age, sex (women have a higher incidence of varicose veins), family history, obesity, and standing or sitting for extended periods of time.

Objective Data

Upon examination, inspect the legs with the patient lying and standing.

Visible distension of veins will be noted. Light palpitation of legs veins may identify additional varicosities. Skin discoloration indicates venous stasis. Other skin abnormalities may include ulcerations, telangiectasis, and micro ulcers. Palpate pulses (femoral, popliteal, posterior tibial, and dorsalis pedis) and note the temperature of extremities.

Additionally, look for signs of deep vein thrombosis (DVT) such as tenderness, unilateral swelling, or palpable cord along a vein.

Laboratory/Diagnostics

A duplex ultrasound tests the leg(s) for reverse or reflux flow of blood.

Non-Pharmacologic Management

No pharmacologic treatment is recommended for varicosities. Compression stockings are the first line treatment for varicose veins. Patients should be encouraged to make lifestyle changes such as eating a healthy diet and exercising for weight management. Extended periods of sitting or standing should be avoided and patients should elevate their legs as needed. Second line treatment for more severe cases includes measures such as sclerotherapy, the use of lasers, vein stripping and endoscopic vein surgery.

Special Considerations

Elderly patients are at a higher risk of developing varicose veins. Pregnancy can also lead to varicose veins due to the increased volume of blood (especially in the third trimester). Additionally, family history plays a role in its development.

Complications

Complications can include ulcers, bleeding, as well as chronic venous insufficiency.

Referrals

A referral to a vascular surgeon may be necessary for some patients.

Chapter 7: Hematology

Iron Deficiency Anemia

Pernicious Anemia

Aplastic Anemia

Sickle Cell Disease

Polycythemia Vera

Leukemia

Diagnosis: Iron Deficiency Anemia

ICD-10 E61.1: Iron deficiency

Adrienne Small, DNP, FNP-C, CNE, CHSE

Pathophysiology

Iron is present in all human cells. Following ingestion, iron is absorbed in the small intestine; 80% of iron is in the form of hemoglobin on red blood cells. The remainder of iron is found in the muscles as myoglobin. Most iron is stored as ferritin, which is transported by the protein transferrin. Transferrin carries oxygen from the lungs in the form of hemoglobin. As myoglobin, iron assists in the storage of oxygen in the muscles. Iron is also part of many vital enzymatic reactions in the body.

The average adult loses 1mg of iron per day through the processes of excretion. Adults absorb 1-2mg of iron per day through dietary intake. Aging or damaged red blood cells are destroyed by macrophage cells; however, the iron from these erythrocytes is stored for further use. Iron deficiency will occur when the amount of iron loss exceeds the amount absorbed. If depleted iron stores are not corrected, iron deficiency will progress to iron deficiency anemia.

Physical Assessment

Subjective Data

A complete medical history should be obtained. Malabsorption disorders such as celiac disease and irritable bowel disease can decrease iron absorption.

Inflammatory conditions such as obesity, cancer and chronic kidney disease can also predispose a patient to iron deficiency. Surgical history identifies excessive blood loss. Patients who have undergone gastric bypass are prone to iron deficiency because the procedure severely decreases the number of sites available for iron absorption. The use of medications such as anticoagulants, aspirin and NSAIDs can cause iron deficiency by increasing bleeding tendencies. Proton pump inhibitors and H2 blockers inhibit intestinal absorption of iron.

A detailed menstrual history should be obtained on females to determine if menstrual blood loss is excessive. Social history should also be obtained, and patients should be questioned about their consumption of iron-rich food and meats. Vegetarian and vegan diets, which restrict meat, can cause iron deficiency. The social history should include the patient's income level and ability to obtain fresh fruits and vegetables. Excessive exercise, such as endurance training, can lead to blood loss.

Patients with iron deficiency may complain of fatigue or activity intolerance, hair loss, breaking nails, and pica. The most common form of pica is ice craving, or pagophagia. Pica is more common in women and children; the cause is poorly understood. Patients may also complain of headaches or irritability.

Objective Data

Physical findings associated with iron deficiency include:

- Pallor of skin, mucous membranes, and nail beds
- Smooth tongue

- Cheilosis
- Hair loss
- Brittle nails
- Restless legs syndrome

Laboratory/Diagnostics

For most patients with new onset of symptoms of iron deficiency, a complete blood count (CBC) will identify a hypochromic microcytic anemia. If resources are limited, a hemoglobin level can be used as an initial screening tool. Perl's staining, which measures the amount of iron in bone marrow aspirate, is the gold standard for diagnosing iron deficiency. However, this method is rarely used because there are cheaper, less-invasive tests that can assess iron stores.

In patients without severe symptoms, iron deficiency can be diagnosed by assessing the response to a therapeutic trial of oral iron therapy. This approach is used during pregnancy and in women with menorrhagia. A therapeutic trial is also useful when iron studies are not readily available. If successful, an adult dose of 100-200mg daily of iron should raise the hemoglobin by 1mg in three to four weeks.

Iron studies are indicated in patients who do not respond to a trial of iron therapy. An initial iron panel consists of a serum iron, serum ferritin, and total iron binding capacity (TIBC). An iron panel should be obtained while fasting.

The serum iron measures circulating iron, which is transported by transferrin. Low serum iron alone is not diagnostic of iron deficiency. Serum ferritin gives an accurate reflection of the body's iron stores. A serum ferritin level below 30 for iron deficiency. The transferrin level is sometimes reported as the TIBC using the following conversion: Transferrin = TIBC x 1.389

Pharmacologic Management

Oral administration of elemental iron is typically first-line treatment.The most common commercially available oral iron preparation is ferrous sulfate 325mg, which contains 65mg of elemental iron.

Parenteral iron has a more rapid onset of action and is administered as a single dose. Intravenous administration is indicated for:

- Inability to tolerate oral iron preparations
- Failure to improve on oral iron therapy
- Malabsorption disorders
- Chronic inflammatory diseases
- Patients with severe physical symptoms

Special Considerations

Pediatrics

Infants should be screened for iron deficiency between 9 and 12 months of age (AAP,2020). Risk factors for iron deficiency include prematurity, poverty, low birth weight and a vegetarian diet. IDA can also occur in breastfeeding infatns who do not receive supplemental iron. There is a link between developmental delay and iron deficiency (Parkin, 2020).

Pre-adolescents may also exhibit asymptomatic iron deficiency during rapid growth spurts, due to increased iron demands. Male and female athletes who are involved in endurance sports may also experience occult blood loss. The pre-participation physical for these adolescents should include screening iron deficiency. Oral iron supplementation for children is dosed at 3 mg/kg given in one dose, taken between meals. Dietary counseling should be given to parents of children who test positive for iron deficiency.

Menstruation and Pregnancy

On average, 1mg of iron is lost per day during menstruation, but more may be lost if menorrhagia exists. Adolescent girls should be screened with either a CBC or hemoglobin level. Uterine fibroids can also cause excessive menstrual bleeding. Symptomatic patients should be screened for iron deficiency.

Iron deficiency is common in pregnancy, as demands are increased during pregnancy and lactation. Pregnant patients should begin taking a prenatal vitamin containing iron as soon as the pregnancy is known. At the first prenatal visit, all patients should receive a CBC to screen for iron deficiency. I the thord trimaester, a CBC should be repeated as the majority of maternal to fetus iron transfer occurs at this time.

Elderly

Individuals over the age of 65 are more likely to have iron deficiency. Common causes include absorption problems, iron-poor diet, and blood loss. Iron deficiency can also cause heart failure or angina . In the absence of a nutritional deficiency or malabsorption problem, every effort must be made to locate the source of occult blood loss.

Complications

Untreated or undertreated IDA is associated with depression, tachycardia, arrythmias, cardiac murmurs, developmental delays in children, and pregnancy complications such as preterm delivery and infant low birth weight.

Referrals

Occult blood loss should always be considered in the absence of obvious sources of bleeding (menstruation, pregnancy, lactation). Occult blood screenings should be conducted. Patients with risk factors for colorectal cancer should be referred for a colonoscopy to rule out a gastrointestinal malignancy. Hematology consult is indicated for iron deficiency that is refractory to treatment.

Diagnosis: Pernicious Anemia

ICD-10 D51: Pernicious anemia, unspecified

Adrienne Small, DNP, FNP-C, CNE, CHSE

Pathophysiology

Pernicious anemia (PA) is an autoimmune disease which causes thinning of the gastric oxyntic mucosa of the stomach's body and fundus. Intrinsic factor binds to dietary B12 and facilitates its absorption in the ileum. Individuals with pernicious have parietal cell autoantibodies and intrinsic factor autoantibodies. These antibodies destroy and attack the sites of the gastric mucosa. Destruction of the gastric mucosa reduces the number of parietal cells, which produce Intrinsic Factor and gastric acid.

Pernicious anemia is a megaloblastic anemia. Megaloblastic anemia, which is a type of macrocytic anemia, occurs because the larger immature red blood cells (called reticulocytes) are prematurely released from the bone marrow without going through the normal process of subdivision. In PA, the MCV is elevated, often greater than 10 fL; and enlarged erythrocytes will be visible on a peripheral blood smear. Other PA manifestations include chronic inflammation of the stomach, and neurologic alterations. Vitamin B12 is crucial for proper cell red blood cell division within the bone marrow.

Physical Assessment

Subjective Data

Symptoms of pernicious anemia tend to develop over the course of several decades, beginning in the stomach body and advancing to severe vitamin B12 deficiencies and neurological deficits. Patients may complain of oral sores, weakness, fatigue headaches, and difficulty concentrating. Early on, patients may experience gastrointestinal symptoms such as abdominal pain and diarrhea, particularly if an underlying malabsorptive disease exists. Elderly patients may also experience chest pain or heart palpitations.

The past medical history should assess for the presence of other autoimmune diseases, such as thyroid disease, type I diabetes, inflammatory bowel disease (IBD), or celiac disease. The majority of these patients will have serum antibodies against parietal cells and intrinsic factor. Patients who have undergone bariatric surgery or gastrectomy are also at risk for pernicious anemia.

The medication history should assess for use of H2 blockers and proton pump inhibitors. These medications, available via prescription or over the counter, interfere with absorption of Vitamin B12 by decreasing the amount of available gastric acid and are commonly taken for gastroesophageal reflux (GERD) and gastritis. Metformin may also inhibit B12 absorption.

The social history should include ethnic background, and other factors that could cause a B12 deficiency. Vitamin B12 deficiency caused by autoantibodies is more common among individuals of northern European descent and is rare in patients of Asian descent. Other possible sources of B12 deficiency such as diet, alcohol consumption, and travel history should be explored. A strict vegan or vegetarian diet, which limits milk, cheese, eggs, and meat, can cause B12 deficiency. Children who are exclusively breastfed by B12 deficient mothers will also be deficient. Alcoholism can cause B12 deficiency and macrocytic anemia.

Objective Data

A general survey of the patient should be conducted, looking for altered mental affect, fatigued appearance and gait.

- EENT: The eyes should be inspected for signs of icterus; the conjunctiva may appear pale if significant anemia is present. The oral mucosa should be inspected for sores, which could indicate decreased replacement of aging epithelial cells.
- Cardiac: assess for tachycardia or murmurs.
- GI: assess for organomegaly.
- NEuro: A late sign of pernicious anemia is demyelination; therefore, a detailed neurologic exam must be performed. Findings could include ataxia, paresthesias, weakness, peripheral neuropathies, sensory deficits, decreased vibratory sense and decreased proprioception.
-

Laboratory/Diagnostics

Initial lab tests include a CBC which will identify megaloblastic anemia. Reticulocyte count and Vitamin B12 level will be decreased. The combination of these three lab results supports a diagnosis of pernicious anemia. Intrinsic factor antibodies will be present.

Pharmacologic Management

The first line treatment for pernicious anemia is Vitamin B12 (Cobalamin), which is a water-soluble vitamin. Vitamin B12 is necessary for erythropoiesis, cell reproduction, protein synthesis and myelin synthesis. B12 forms a complex with intrinsic factor. It attaches to receptor sites in the ileal mucosa where it eventually enters the plasma; it is stored in the bone marrow and is stored in the liver as coenzyme B12.

Suggested dosing of Vitamin B12 is:

- 1,000mcg intramuscular (IM) or subcutaneous (SC) once a week for eight weeks followed by 1,000mcg once a month for life
- 1,000mcg IM or SC every day or every other day for one week, followed by 1000mcg every week for four weeks, then 1000mg every month for life
- 500mcg intranasally into 1 nostril once weekly
- 1,000 to 2,000mcg/day by mouth for life

Special Considerations

Infants born to mothers with vitamin B12 deficiencies will also have deficiencies, as there are no B12 stores in the bone marrow or liver. These infants do not necessarily have pernicious anemia, which is diagnosed by the presence of parietal and Intrinsic Factor antibodies accompanied by gastric body atrophy. However, infants born to mothers with vitamin B12 deficiency should be tested for antibodies to allow for early diagnosis and treatment.

Complications

Untreated or undertreated PA can lead to heart and lung damage, nerve damage, memory loss, gastrointestinal issues, and increased risk of stomach cancer. Lifelong treatment is necessary.

Referrals

Up to 10% of patients with autoimmune gastritis may be predisposed to bowel cancers. These patients may benefit from gastroenterology referral with periodic screenings. A hematology referral is indicated for patients who do not respond to B12 replacement.

Patients with pernicious anemia should receive an annual CBC, ferritin level, and serum cobalamin to monitor for iron deficiency and to assess the effectiveness of B12 replacement therapy.

Diagnosis: Aplastic Anemia

ICD-10 D61.9: Aplastic anemia, unspecified

Michelle Krawczyk, DNP, ARNP-BC, CNE

Introduction

Aplastic Anemia (AA) is a rare disease, estimated to affect one in 500,000 people in North American and Europe. The incidence is two to three times higher in Asian countries, which is likely due to environmental or genetic factors. All ages can be affected; however, it is most diagnosed between the age of 15 and 25 years of age. The disease also peaks again in patients over the age of 60 year. There is no difference in incident between genders.

Pathophysiology

In patients with AA, damage has occurred to the bone marrow through chemotherapy, radiation therapy, chemical and medication exposure, and viruses (such as Epstein-Barr virus, Hepatitis or Human Immunodeficiency virus [HIV]). Although most cases are idiopathic, autoimmune disease and pregnancy can also be a cause, although rare. If the cause is related to drug exposure, the aplastic anemia will generally resolve after removing the precipitating drug.

The cause of the AA is lymphocyte destruction of immature hematopoietic cells. This destruction causes fatty replacement and cellular depletion within the bone marrow. There is often an increase production of growth factors such as granulocyte- stimulating factor (G-CSF) and granulocyte-macrophage colony-stimulating factor([GM-CSF); however, these growth factors are not able to correct the cytopenia.

Assessment

Subjective

Patients may report feelings of fatigue, shortness of breath, bruising, bleeding (particularly in the skin, mucous membranes, menorrhagia, and epistaxis), palpitations, and headaches.

Objective

Upon examination, patients may be pale, have bruising or petechiae. However, some patients may present with a normal physical examination, as symptoms might not present until the aplastic anemia is severe. Splenomegaly and hepatomegaly are usually not present.

Laboratory/Diagnostics

The following laboratory findings will be seen for patients with AA:

- CBC will demonstrate pancytopenia in at least two out of the three cell lines.
- Serum iron and transferrin saturation will be increased, as the iron is not being used for erythropoiesis.
- Liver function tests (LFT) will be normal unless the cause of the AA is hepatitis.
- Bone marrow biopsy with flowcytometry is the hallmark for diagnosis of AA. Bone marrow biopsy will show marked hypocellularity with fatty replacement.

Management

Patients with AA should be managed by Hematology and Oncology practitioners.

Hematopoietic stem cell transplant (HSCT) is the first choice of treatment if a match donor is present, such a sibling. HSCT treatment has been shown to have a 65-90% long term survival, with the higher range more common in children.

If HSCT is not an option due to patients' condition or the lack of a donor, immunosuppressive therapy is the treatment of choice. However, success rates for this treatment are lower than HSCT.

Blood product transfusion should be administered sparingly. Platelet transfusions should only be administered if the patient is actively bleeding or if the platelet counts are less 10,000 *u*L. Blood transfusions should only be given if the patient is symptomatic from the anemia.

Special Considerations

Pregnant patients should be managed by a hematology specialist and high-risk maternal fetal practitioners.

Complications

Complications of AA are related to the patient's pancytopenia and possible treatment. The most prevalent complications are associated with anemia (fatigue, shortness of breath, cardiac, etc.), neutropenia (increased risk of infection) and thrombocytopenia (bleeding and easy bruising).

Referrals

Referral should be made to hematology practitioners as soon as pancytopenia is identified. For pregnant patients with AA, referral to high-risk maternal fetal practitioners is recommended.

Diagnosis: Sickle Cell Anemia

ICD-10 D57.1: Sickle-cell disease without crisis

ICD-10 D57.219: Sickle-cell/Hb-C disease with crisis, unspecified

Michelle Krawczyk, DNP, ARNP-BC, CNE

Introduction

Sickle cell disease is a term that refers to a group of genetic disorders involving abnormal hemoglobin S (HbS). Patients most affected by this genetic disorder are of African descent, especially central and west Africa, as well as parts of India, Asia, and the Mediterranean. Approximately a million people worldwide are affected, with 1000,000 people in the United States.

Pathophysiology

The hallmark of sickle cell anemia is the presence of HbS. When properly oxygenated, HbS does not cause a problem for patients. However, when the HbS deforms into a sickle shape, the patient can become symptomatic. Sickling can result from dehydration, deoxygenation or a decrease in pH. The sickling of the HbS cells can be reversed if caught early enough, however repeated sickling over time can cause permanent damage to the vessel membrane. In addition to the sickling of the HbS cells, the rigid sickled red blood cell can cause additional dehydration that can cause hemolytic anemia as well as vaso-occlusion (Hsieh et al., 2019). Vaso-occlusion then increases the number of sickled cells through oxygen tension and decrease in pH, causing the cycle to perpetuate. This sickling process causes significant pain for the patient as a result of deoxygenation and tissue damage.

The typical lifespan of a normal red blood cell is about 120 days; however, the sickled red blood cell has a significant shorter life span of about 10 to 20 days. The lifespan of the sickled cell is greatly diminished as a result of chronic hemolytic anemia, even without clinical symptoms. The spleen filters the sickled cells at a higher rate than normal red blood cells, while other sickled HbS cells are destroyed by force as they circulate through the vessels. This hemolysis activated inflammatory mediators such as platelet-activating factor, interleukin-2, thrombin, and tumor necrosis factor-alpha.

Physical Assessment

Subjective Data

Patients with sickle cell anemia may report the following symptoms:

- Fatigue, malaise
- Shortness of breath
- Joint pain
- Dizziness

Objective Data

Patients may be jaundiced (skin and/or whites of the eyes), be small in stature, have a retinal hemorrhage, and present with a fever. Cardiac examination may reveal a heart murmur or tachycardia. Patients may also be coughing, wheezing and experience tachypnea. Hepatosplenomegaly (HPM) may be present, as well as priapism in males (prolonged erection of the penis). Patients may demonstrate stroke symptoms and have leg ulceration.

Laboratory/Diagnostic

Screening for all newborns is conducted in the United States, regardless of race or ethnic background. This screening is required by law in all 50 states in the nation.

Laboratory data associated with sickle cell disease includes:

- Complete blood count (CBC): Hemoglobin (Hgb) usually ranges between 6-8 g/dL (normocytic, normochromic), leukocytosis with a shift to the left, thrombocytosis
- Comprehensive metabolic profile (CMP) to evaluate liver and kidney function
- Reticulocyte count is usually 5%-20% (although decreases during an acute crises)
- Peripheral smear demonstrates sickled cells, fragmented red cells, nucleated red cells.
- Hemoglobin (HgB) electrophoresis: Definitive test
- Measurement of hemoglobin A2 and fatal hemoglobin (HbF)
- Bone marrow biopsy demonstrates erythroid hyperplasia (except during a crisis)

Pharmacologic Management

Treatment for sickle cell generally focuses upon avoidance of pain, as well as preventing complications. This includes hydration of the patient, prevention of infection, and early intervention for acute vaso-occlusion crises.

The first line treatment for sickle cell is Hydroxyurea (Hydrea), which is an antineoplastic drug whose mechanism of action is poorly understood; however, in rat studies it has shown to inhibit DNS synthesis. Dosing of hydroxyurea is 15 mg/kg/day for adults (reduced for patients with chronic kidney disease [CKD]) for adults. For children/pediatrics, dosing is 20 mg/kg/day Clinical response may take up to six months and it is vital to monitor patient laboratory data during treatment.

Special Considerations

Pediatric patients are usually diagnosed through newborn screening; however, if not screened, symptoms present with symptoms between 6-24 months of age. Sickling rarely occurs before this time because of their increased Hgb levels. Children most frequently present with failure to thrive, hemolytic anemia, infection and painful swelling in the extremities. Life expectancy of children with sickle cell disease has improved due to improved medical care.

For women, contraception and prepregnancy genetic counseling should be performed. There are generally no restrictions on contraception unless the patient has had a cerebral vascular accident (CVA); if patients have a history of CVA, estrogen contraception would be contraindicated. Pregnant patients with sickle cell disease are at higher risk for venous thromboembolism, maternal mortality, and preeclampsia.

Complications

Patients with sickle cell are at an increased risk for inflection such as pneumococcal and meningococcal infection, as well as influenza.

Referrals

Patients with sickle cell disease should be referred to a hematologist for follow-up. Patients who are pregnant need a referral to a maternal fetal specialist; inpatient services are needed for this in acute vaso-occlusive crisis.

Diagnosis: Polycythemia Vera

ICD-10 D75.0: Polycythemia, familial

ICD-10 D75.1: Polycythemia, secondary

Michelle Krawczyk, DNP, ARNP-BC, CNE

Introduction

Polycythemia Vera (PV) is a disorder characterized by a spontaneous overproduction of erythroid, granulocytic and megakaryocited. The medium age of onset is 60 years old with a slightly higher incidence in men. The disease is more common in persons of Eastern European descent and Jewish individuals. The patient may be asymptomatic during early phases of the disease; diagnosis can often be made with routine blood work.

Pathophysiology

The increased production of mature blood line cells results in increases in hemoglobin, hematocrit, erythrocytosis, and thrombocytosis. While the etiology is unclear, patients with PV have a defect in the pluripotential stem cell. The pluripotential stem cell can differentiate into either red blood cells, while blood cells or platelets. Most patients (approximately 96%) have been found to be positive for the JAK2 mutation. This mutation causes production of blood cells independently of erythropoietin.

Diagnosis is based on excluding other potential causes of pancytosis. Other causes of erythrocytosis can be hypertension, smoking, the use of drugs and alcohol, high altitudes, sleep apnea, tumors, and kidney disease. The increase in blood viscosity can lead to an increased risk of thrombosis or an increased risk of bleeding.

Physical Assessment

Subjective Data

Patients with PV may present with a headache, lightheadedness, blurred vision, fatigue, epistaxis, bruising, pruritis (especially after warm showers), weakness, sweating, joint pain, weight loss, tinnitus, and paresthesia.

Objective Data

Upon examination patients may be hypertensive and have a ruby or red complexion (plethora). Splenomegaly is common; hepatomegaly and ulcerations may be present. Examination features can be related to secondary complications such as thrombosis or bleeding.

Laboratory/Diagnostics

Laboratory data for patients may demonstrate the following:

- CBC: Pancytosis: increase in WBC, RBC/Hgb/Hct, Platelets
- RDW (red cell distribution width): elevated
- RCM (red cell mass): increased
- Retic count: normal or slightly elevated
- Erythropoietin: decreased
- Serum B12: increased
- LAP (Leukocyte alkaline phosphatase): elevated

- Bone Marrow Biopsy: hypercellular with hyperplasia. JAK2 mutation usually present, increased reticulin or fibrosis
- O2 Saturation: normal

Pharmacologic Management

Patients with PV may benefit from lifestyle modifications including exercise, skin care, smoking cessation, and avoidance of extreme temperatures.

First line treatment is always therapeutic phlebotomy with a target hematocrit value of less than 45% for men and less than 40% for women. Additional pharmaceutical interventions should be prescribed by hematology experts.

Special Considerations

Pregnancy can pose additional complication because of the increased blood volume during pregnancy. Therefore, pregnant women should be monitored by high risk maternal fetal practitioners.

Complications

Patients are at risk for clotting, which can lead to stroke or heart attacks. Development of splenomegaly can lead to infection.

Referrals

Patients with PV should be referred to a hematologist for follow-up. Pregnant women should be monitored by high risk maternal fetal practitioners.

Diagnosis: Leukemia

ICD-10 C95.91: Leukemia, unspecified, in remission

Michelle Krawczyk, DNP, ARNP-BC, CNE

Introduction

Leukemia is characterized by an abnormal proliferation of hematopoietic tissue that replaces normal bone marrow elements with neoplastic blood cells. There are four different main types of leukemia; acute myeloid leukemia (AML), acute lymphoblastic lymphocytic leukemia (ALL), chronic lymphocytic leukemia (CLL) and chronic myeloid leukemia (CML).

Pathophysiology

Acute Myeloid Leukemia (AML) is characterized by proliferation of myeloid progenitor cells, which replace normal hematopoiesis. There are diverse underlying genetics that cause AML. Acute lymphoblastic leukemia (ALL) is the most common pediatric malignancy. This type of leukemia results from a mutation of lymphoid precursor cells in the bone morrow of thymus.

Chronic lymphocytic leukemia (CLL) manifests with incompetent B lymphocytes. There is an increase in the incompetent B lymphocytes in the lymphatic tissue, blood and bone marrow. This is the most common type of leukemia in Western countries. B cells are responsible for B symptoms such as night sweats, weight loss and fever.

The hallmark for chronic myelogenous leukemia (CML) is being positive for BRC-ABLE. This is referred to as a Philadelphia chromosome. T cells are not affected for this type of leukemia. CML generally progressed to acute leukemia with increased blast cells in the blood and bone marrow. CML was the first type of leukemia that used targeted gene therapy as treatment. Table 7.1 further describes the various types of leukemia.

Table 7.1: Types of Leukemia

	ALL	**AML**	**CLL**	**CML**
Cell line affected	Malignancy of immature lymphocytes	Increase number of immature myeloid cells	Disorder of B cells.	Characterized by Philadelphia chromosome; reciprocal chromosomal translocation (Jain, 2013)
Incidence	10.8-1.5 per 100,000	4.1 per 100,000	4.6 per 100,000; >20/1000,000 in persons older than 65 yo.	1.5 in 100,000
At risk patients	Children <5 yo, followed by >55yo; Down syndrome	Survivors of childhood & young adult cancer; Down syndrome	Older adults. Median age of diagnosis is 72yo.; twice as frequent in men than women	Incident increases with age. Rare in children.
CBC	Lymphoblasts in blood and bone marrow	Anemia, neutropenia, thrombocytopenia, and myeloid blasts	Anemia, thrombocytopenia, increased lymphocytes	Leukocytes elevated, mild anemia, plt count normal or slightly elevated.

Physical Assessment

Subjective Data

Symptoms generally depend on the type of leukemia. Patients with leukemia may present with chest pain, bruising/bleeding, shortness of breath, coughing, lymphadenopathy, night sweats, fatigue, headache, fever, bone pain, petechiae, abdominal pain, nausea/vomiting/diarrhea, and unplanned weight loss.

Objective Data

Upon examination patients may demonstrate fever and pallor. Lymphadenopathy and hepatosplenomegaly, as well as ecchymosis and petechia may be present.

Laboratory/Diagnostics

A bone marrow biopsy may be used to assist in diagnosis. Laboratory data in patients with leukemia may demonstrate the following:

- CBC: Increased WBC, anemia, thrombocytopenia
- CMP: Hyperuricemia, increased blood urea nitrogen and creatinine, hypokalemia
- Uric Acid: Lactic acidosis
- Lactate dehydrogenase (LDH): Elevated

Pharmacologic Management

Treatment is administered by oncology providers and may include chemotherapy, radiation therapy, bone marrow transplant and immunotherapy.

Special Considerations

Leukemia is the most common childhood cancer; particularly ALL and AML. ALL has an approximate survival rate of 92% versus 69% for AML.

Complications

Complications of leukemia include an increase in infections and bleeding.

Referrals

Patients with leukemia require a referral to an oncologist for management.

Chapter 8: Gastrointestinal and Liver Disease

Peptic Ulcer Disease

Gastroenteritis

Cholecystitis

Appendicitis

GERD

Hepatitis

Diverticular Disease

Pancreatitis

Pancreatic Cancer

Diagnosis: Peptic Ulcer Disease (PUD)

ICD-10: K27.9 Peptic ulcer, site unspecified, unspecified as acute or chronic, without hemorrhage or perforation

Yvette T. Wilson, DNP, APRN, FNP-BC

Pathophysiology

The most common causes of Peptic Ulcer Disease (PUD) include *H. Pylori* infection and the use of NSAIDs drugs. *H.Pylori* can be communicated through person to person contact and contaminated food and water. NSAIDs can cause erosions and weakening of the gastrointestinal lining allowing *H.Pylori* to penetrate. There are two major classifications of Peptic Ulcers: Gastric and Duodenal. Both types will be compared.

Assessment

Diagnosis	Gastric Ulcer	Duodenal Ulcer
Subjective findings	Epigastric pain, belching, bloating Burning sensation **immediately** after a meal OTC antacids provide **little relief**	Epigastric pain, belching, bloating Burning sensation **2-3 hours after** a meal OTC antacids **relieves the pain** Pain worse at night
Objective findings	Nonspecific but may include: Epigastric tenderness Guaiac positive stool	Nonspecific but may include: Epigastric tenderness Guaiac positive stool

Laboratory/Diagnostics

- Urea breath test- positive for *H.Pylori*
- Stool antigen- positive for *H.Pylori*

An Endoscopy to rule out malignancy should be considered for the following:

a. Patients over age 55
b. One or more alarm symptoms:
   Persistent vomiting, weight loss, difficulty swallowing, bloody stools

Pharmacologic Management

First line treatment

Triple Therapy: Proton Pump Inhibitor (PPI) + Amoxicillin + Clarithromycin

Or

Triple Therapy: PPI + Clarithromycin + Metronidazole

Second line treatment

Quadruple Therapy: PPI + Bismuth + Tetracycline + Metronidazole

Third line treatment: Dependent on treatment failure and/or antibiotic resistance.

Special Considerations

Older persons are at a higher for complications related to possible use of antiplatelet, warfarin and SSRI medications. Providers should also discourage the overuse of NSAIDS.

Complications

Complications of PUD include bleeding, perforation, gastric outlet obstruction and gastric cancer.

Referrals

Patients diagnosed with PUD should be referred to a gastroenterologist.

Diagnosis: Gastroenteritis

ICD-10 K52.9: Noninfective gastroenteritis and colitis, unspecified

Yvette T. Wilson, DNP, APRN, FNP-BC

Pathophysiology

Gastroenteritis is an inflammatory process that involves the stomach and the intestines. The inflammatory process can be related to a bacterial infection, parasitic infection, viral infection or an allergic reaction to food or medications. When there is inflammation of the gastric mucosa, the vomiting center of the medulla is stimulated; when the lining of the intestines is inflamed, this can result in diarrhea and increased motility. Most cases of gastroenteritis are mild and self-limiting. Serious illness can result when the host is immunocompromised, or the infectious agent is more virulent.

Assessment

Subjective Data

Patients with gastroenteritis may report symptoms such as:

- Nausea/vomiting/diarrhea
- Abdominal cramping and pain
- Low-grade fever
- Malaise

Objective Data

Patients with gastroenteritis may exhibit signs of dehydration (tachycardia, threaded pulse, hypotension, and weight loss), abdominal pain and tenderness, guarding and an elevated temperature.

Laboratory/Diagnostics

Common pathogens associated with viral enteritis include norovirus and rotavirus. No labs are recommended in the diagnosis of viral enteritis.

Bacterial gastroenteritis is due to C. *difficile, Rotavirus, Salmonella, Shigella* and *Campylobacter*. A CBC may reveal an elevated WBC, blood cultures will identify the bacteria. Abdominal imaging may be ordered if obstruction or perforation is suspected.

Giardia and cryptosporidium are found with parasitic causes of gastroenteritis. For suspected parasitic gastroenteritis, a CBC may note a low WBC count, blood cultures or stool studies (ova and parasites) will identify the organism. Abdominal imaging may be ordered if obstruction or perforation is suspected.

Pharmacologic Management

First line treatment includes the promotion of patient hydration, rest, replacement of electrolytes, management of pain/fever, and observation. Antidiarrheals and antiemetics are not recommended, especially if the patient's gastroenteritis is caused by *Clostridium Difficile* or *E. coli*, as these medications can prevent the patient from ridding their body of the toxins, prolonging infection. Antibiotic therapy with use of Azithromycin, Vancomycin, Metronidazole or Fidaxomicin may be needed for severe bacterial or parasitic infections.

Complications

Complications of gastroenteritis include dehydration, metabolic acidosis from excessive diarrhea, metabolic alkalosis due to vomiting, septic shock, and death.

Referrals

Patients requiring a higher level of care due to complications may need to be referred to a gastroenterologist, the emergency department and/or admitted as an inpatient in the hospital for management.

Diagnosis: Cholecystitis

ICD-10 K81.0: Cholecystitis, unspecified

Yvette T. Wilson, DNP, APRN, FNP-BC

Pathophysiology

Cholecystitis is inflammation of the gallbladder that typically manifests over hours due to blockage of the cystic duct by a calculi (gallstone). The primary function of the gallbladder involves the storage and transportation of bile, which is an enzyme produced in the liver used to break up and digest fatty foods in the small intestine. Approximately 95% of patients presenting with signs and symptoms of cholecystitis have cholelithiasis. The incidence of gallstones increases with age; patients with a history of diabetes, who are obese, are female, and persons taking hormones or contraception, as well as patients with a history of rapid weight loss are at a higher risk for developing gallstones.

Assessment

Subjective Data

Patients may report abdominal pain lasting more than six hours, as well as right upper quadrant abdominal tenderness. Patients may experience nausea and vomiting, a low-grade fever, and chills. Signs and symptoms often occur after meals; especially meals that are fatty or large.

Objective Data

Upon examination, patients will have a positive Murphy's sign and demonstrate right subcostal tenderness. Additionally, patients may exhibit abdominal guarding, as well as diffuse abdominal pain (suspect gallstone pancreatitis).

Laboratory/Diagnostics

To assist in diagnosis of cholecystitis, the practitioner may order a CBC (elevated leukocytes may be present). A computerized tomography (CT) scan may be beneficial to identify a suspected perforation and/or pancreatitis. An abdominal ultrasound may reveal cholecystitis or gallstones in the gallbladder or bile ducts. Additionally, a liver function test (LFT) may show elevated levels of bilirubin, amylase, and lipase for patients with cholecystitis.

Pharmacologic Management

Analgesics (Ibuprofen) and antispasmodics (Scopolamine) are the first line treatment for patients with cholecystitis. Analgesics decrease inflammation by inhibiting prostaglandin release; while antispasmodics are an anti-cholinergic agent that help to decrease spasms of the gallbladder.

Special Considerations

Cholelithiasis occurs frequently in pregnant women due to pregnancy hormonal changes. This condition does not harm the fetus but can be uncomfortable for the mother. Expectant management is often chosen to avoid surgery during pregnancy.

Complications

Complications stemming from cholecystitis include perforation of the gallbladder, peritonitis, Mirizzi syndrome (rare), and gallstone pancreatitis.

Referrals

Referral to a gastroenterologist or general surgeon is recommended for patients with cholecystitis. A laparoscopic cholecystectomy is the recommended surgical procedure.

Diagnosis: Appendicitis

ICD-10 K35.8: Unspecified acute appendicitis

Yvette T. Wilson, DNP, APRN, FNP-BC

Pathophysiology

Appendicitis is inflammation of the appendix resulting from an obstruction in the appendiceal lumen, which is commonly seen in patients 10-30 years of age. The luminal obstruction results in bacteria build up leading to inflammation and potential for abscess formation and perforation.

Assessment

The diagnosis of acute appendicitis is made clinically and requires a thorough history and physical examination.

Subjective Data

Symptoms often appear suddenly and can include the following:

- Mild to severe colicky pain aggravated by walking or coughing
- Vague epigastric or periumbilical pain initially which localizes to the right lower quadrant (RLQ) over time
- Nausea with or without vomiting
- Mild fever 99-100 degrees F
- Shaking chills (consider perforation/emergency)

Objective Data

Upon abdominal examination, patients may have a positive McBurney's sign (RLQ pain with palpation) and a positive obturator sign (RLQ pain on rotation of a flexed right leg and knee). Patients with appendicitis may have a positive Psoas sign (RLQ pain when lifting right leg against slight pressure), as well as a positive Rovsing's sign (RLQ after deep palpation of the left lower quadrant [LLQ]).

Laboratory/Diagnostics

A CBC may indicate leukocytosis. An abdominal ultrasound can help to confirm diagnosis; a CT scan or MRI can be used if the ultrasound is inconclusive.

Pharmacologic Management

First line treatment for acute presentations of appendicitis include bed rest, IV hydration, antibiotics and NPO status. The standard of care for acute appendicitis is surgical removal. Anti-infective agents such as Ampicillin, Gentamycin, Metronidazole, and Ampicillin-sulbactam are commonly prescribed for patients with appendicitis..

Complications

Complications of appendicitis include perforation and peritonitis. Patients who report a sudden relief of pain may have a ruptured appendix, which is life-threatening and requires immediate surgical intervention. Patients on anti-infective agents should avoid laxatives and narcotics; laxatives can cause the appendix to rupture and narcotics can hide the presentation of a perforation

Referrals

Patients with appendicitis should be referred to a gastroenterologist or general surgeon for management.

Diagnosis: Gastroesophageal Reflux Disease (GERD)

ICD-10 K21.9: Gastro-esophageal reflux disease without esophagitis

Yvette T. Wilson, DNP, APRN, FNP-BC

Pathophysiology

Gastroesophageal reflux disease (GERD) is a syndrome that results from the the backward flow of stomach gastric acid into the esophagus due to a weakened lower esophagus sphincter (LES), or relaxation of the LES. If the LES loses its tone, stomach contents and gastric acid can reflux backwards into the esophagus. Hiatal hernias are often isolated as a cause of GERD. Other conditions that could lead to a weakened LES tone include cigarette smoking, caffeine, fatty foods, and alcohol intake. Obesity and delayed gastric emptying can lead to increased abdominal pressure, which also has a direct relationship on the LES tone.

Assessment

Subjective Data

Patients with GERD may report the following symptoms:

- Burning epigastric sensation (heartburn) , worse after meals or lying down
- Bitter/sour taste in the mouth
- Dysphagia
- Hoarseness
- Belching
- Chronic cough (due to vagal innervation)

Objective Data

Upon examination clients may report tenderness upon palpation to the epigastric region. Dental erosions may be noted as well as oral erythema from gastric acid exposure. Otherwise, the physical examination may be normal. Possible positive stool guaiac will occur if erosions are present.

Laboratory/Diagnostics

If the patient has no relief after an eight-week trial of medications, the following testing is recommended:

- Upper GI series
- Endoscopy
- Esophageal Manometry
- Esophageal pH

Pharmacologic Management

An eight-week trial of a Proton Pump Inhibitor (PPI) such as Omeprazole, Lansoprazole, or Pantoprazole is recommended. PPI can reduce the production of acid by blocking the enzyme in the wall of the stomach that produces acid.

Complications

Chronic GERD may lead to esophageal/peptic strictures, Barrett's esophagus (pre-cancerous changes), and esophageal cancer.

Referrals

A referral to a gastroenterologist is suggested for patients with GERD.

Diagnosis: Hepatitis

ICD-10 B19: Acute viral hepatitis, unspecified

ICD-10 B15: Acute hepatitis A

ICD-10 B16: Acute hepatitis B

ICD-10 B17: Other acute viral hepatitis

ICD-10 B18: Chronic viral hepatitis

ICD-10 K73.9: Chronic hepatitis, unspecified

Vannessa Davis, DNP, APRN, FNP-C, CNN

Pathophysiology

Hepatitis refers to inflammation of the liver. Hepatitis is classified by the name of the causative virus. Hepatitis is classified as: hepatitis A virus (HAV), hepatitis B virus (HBV), hepatitis C virus (HCV), the HBV-associated delta agent or hepatitis D virus (HDV), and hepatitis E virus (HEV). With the exception of hepatitis B, which is a DNA virus but replicates like a retrovirus, all the other hepatitis viruses are RNA viruses. Drug or alcohol use can also cause hepatitis. Hepatitis can be acute or chronic in nature. The properties and clinical characteristics of hepatitis are explained in Table 8.1

Table 8.1: Properties and Clinical Characteristics of Viral Hepatitis

	Hepatitis A	Hepatitis B	Hepatitis C	Hepatitis D	Hepatitis E
Virus size	27nm	42nm	32nm	36nm	32-34nm
Length	7.5kb	3.2kb	10kb	1.7kb	7.6kg

Genome	RNA	DNA	RNA	RNA	RNA
Incubation	14-49 days	30-180 days	14-160 days	21-42 days	21-63 days
Transmission	Fecal-oral	Percutaneous, sexual, perinatal	Percutaneous, (especially injection drug user), sexual (rare), perinatal (rare)	Percutaneous and intrafamily	Fecal-oral
Vaccine	Available	Available	None	None but hepatitis B vaccine protects against acute hepatitis D	Available outside the United States
Severity of illness	Usually mild, particularly in children	Adults: 70% subclinical, 30% clinical, <1% severe Newborn: subclinical	Usually subclinical, 1% severe	May be severe	May be severe; 20% mortality in pregnancy
Chronic infection	None	90% neonatal, 50% infants, 20% children, <1% healthy adults	>85%	5% with HBV coinfection, >90% with HBV superinfection	May occur in immunocompromised hosts

Physical Assessment

All types of viral hepatitis produce clinically similar illnesses although they are distinguished by their molecular and antigenic properties (Ghany, & Morgan, 2020). Chronic viral hepatitis is often asymptomatic; most patients are unaware of their condition until the diagnosis is made incidentally or until progression to advanced liver disease results in systemic symptoms and clinical features of hepatic dysfunction. Subjective and objective findings vary between acute and chronic viral hepatitis (see Table 8.2).

Table 8.2: Subjective and Objective Findings

	Acute Viral Hepatitis	Chronic Viral Hepatitis
Subjective Data	• Symptoms are usually nonspecific • Malaise • Fatigue • Nausea • Vomiting • Anorexia • Arthralgias. • Fever, if present, is usually low grade. • Pruritus, with disease progression, • Dark urine • Clay colored stool • Arthralgias • Myalgias • Headache • Photophobia • Pharyngitis • Cough • Coryza	• Fatigue • Anorexia • Pruritus • Dark urine
Objective Data	• Scleral icterus • Jaundice • Splenomegaly • Cervical adenopathy • Neutropenia • Transient Lymphopenia • Lymphocytosis • Serum aminotransferase levels typically exceed 500 units/L and often 1000 units/L, with alanine aminotransferase (ALT)	• Severe liver damage • Elevated liver enzymes with ALT >AST • Jaundice • Splenomegaly • Cervical adenopathy • Neutropenia • Transient Lymphopenia • Lymphocytosis • Elevated bilirubin • Prolonged prothrombin

	higher than aspartate aminotransferase (AST). • Elevated bilirubin • Prolonged prothrombin time (PT)	time (PT)

Laboratory/Diagnostics

Serologic tests are available routinely to establish a diagnosis of hepatitis A, B, D, and C. Tests for fecal or serum HAV are not routinely available; therefore, a diagnosis of hepatitis A is based on the detection of IgM anti-HAV during acute illness. HBV infection is usually diagnosed by the detection of HBsAg in serum. Note that HBsAg levels may be too low to be detected during acute HBV infection; as such, the diagnosis can be established by the presence of IgM anti-HBc.

Diagnostic tests appropriate to different clinical situations detect specific viral antigens and antibodies in serum by sensitive immunoassay and viral DNA/RNA by sensitive amplification assays (polymerase chain reaction [PCR]). Ultrasound, computed tomography (CT), or magnetic resonance imaging (MRI) are useful to evaluate liver parenchyma and to assess for the existence of varices, reversal of portal hepatic flow, ascites, splenomegaly, and other signs of portal hypertension; hepatic vein occlusion and other vascular abnormalities; and focal mass lesions.

Pharmacologic Management

Most people with acute hepatitis (especially A, B, and E) recover spontaneously and do not require specific antiviral therapy. Antiviral therapy with a nucleoside analogue (entecavir or tenofovir, the most potent and least resistance-prone agents) is recommended for severe, but not mild–moderate, acute hepatitis B. Treatment should continue until 3 months after HBsAg seroconversion or 6 months after HBeAg seroconversion (Kasper et al., 2018). First line treatment is Entecavir, an anti-HBV reverse transcriptase inhibitor, which inhibits reverse transcription, DNA replication and transcription in the viral replication process of HBV.

Special Considerations

Elderly persons with serious underlying medical disorders may have a prolonged course and are more likely to experience severe hepatitis. Patients who present initially with ascites, peripheral edema, and symptoms of hepatic encephalopathy have a poorer prognosis.

Prolonged prothrombin time (PT), low serum albumin level, hypoglycemia, and very high serum bilirubin values suggest severe hepatocellular disease. Neonates, persons with Down's syndrome, hemodialysis patients, and immunosuppressed patients may remain chronically infected after acute HBV infection.

Complications

Complications associated with hepatitis include:

- Cholestatic hepatitis
- Encephalopathy
- Portal hypertension
- Hepatic vein occlusion
- Other vascular abnormalities

- Focal mass lesions
- Hepatocellular carcinoma
- Chronic liver disease
- Cirrhosis

Referrals

Patients with hepatitis may benefit from referral to a gastroenterologist and/or an infectious disease specialist.

Diagnosis: Diverticular Disease

ICD-10 K57.20: Diverticulitis of intestine part unspecified, without perforation or abscess without bleeding

ICD-10 K57.90: Diverticulosis of intestine, part unspecified, without perforation or abscess without bleeding

Cameron Duncan DNP, MS, APRN, FNP-C, PMHNP-BC

Introduction

Diverticulosis is the eighth most common condition in the United States and is the most common gastrointestinal reason for an emergency room visit (Rezapour, Ali & Stollman, 2018; Wheat & Strate, 2016). Diverticular disease is broad term referring to disease of the diverticula of the colon, which includes asymptomatic diverticulosis and symptomatic diverticulosis. Asymptomatic diverticulosis is often found incidentally during a routine colonoscopy and does not require further monitoring or treatment. However, symptomatic diverticulosis can present in several ways and requires further, specialized treatment (Rezapour et al., 2018). There are three presentations of illness: diverticulitis, uncomplicated diverticular disease, and segmental colitis. Diverticulitis is the most common presentation and requires the most attention by the FNP.

Pathophysiology

Diverticulitis is inflammation of the diverticula and can present as an acute or chronic problem. Diverticula are small pouches that are believed to be caused by increased pressure in specific areas of wall of the diverticulum. Older evidence suggested that these pouches would become irritated by food or stool trauma, ischemia, or other complications including diverticulitis. However, more recent research describes diverticulitis as a result of genetics, changes in the microbiome, decreased bowel motility, and chronic, microscopic inflammation (Tursi et al., 2018).

Physical Assessment

Subjective Data

Patients with diverticulitis may present with left lower quadrant (LLQ) and/or abdominal pain, nausea, and vomiting, as well as fever and chills. If inflammation of the diverticulum is near the bladder, the patient may complain of dysuria, polyuria, and/or urgency.

Objective Data

Upon examination, there may be decreased or absent bowel sounds. Additionally, patients may exhibit guarding, LLQ tenderness, as well as a LLQ mass.

Laboratory and Diagnostics

If diverticulitis is suspected based on a thorough subjective assessment and physical examination, imaging is necessary to diagnose the disease. A CT scan is recommended because of its sensitivity and specificity, and high predictive accuracy compared to an ultrasound (You, Sweeny, Cooper, Von Papen & Innes, 2019). The CT will assist in confirming the diagnosis of diverticulitis, identify the severity of the disease, and will guide management plans.

C-reactive protein (CRP) is the most powerful lab test used to predict diverticulitis versus other abdominal complications (You et al., 2019). Together, an elevated CRP and elevated cell counts can help determine disease severity. However, lab values alone cannot confirm the diagnosis of diverticulitis.

Management

Diverticulitis can be managed in an outpatient setting depending on the severity of the illness. If the patient presents afebrile and without a cyst, and uncomplicated diverticulitis, outpatient care is recommended. Nonpharmacological treatment consists of a clear liquid diet for 2-3 days, and a low fiber diet until pain improves.

Pharmacologic treatment includes the use of acetaminophen and antispasmodics for pain, as well as the use of antibiotics if needed. For mild to moderate symptoms, antibiotics include Trimethoprim/sulfamethoxazole DS or Ciprofloxacin (Cipro). If the patient is immunocompromised, antibiotics should be considered in an uncomplicated case of diverticulitis.

In an immunocompetent patient, antibiotic therapy is not recommended. In complicated diverticulitis (presence of an abscess on CT imaging), intravenous, broad-spectrum antibiotics and bowel rest are recommended and should be administered in the inpatient setting.

Complications

Patients with acute diverticulitis are at risk for developing fistulas, bowel blockage, abscess, or peritonitis

Referrals

Appropriate referrals and collaborative care are determined by the severity of the disease. Asymptomatic diverticulosis can be managed in the primary care setting; diverticulitis can be managed in the outpatient setting by a gastroenterologist, depending on the severity of the disease. Complicated diverticulitis may require a referral to the emergency department.

Diagnosis: Pancreatitis

ICD-10 K85.0: Idiopathic acute pancreatitis

ICD-10 K85.1: Biliary acute pancreatitis

ICD-10 K85.2: Alcohol induced acute pancreatitis

ICD-10 K85.3: Drug induced acute pancreatitis

ICD-10 K85.9: Acute pancreatitis, unspecified

ICD-10 K86.1: Other chronic pancreatitis

Shay A. Schroetter DNP, APRN, ANP-BC

Pathophysiology

Pancreatitis is an inflammatory condition that can lead to necrosis and/or infection of the pancreatic parenchyma. The two primary causes of pancreatitis are a blockage of the pancreatic duct (by either gallstones or pancreatic stones) or long-term alcohol use. Other causes and risk factors for pancreatitis include use of drugs, abdominal trauma, autoimmune conditions, infections (viral, bacterial, fungal, and parasitic), tumors, hypertriglyceridemia, hypercalcemia, and vascular abnormalities. Rarely, acute pancreatitis can be an indicator of pancreatic cancer (Kornusky & Caple, 2018). Etiology can also be idiopathic.

Physical Assessment

Subjective and objective findings associated with pancreatitis depend upon whether it is acute or chronic in nature and level of severity. (see Table 8.3)

Table 8.3: Subjective and Objective Findings

	Acute Pancreatitis	**Chronic Pancreatitis**
Subjective	• Sudden onset abdominal pain (left lower quadrant, periumbilical, and/or epigastrium). • Pain worse after eating ("postprandial pain") and drinking (especially fatty foods) • Pain becomes constant over time • Nausea and vomiting	• Ongoing abdominal pain in most patients (can range from occasional to debilitating); few patients may have no pain • Pain can radiate to back • Pain might be relieved with sitting upright or leaning forward • Nausea and vomiting
Objective	• Fever • Hypotension • Tachycardia • Tachypnea • Diaphoresis • Abdominal tenderness • Abdominal guarding • Abdominal distention • Decreased bowel sounds • Jaundice • Altered mental status • Weight loss • Cullen sign (edema & ecchymosis around umbilicus) • Grey Turner sign (ecchymosis of the flank)	• Abdominal tenderness (typically epigastric) Jaundice • Pallor • Bruising • Epigastric mass (suggestive of pseudocyst) • In mild cases, exam may be normal • Advanced disease, steatorrhea and physical signs of malnutrition may be present (loss of subcutaneous fat, temporal wasting)

The APACHE II scale or the HAPScore can be used to classify severity of illness.

Laboratory / Diagnostics

Two of the following three criteria are required to diagnose acute pancreatitis: characteristic abdominal pain, elevated serum amylase, and lipase (two to four times above the upper limit of normal), and radiologic evidence of pancreatitis on ultrasound or computerized tomography (CT).

Pharmacological Management

Acute Pancreatitis

Mild pancreatitis can be treated outpatient. Management of acute pancreatitis is typically supportive and includes fluid resuscitation, pain management, and nutrition support. If the patient presents with no ileus, nausea, or vomiting, then start a low residue, low fat, soft diet. Antibiotic therapy is not needed if cultures are negative and no source of infection is identified. Cessation of alcohol and tobacco use strongly encouraged.

Chronic Pancreatitis

Management is supportive and pain control is necessary. Small, low fat meals should be encouraged. Pancreatic enzyme supplements may help to reduce pain. Steroid therapy may be used for autoimmune pancreatitis. Cessation of alcohol and tobacco use is strongly encouraged. Additionally, consider screening for depression and treat as indicated (Barry, 2018).

Special Considerations

The causative factor must be identified quickly in order to reduce morbidity and mortality. Patients with severe acute pancreatitis need hospital admission; approximately 50% of patients ultimately require surgery such as decompression or resection (Barry, 2018).

Cholelithiasis is the most common cause of pancreatitis in pregnancy, occurring most often in the third trimester. This is often misdiagnosed as hyperemesis gravidarum.

Complications

Serious complications are associated with pancreatitis, including:

- Pseudocyst formation
- Pancreatic necrosis and infection
- Acute pancreatitis can transition into chronic pancreatitis
- Malnutrition
- Gastric varices
- Ileus
- Disseminated intravascular coagulation
- Acute renal failure
- Acute respiratory distress syndrome
- Systemic inflammatory response syndrome (SIRS)
- Sepsis
- Death

Referrals

Patients with pancreatitis may be referred to a gastroenterologist, general surgeon, as well as pain medicine specialist.

Diagnosis: Pancreatic Cancer

ICD-10 C25.9: Malignant neoplasm of pancreas, unspecified

Cara Wallace PhD, RN

Pathophysiology

Pancreatic cancer begins when mutations occur in the cells of the pancreas. The mutations can grow uncontrollably, leading the pancreatic cells to form into tumors. The tumors can be either exocrine or neuroendocrine (endocrine). Knowing the type of tumor is important for the practitioner, as the type is unique and responds differently to treatment. Adenocarcinoma is the most common, and most aggressive, type of pancreatic cancer.

Individuals over the age of 65 are at a higher risk of developing pancreatic cancer. Other risk factors include a history of diabetes, obesity, smoking, chronic and hereditary pancreatitis. Additionally, African Americans and persons of Ashkenazi Jewish heritage are at an increased risk to develop pancreatic cancer.

Physical Assessment

Symptoms of pancreatic cancer may be initially be vague, which results in it being difficult to diagnose early on given symptoms generally occur once the cancer has metastasized. Patients with pancreatic cancer may present with the following:

- Pain in the abdomen radiating to the back

- Unexpected weight loss, loss of appetite
- Jaundice (yellowing of the skin, eyes or both) with or without itching
- Fatigue
- Light-colored stools, dark-colored urine
- Uncontrolled diabetes or recent-onset diabetes

Laboratory/Diagnostics

Given the vague symptomology of pancreatic cancer can be subtle, it is often difficult to detect early. Image modalities such as computed tomography (CT) scans, magnetic resonance imaging (MRI) and positron emission tomography (PET) scans may be beneficial in the diagnosis of pancreatic cancer.

A biopsy may be collected, as well as the tumor marker CA19-9,which is elevated in patients with pancreatic cancer. Note some patients may not have an elevated CA19-9, which can make the marker unreliable for some patients.

Management

Treatment options for pancreatic cancer may include a combination of surgery, chemotherapy, and radiation therapy. Palliative care may be used to provide pain relief, as well as address other symptoms the patient is experiencing. For late stage pancreatic cancer, it may be necessary to admit the patient to Hospice care.

Complications

Upon progression of the cancer, complications such as weight loss due to malabsorption may occur. Additional complications include pain resulting from the growing tumor, jaundice due to blockage of the bile duct, as well as obstruction of the bowel secondary to blockage of the duodenum.

Referrals

Patients with pancreatic cancer should be referred to an oncologist for management. Additional referrals may include general surgery, radiation oncology, palliative care, and hospice care.

Chapter 9: Renal/Urinary

Cystitis

Urethritis

Pyelonephritis

Glomerulonephritis

Urolithiasis

Benign Prostatic Hypertrophy

Renal Failure

Diagnosis: Cystitis

ICD-10 N30.90: Cystitis, unspecified without hematuria

Pamela Porter DNP, APRN, FNP-BC, CNS, PA-S

Pathophysiology

Cystitis is inflammation of the bladder. Cystitis is most often cause by a urinary tract infection (UTI), which occurs when bacteria ascends the urinary tract system causing an infection. Cystitis is more common in women due to anatomy, as the shorter urethra and the proximity of the vagina and anus can contribute to cystitis. Table 9.1 identifies the pathogens, which cause UTI.

Table 9.1: UTI Pathogens

Gram-Negative Pathogens	Gram-Positive Pathogens
• Escherichia coli- (most common) • Klebsiella species • Proteus species • Pseudomonas aeruginosa	• Enterococcus species • Staphylococcus (more common in younger women)

Physical Assessment

Subjective Data

Patients with cystitis may present with dysuria, urgency, frequent urination, and gross hematuria. Patients may also report different smelling urine, suprapubic pain, as well as a low-grade fever.

Objective Data

Upon physical examination, patients with cystitis may demonstrate suprapubic tenderness, as well as urethral discharge. Patients may also be febrile.

Laboratory/Diagnostics

A clean-catch midstream sample urine collection or a urine sample collected by bladder catheterization are suitable for culture.

The following laboratory and diagnostic testing may be beneficial in diagnosing cystitis:

- **Urine dipstick -** Findings suggestive of infection include positive leukocyte esterase, positive hemoglobin, positive nitrates. Positive nitrates are present if there is an infection from Enterobacteriaceae, E. Coli, and are formed from the breakdown of nitrate to nitrite.
- **Urinalysis** - Findings in infection include pyuria (elevated white blood cells (WBC), hematuria, and bacteria casts indicate pyelonephritis while epithelial cells indicate a contaminated sample.
- **Urine culture and sensitivity -** Identifies pathogen. Infection is determined by the amount of colony-forming units (CFU)/mL. In midstream, clean-catch sample has bacteria with >1x105 CFU/mL and for a catheterization sample has >1 x 102 CFU/mL. Urine sensitivity establishes the most effective antibiotic to treat the UTI and identifies resistant strains of bacteria.
- **Sexually Transmitted Infections** (STI)- Gonorrhea and chlamydia urine sample for both male and female

- **Imaging Studies** – Ultrasound or cystoscopy may be used.

  Order if any anatomical anomaly is suspected.

Pharmacologic Management

Nitrofurantoin and Trimethoprim-sulfamethoxazole are considered first line treatment for initial cystitis. Nitrofurantoin is an antimicrobial that inactivates or alters bacterial ribosomal proteins, inhibiting protein synthesis, aerobic energy metabolism, DNA, RNA, and cell wall synthesis. Trimethoprim-sulfamethoxazole is a folate synthesis inhibitor that interferes with bacterial folic acid synthesis and growth; inhibits dihydrofolic acid reduction to tetrahydrofolate resulting in sequential inhibition of enzymes of the folic acid pathway.

Lifestyle modifications may be beneficial and address patient discomfort. Patients should be encouraged to hydrate, avoiding caffeinated drinks, as well as alcohol. Additionally, patients may benefit from use of a heating pad on their abdomen to address pain or discomfort.

Special Considerations

Not all persons present with the classic signs and symptoms of UTIs. For example, very young children and pregnant women may be febrile. Pregnant females may present with asymptomatic bacturiuria not on routine urinalysis which must be treated. Elderly patients may exhibit sudden onset confusion.

Persons with recurrent cystitis require follow-up for potential kidney stones and fistulas. Postmenopausal women with frequent UTIs require evaluation for genitourinary syndrome of menopause (GSM).

Complications

Untreated or undertreated cystitis can ascend to the upper urinary tract and may result in pyelonephritis and kidney damage.

Referrals

Patients with recurring or non-resolving cystitis should be referred to a urologist or gynecologist for follow-up and medical management.

Diagnosis: Urethritis

ICD-10 N34.1: Non-specific urethritis

Nicole Sinkler, DNP, MS, APRN, FNP-C

Pathophysiology

Urethritis is inflammation of the urethra and occurs in both men and women. The inflammation is typically from a sexually transmitted infection (STI) and is categorized as gonococcal urethritis (GU) or nongonococcal urethritis (NGU). Chlamydia trachomatis and Neisseria gonorrhoeae are the infection-causing organisms that contribute to urethral discharge. Organisms that can cause urethritis, from most common to the least common, include:

- *Neisseria gonorrhoeae*
- *Chlamydia trachomatis*
- *Mycoplasma genitalium*
- *Ureaplasma urealyticum*
- *Trichomonas vaginalis*
- *Treponema pallidum*
- *Haemophilus species*
- *Lymphogranuloma venereum* (a type of chlamydia infection)
- *Herpes* simplex
- Noninfectious-reactive arthritis

Physical Assessment

Subjective Data

Many patients are asymptomatic. Patients usually complain of mucopurulent or purulent discharge from the urethra. Men will report burning on urination and increased urethral pain over time, as well as profuse discharge. A detailed medical and sexual history including current partners and a prior history of sexually transmitted diseases (STDs) is vital.

Objective Data

Upon examination, patients with urethritis will exhibit normal vital signs and external genitalia examinations should be unremarkable.

Laboratory/Diagnostics

The following laboratory and diagnostic testing will be beneficial in the diagnosis of urethritis:

- Urethral smear -identify organism
- Gram stain >5 WBC per high power field. gram-negative intracellular diplococci present with gonorrhea
- First voided urine to detect for the presence of leukocyte esterase on urine dipstick or white blood cells (WBCs) on microscopy
- Polymerase chain reaction assays for Chlamydia and Gonorrhea
- Wet prep to detect trichomonas organism
- Rapid plasma reagin (RPR) or syphilis, Human Immunodeficiency Virus

- Pregnancy testing should be offered to women who have engaged in unprotected sexual intercourse

Pharmacologic Management

It is important to administer antibiotics that cover both GU and NGU. The first line treatment is cceftriaxone plus azithromycin. Ceftriaxone is a third-generation cephalosporin that inhibits cell wall mucopeptide synthesis; azithromycin is macrolide antibiotic, which works to stop bacterial protein synthesis.

Special Considerations

The sexual partners of patients with urethritis should also be treated. After one week of antibiotics, patients should be evaluated to determine the effectiveness of the therapy. Infection at the time of delivery can result in potential transmission to the newborn.

Complications

Complications in men include urethral stricture or stenosis, prostatitis, infertility, acute epididymitis, proctitis, and abnormal semen. For women, complications may include pelvic inflammatory disease (PID), infertility, and ectopic pregnancy.

Referrals

Male patients with urethritis should be referred to urology for further evaluation and treatment. Note any STI needs to be reported to the public health department.

Diagnosis: Pyelonephritis

ICD-10 590.80: Pyelonephritis, unspecified

Vannessa Davis, DNP, APRN, FNP-C, CNN

Pathophysiology

Pyelonephritis also known as kidney infection is an ascending urinary tract infection (UTI), which commonly begins in the urethra or bladder and migrates upstream to one or both kidneys. Pyelonephritis can also be caused by seeding of the kidneys from bacteremia. Some cases of pyelonephritis are associated with seeding of the kidneys from bacteria in the lymphatics. In a kidney with pyelonephritis, scarring is common, which can cause resistance leading to hypertension.

Physical Assessment

Subjective

Patients with pyelonephritis may report the following symptoms:

- Fever
- Chills
- Cloudy urine with foul odor
- Back, side (flank) pain or groin pain on affected side
- Frequent urination
- Urgency
- Dysuria
- Nausea and vomiting

- Hematuria
- Foul smelling or cloudy urine
- Abdominal pain

Objective

Upon examination, patients may demonstrate the following:

- Fever
- Costovertebral angle tenderness on affected side
- Pelvic or perineal pain in men, which can suggest accompanying prostatitis
- Hypertension

Laboratory/Diagnostics

- **Urine dipstick -** Findings suggestive of infection include positive leukocyte esterase, positive hemoglobin, positive nitrates. Positive nitrates are present if there is an infection from Enterobacteriaceae, E. Coli, and are formed from the breakdown of nitrate to nitrite. Hematuria may be present.
- **Urinalysis** - Findings in infection include pyuria (elevated white blood cells (WBC), hematuria, and bacteria casts indicate pyelonephritis while epithelial cells indicate a contaminated sample.
- **Urine culture and sensitivity -** Identifies pathogen. Infection is determined by the amount of colony-forming units (CFU)/mL. In midstream, clean-catch sample has bacteria with >1x105 CFU/mL and for a catheterization sample has >1 x 102 CFU/mL. Urine sensitivity establishes the most

effective antibiotic to treat the UTI and identifies resistant strains of bacteria.

- **Imaging-** Ultrasound will show any enlargement of the affected kidney and signs of hydronephrosis. CT scan will show renal abscess, obstruction, renal enlargement, and inflammation.

Pharmacologic Management

Antibiotics, specifically Fluoroquinolones (Norfloxacin, Ciprofloxacin, Ofloxacin, and Levofloxacin), are the first line of treatment for pyelonephritis. Treatment for obstructive pyelonephritis includes antipseudomonal carbapenem (imipenem, meropenem or doripenem) in addition to vancomycin.

Fluoroquinolones act by inhibiting two enzymes involved in bacterial DNA synthesis, both of which are DNA topoisomerases that human cells lack and that are essential for bacterial DNA replication, thus enabling these agents to be both specific and bactericidal.

Special Considerations

Pyelonephritis is treated outpatient or inpatient depending on severity.

Diabetics and immunocompromised people are at increased risk for pyelonephritis.

Pregnant women have an increased risk; pregnant women with a UTI should be assessed and treated as soon as possible. Patients with spinal cord injury and neurogenic bladder can present with autonomic dysreflexia and increased spasticity. Elderly or debilitated patients may present with more generalized signs or symptoms of infection (such as fever and chills) without clear symptoms localizing to the urinary tract; often, confusion may be the only presenting symptoms.

Fluoroquinolones are associated with disabling and potentially irreversible serious adverse reactions including tendinitis and tendon rupture, peripheral neuropathy, and CNS effects. Therefore, discontinue their use immediately if any of these symptoms occur.

Complications

If left untreated, pyelonephritis can lead to potentially serious complications including:

- Kidney scarring, which can lead to chronic kidney disease, high blood pressure and kidney failure.
- Pyelonephritis can cause the bacteria to spread through your bloodstream leading to septicemia.
- Complications during pregnancy include babies who have a low birth weight.
- Kidney failure
- Death

Referrals

Patients with pyelonephritis should be referred to a nephrologist or a urologist for further evaluation.

Diagnosis: Glomerulonephritis

ICD 10 N05.2: Unspecified nephritic syndrome with diffuse membranous glomerulonephritis

Mary Sizemore DNP, APRN-FNP

Pathophysiology

There are two types of glomerulonephritis-acute and chronic. Both types of glomerulonephritis have different pathophysiological considerations. Regardless of the type, glomerulonephritis is a type of kidney disease caused by damage to the glomeruli.

Acute glomerulonephritis occurs after infections such as strep throat and are referred to as acute poststreptococcal glomerulonephritis (APSGN). Antistreptococcal antibodies are produced in response to the streptococcal infection, creating the antigen-antibody complex (type III hypersensitivity reaction). The antigen-antibody complex lodges in the glomerular capillaries that initiates the body's complement system and results in an inflammatory response in the glomeruli of both kidneys. Once inflamed, glomeruli start leaking significant protein and erythrocytes into the filtration. Acute glomerulonephritis can also occur with other IgA nephropathy, systemic lupus erythematosus (SLE), vasculitis, and amyloidosis.

Chronic glomerulonephritis can be caused by hypertension (HTN), diabetes mellitus (DM), and cancer.

If the damage progresses quickly, the patient may be diagnosed with acute glomerulonephritis. However, if progression occurs slowly, it is classified as chronic glomerulonephritis.

Physical Assessment

The signs and symptoms, both subjective and objective, of glomerulonephritis vary according to whether it is acute or chronic in nature (see Table 9.2).

Table 9.2: Signs and Symptoms of Glomerulonephritis

	Acute	**Chronic**
Subjective	• Abdominal pain • Decreased urinary output • Edema to face and ankles	• Decreased urinary output • Edema to face and ankles • Fever, chills, weight loss, night sweats, and fatigue • Rash • Muscle aches • Frequent nighttime urination • Bubbly or foamy urine
Objective	• Hematuria • Proteinuria • Hypertension • Edema	• Hematuria • Proteinuria • Hypertension • Edema • Hypercoagulability

Laboratory and Diagnostic Testing

- urinalysis- proteinuria, hematuria and erythrocyte casts
- CMP (Comprehensive Metabolic Profile)- elevated serum urea, creatnine, pH
- GFR (Glomerular Filtration Rate)-decreased

Additional laboratory evaluation should be based on the cause of the symptoms and other disease processes such as systemic lupus erythematosus.

Pharmacologic Management

Treatment for glomerulonephritis is based on the cause, symptoms, severity, and progression of the disorder. The first line treatment for acute glomerulonephritis is penicillin, which is a bactericidal. If the patient has moderate to severe disease, the treatment should be aimed at reduction in blood pressure with an ACE inhibitor or angiotensin II receptor antagonists. If the patient has fluid retention, then a diuretic such as furosemide could be utilized. For cases involving nephrotic syndrome the patient may be prescribed prednisone with a possibility of additional immunosuppressants such as cyclophosphamide and azathioprine.

Special Considerations

Special considerations are associated with the treatment of glomerulonephritis. It is important to note that penicillin may be used during pregnancy and while breastfeeding; however, ACE Inhibitors or Angiotensin II Receptor Blockers (ARBs) must be avoided. Additionally, the safety of furosemide, a loop diuretic, has not been established in obstetric or lactating patients. There is an increased risk of adverse side effects associated with the use of furosemide in elderly patients, while its use in pediatric patients can lead to an increased risk of renal calculi.

Complications

Complications can occur if patients do not receive the appropriate treatment. Improperly or untreated glomerulonephritis can lead to reduced renal function, end stage renal disease and chronic renal failure.

Referrals

Patients with glomerulonephritis should be referred to a nephrologist.

Diagnosis: Urolithiasis

ICD-10 N20.0: Calculus of kidney

Vannessa Davis, DNP, APRN, FNP-C, CNN

Pathophysiology

Urolithiasis is the formation of stones anywhere in the urinary system involving the kidneys, urinary tract or bladder. Stones usually form in the renal pelvis, and symptoms occur with passage of the stone into the ureter. While the male to female ratio of occurrence is 3:1, stone incidence is highest among whites with a peak incidence between ages 20 and 50. Bladder stones are less common, and patients may present with hematuria or intermittent urinary obstruction.

Stones can form either from solutes that accrete upon a nidus (usually calcium oxalate, but also uric acid) or as a result of chronic urinary tract infections with urea-splitting organisms (struvite stones). Microscopic or gross hematuria may be present intermittently, but most stones are asymptomatic until they cause obstruction to a ureter or bladder outlet. The types of renal stones, in order of decreasing prevalence, include:

- Combination of calcium oxalate and calcium phosphate
- Calcium oxalate
- Struvite
- Calcium phosphate
- Uric acid

- Cystine

Physical Assessment

Subjective Data

Patients occasionally present as asymptomatic. There may be a sudden onset of unilateral flank pain that radiates to the ipsilateral lower quadrant, groin, scrotum, or labia. Patients may also experience:

- Intermittent gross hematuria
- Colicky loin pain with or without radiation to groin or testis
- Vasovagal syncope caused by pain
- Nausea and vomiting

It is important to obtain a previous medical history, inquiring about a history of similar attacks or a predisposing condition (such as previous documented urolithiasis, gout, hypercalcemia, or anatomic urinary system variants).

Objective Data

Upon examination, vital signs may be normal in the absence of infection. Patients may present with tachycardia from pain, as well as costovertebral angle tenderness. Additional symptoms may include:

- Microscopic hematuria
- Signs and symptoms of pyelonephritis if complicating infection is present
- Bradycardia from vagal hypertonicity

- External genitalia examinations should be unremarkable in cases of urolithiasis

Laboratory/Diagnostics

Laboratory and diagnostic testing for urolithiasis includes:

- Complete urinalysis: assess for blood, nitrites and WBS are indicative of infection
- Urine culture if suspecting an infected stone by bacteriuria and fever.
- Blood urea nitrogen and serum creatinine, calcium, magnesium, phosphorus, and uric acid levels to assess for metabolic causes of stone formation.
- Urine qualitative pregnancy test or a serum human chorionic gonadotropin level for all females of childbearing age.
- Imaging studies may be helpful to identify stone location and size these include non-contrast enhanced helical CT, plain kidney, ureter and bladder (KUB) radiography, intravenous urogram also known as intravenous pyelogram, kidney ultrasound
- Two 24-hour urine collections on normal day while on a normal diet for patients with recurrent stones

Pharmacologic Management

Opioids and antiemetics are the first line of treatment. Ketorolac, a nonsteroidal anti-inflammatory drug (NSAID), is as equipotent as mild narcotic analgesics. Ketorolac provides analgesia, and given its antiprostaglandin effects, can decrease the inflammatory response, promote relaxation of the ureteral spasm, and alleviate capsular distention. Additionally, it inhibits prostaglandin synthesis by competitive blocking of the enzyme cyclooxygenase (COX).

Special Considerations

NSAIDs can cause an increased risk of serious cardiovascular thrombotic events, including myocardial infarction (MI) and stroke, which can be fatal. This risk occurs early in treatment and may increase with the duration of use.

Ketorolac is contraindicated in coronary artery bypass graft (CABG) surgery, as well as patients with active peptic ulcer disease, recent GI bleeding or perforation, and a history of peptic ulcer disease or GI bleeding. Additionally, it is also contraindicated for intrathecal or epidural administration due to its alcohol content. Overall, it is vital to consider counteracting measures when administering the first dose of ketorolac injection since hypersensitivity reactions ranging from bronchospasm to anaphylactic shock may occur.

Complications

Stones can lead to pelviuteric junction or ureter obstruction, which can cause hydronephrosis or pyelonephritis. Progressive renal failure may also occur.

Referrals

Patients should be referred to a urologist within 24–48 hours for further evaluation and treatment. A referral to a nephrologist is needed if renal failure occurs.

Diagnosis: Benign Prostatic Hypertrophy and Malignant Disease

ICD-10 N40.1: Benign prostatic hyperplasia with lower urinary tract symptoms

ICD-10 C61: Malignant neoplasm of prostate

Joel Regalado, DNP, ACNP-BC, CCRN-CMC, PCCN

Pathophysiology

The prostate is a small gland about the size of a walnut, which sits under the bladder in front of the rectum. The prostatic urethra goes through the prostate before reaching the penis. The prostate is covered by a capsule of connective tissue and smooth muscle; the inside of the capsule is made up of layers or zones. The transitional zone, as the term applies, contains transitional cells that are also found in the bladder. The transitional zone undergoes hyperplasia with increasing age, often leading to the compression of the urethra. This is called Benign Prostatic Hypertrophy (BPH) and is considered a typical occurrence in aging.

The prostate is made up of tiny glands surrounded by a basement membrane; inside the membrane lies basal cells. Beneath the basal cells are the neuroendocrine cells and luminar columnar cells. Luminar cells secrete substances that make the fluid slightly alkaline, which helps sperm to survive in the acidic environment. The luminar cells also produce prostate specific antigen (PSA), which help liquefy semen after ejaculation, thereby allowing the sperm to swim freely.

The basal cell and luminal cells rely on androgens for survival. Androgens and testosterone are produced from the testicles; androstenedione is produced by the adrenal glands; and dihydrotestosterone is converted by the enzyme 5-α reductase from testosterone. Without androgens, the prostate cells, in particular the luminar cell, will undergo apoptosis.

Prostate adenocarcinoma results from a genetic mutation in the luminal or basal cells resulting in the cell dividing uncontrollably. Mutations in two genes that have been linked specifically to prostate cancer are the breast cancer gene one and two, which are known as BRCA1 and BRCA2 (both also cause breast cancer). Once the mutation occurs, the affected cells begin to grow and replicate forming a tumor. Transitional cell carcinoma arises from cells in the transitional zone, whereas small cell prostate cancer arises from neuroendocrine cells (Kasper et al., 2015).

Physical Assessment

Subjective Data

In early or gradual enlargement of the prostate there may be no symptoms because the detrusor muscle can compensate for increased urethral resistance. However, as the prostate enlarges, patients may report symptoms such as:

- Hesitancy
- Diminished forced and amount of urine stream
- Terminal dribbling

- Sensation of incomplete emptying of the bladder
- Urinary retention, urgency, frequency and nocturia
- Hematuria
- Hip or lower back pain

Objective Data

Upon examination, patients may present with hematuria. Additionally, there may be a diminished force of urine stream or a decreased amount of urine during micturition.

Laboratory/Diagnostics

A digital rectal exam should be performed to evaluate the size, texture, and consistency of the prostate. A urinalysis can be used to rule out hematuria and infection. Additional testing may include:

- Serum creatinine and BUN (blood urea nitrogen) to evaluate for renal function
- Serum PSA to rule out cancer; may also be elevated in BPH
- Transrectal ultrasound or MRI to image the prostate
- Biopsy of the prostate to grade cells based on the Gleason Grading System where the two most common cell patterns are scored from 1 to 5. Once the primary and secondary patterns are graded, these two numbers are added resulting in a total score of anywhere between two and 10. Where two means low-grade tumors and 10 mean high-grade tumors. There is also the

Prostate cancer TNM staging to help guide treatment (American College of Surgeons, 2017).

Management

Symptom relief and the prevention of obstructive uropathy are the primary goals of treatment. For prostate adenocarcinoma, active surveillance is warranted when the tumor is confined to the prostate; this includes routine tumor marker measurement and imaging to confirm that the tumor is not progressive. If the tumor spreads, options may include surgery, radiation therapy, chemotherapy, and hormonal therapy.

Pharmacological management includes the use of Flomax (tamsulosin), an alpha blocker whose mechanism of action selectively antagonizes prostate alpha 1-α adrenergic receptors, relaxing smooth muscle and improving urine flow (Vallerand & Sanoski, 2019). Proscar (finasteride), a 5- α reductase inhibitor, is also used. The drug inhibits 5- α reductase, an intracellular enzyme that converts the androgen testosterone into 5α dihydrotestosterone (Vallerand & Sanoski, 2019).

Special Considerations

There is no specific numerical PSA threshold that accurately determines the presence of prostate cancer. As such, the American Urological Association (AUA) in their published guidelines for early detection of prostate cancer (2018) does not recommend PSA screening in men under 40 years old because of low prevalence in this age group. Men between 40-54 years of age should be evaluated based on risk factors such as being of African American race and those with a family history of metastatic cancer. The greatest benefit of screening occurs between the ages of 55-69; however, this should be a shared decision-making process between the patient and provider. A routine screening interval of two years or more may be preferred over annual screening in men who have participated in shared decision-making and decided on screening. Routine PSA screening is not recommended for men over 70 years old or any man with less than 10-15 years life expectancy. Similarly, a prostate biopsy is not warranted if patient has significant comorbidities that limit life expectancy.

Complications

Complications of BPH include renal stones, hydronephrosis, obstructive uropathy, as well as renal failure.

Referrals

For BPH, patients should be referred to a urologist or a nephrologist. Patients with suspected malignancy should be referred to an oncologist for follow-up and treatment.

Diagnosis: Renal Failure

ICD-10 N17: Acute renal failure

ICD-10 N19: Unspecified renal failure

ICD-10 N18: Chronic kidney disease

☐ Susan A. Simmons DNP, FNP-C

Pathophysiology

Acute Renal Failure

Acute renal failure occurs when the blood flow to the kidneys is reduced from an insult. This causes a rapid decline renal profusion and glomerular filtration; as a result, nitrogenous waste (azotemia, high serum creatinine, and fluid retention) products accumulate in the body. Acute renal failure is divided into the phases of onset, oliguria, diuresis, and recovery (See image below for a description of phases). Interventions can be implemented to reverse the acute renal failure within 2 weeks to 3 months of the initial insult occurring.

Chronic Renal Failure

Chronic renal failure is irreversible and has an insidious gradual onset based on the cause. The onset may take months to years according to cause for the nephrons to be affected; thus, progressing to end-stage renal failure where the kidneys are unable to excrete the nitrogenous waste making dialysis or kidney transplant options to support life. Stages of chronic renal failure, as determined by the National Kidney Foundation, are shown in Table 9.3.

Table 9.3: Stages of Chronic Renal Failure

Stage 1: kidney damage with normal or increased GFR (greater than 90 mL/min)
Stage 2: mild reduction in GFR (60 to 89 mL/min)
Stage 3: moderate reduction in GFR (30 to 59 mL/min)
Stage 4: severe reduction in GFR (15 to 29 mL/min)
Stage 5: kidney failure (GFR lower than 15 mL/min)

End Stage Renal Failure

End stage renal failure occurs when the kidneys deteriorate with widespread effects of uremia (urine in the bloodstream). The nephrons can no longer preform their function of filtration of the blood. Such functions include blood pressure maintenance, erythropoietin synthesis, and acid base balance. Dialysis and/or renal transplant are necessary and only options for survival

Physical Assessment

Subjective and objective assessment findings are specific for patients with acute, chronic or end-stage renal failure. Table 22 outlines the various symptoms patients may experience based on the type of renal failure they have.

Table 9.4: Subjective and Objective Assessment Findings

	Acute Renal Failure	**Chronic Renal Failure**	**End-Stage Renal Failure**
Sub jective	• Feeling tired • Nausea • Shortness of breath • Pain	• Fatigue/weakness • Trouble concentrating • Difficulty sleeping • Muscle twitching • Puffiness around eyes, especially in the morning • Swollen ankles and feet • Persistent itching, dry skin • Urinary frequency, nocturia • Muscle cramping at night • Poor appetite	• Itching • Nausea/vomiting • Weight loss • Muscle cramps • Loss of appetite • Too much or not enough urine • Trouble catching breath • Difficulty sleeping • Rash
Ob jective	• Dependent and periorbital edema • Seizures • Tachycard ia • Hypertens ion • Decreased urinary output • Electrolyt e imbalance	• Swelling of feet and ankles • Decreased mental status • Weight gain • Poorly controlled hypertension • Elevated serum creatinine • Seizures	• Weight gain • Tachycardia • Hypertension • Edema • Seizures • Electrolyte imbalance

Laboratory/Diagnostics

Laboratory analysis for symptoms suggestive of renal failure should include a urinalysis, CBC, CMP (BUN and creatinine), lipid profile. Additional laboratory evaluation, such as a GFR and ABG, should be based on the cause of renal failure, symptoms, and extent of renal failure.

Diagnostic testing may include a renal ultrasound or X-ray of the kidneys. Further imaging tests include a CT and MRI to evaluate the kidneys.

Pharmacologic Management

Pharmacologic management is aimed at treating the underlying cause of the renal failure and the progression of the renal failure. First line treatment includes fluid administration for prerenal acute renal failure. At the point of oliguria, diuretics such as Lasix are indicated with caution.

Fluid and electrolyte replacement, blood pressure (antihypertensive), and erythropoietin stimulating medications may also be necessary. Once the GFR is lower than 10 to 20 mL/min, dialysis is initiated and possible evaluation for kidney transplant.

Complications

Complications of renal failure include respiratory compromise due to fluid overload. Additionally, uremic coma or death may result.

Referral

Patients with renal disease should be referred to a nephrologist for follow-up and treatment.

Chapter 10: Allergy, Immunology, Rheumatology

Allergic Rhinitis

Food Allergies

Atopic Dermatitis

Anaphylaxis

Systemic Lupus Erythematosus

HIV/AIDS

Diagnosis: Allergic Rhinitis

ICD-10 J30.9: Allergic rhinitis, unspecified

Claudia Griffin, DNP, CPNP

Pathophysiology

When the nasal airways come in contact with an irritant, a hypersensitivity reaction occurs as an immune response which is mediated by Immunoglobulin E (IgE). Hypersensitivity allergic reaction takes place within minutes when a person is in contact with an allergen trigger that the body has previously been sensitized to. Rhinitis symptoms are an IgE-mediated inflammatory response due to exposre to inhaled irritants.

Assessment

Subjective Data

Patients with allergic rhinitis may experience the following symptomology:

- Runny nose
- Nasal congestion
- Red, itchy eyes
- Headaches
- Coughing and wheezing
- Postnasal drip
- Watery nasal discharge
- Sore throat (due to secretations)

Objective Data

- Reddend sclera nd conjunctiva
- edematous turbinates
- pale and boggy mucosa
- watery, clear nasal discharge
- erythematous pharynx
- cervical lymph nosdes not enlarged

Laboratory/Diagnostic

Patients with an unremarkable history do not need diagnostic testing unless there is consideration for allergen immunotherapy. Skin testing or serum IgE may be performed to confirm allergens. Skin testing is generally more sensitive, although serum testing continues to improve. If drawn, a CBC with note eosinophilia.

Pharmacologic Management

In situations where an allergen cannot be avoided, medications may be used to alleviate symptoms.

First line therapy often includes nasal corticosteroids and oral or nasal antihistamines. Antihistamines such as loratadine block the peripheral effects of histamine that is released during an allergic reaction. Decongestants are sometimes used but can lead to increased blood pressure. Decognestants can create a rebound effect when discontinued, they are not to be used for long-term treatment.

Special Considerations

Individuals with asthma may have an increased risk of developing allergic rhinitis. Additionally, family history, exposure to allergens, as well as exposure to smoking during the first years of life can increase the risk of allergic rhinitis.

Complications

Complications include interrupted or poor sleep patterns, which can lead to general feelings of malaise. Allergic rhinitis can worsen symptoms of asthma and increase coughing, as well as wheezing.

Referrals

Patients with allergic rhinitis may benefit from referral to an allergist or immunologist.

Diagnosis: Food Allergies

ICD-10 Z91.0: Food allergy status

ICD-10 Z91.018: Allergy to other foods

Claudia Griffin, DNP, CPNP

Introduction

Food allergies occur when the body ingests a food, or a substance in the food, and the body treats the protein in the food as if it is an invader. The body producces chemicals to defend against the invader, which can lead to symptoms. According to the American College of Allergy, Asthma, and Immunology (ACAAI, 2021), food allergies affect 8% of children and 4-6% of adults. 90% of all food allergies are attributed to eight foods, including: eggs, milk, peanuts, tree nuts, fish, shellfish, wheat, and soy (Centers for Disease Control and Prevention, 2021).

Assessment

Food allergies affect individuals differently and may involve one or more body system. A family history of food allergies, being a male, and having other allergies can increase an individual's risk of having a food allergy.

Subjective and Objective Data

Patients with a food allergy may exhibit any of the following symptoms:

- Swelling of the lips, face, tongue, throat
- Abdominal pain, diarrhea
- Nausea and vomiting with exposure to allergan
- Tingling feeling in the mouth

Anaphylaxis may occur in patients with severe food allergies; therefore, it is paramount to react accordingly if a patient presents with airway constriction/difficulty breathing, shock, or severe hypotension.

Diagnostic Testing

Confirmation of a food allergy may depend upon the subjective details provided by the patient or parent. A food diary can be beneficial and provide insight into what food or foods lead to symptoms. Foods suspected of causing symptoms may be eliminated on a trial basis; however, elimination of the food may not be demonstrative of an allergy, as the patient might simply have food sensitivity. Therefore, allergy testing might be warranted.

Management

Avoidance of the food or food substance is the only preventative measure. In cases of anaphylaxis injectable epinephrine is imperative and the only proven medication. Immunotherapy for foods is now considered a recognized therapy and can occur via skin patches or forms of oral therapy (but not injectables).

Special Considerations

Peanut allergies pose an increased risk for school-aged children. Parents should be provided education about making the school aware of any food allergies their child has. Most food allergies appear before the child is three years old and the child usually outgrows most food allergies by the time they are adults. Children with food allergies may also present with asthma and/or eczema.

Introducing solid foods in infants before four months of age increases the risk of food allergies. The American Academy of Pediatrics (2019) recommends introducing allergenic foods to an infant as early as 4-6 months to help prevent the development of food allergies.

Complications

Patients with food allergies can have life-threatening reactions, which can lead to anaphylaxis. Skin reactions, such as eczema, may also result from food allergies.

Referrals

Referral to an allergist or immunologist is recommended for patients with suspected food allergies.

Diagnosis: Atopic Dermatitis

ICD-10 L20.9: Atopic dermatitis, unspecified

Claudia Griffin, DNP, CPNP

Introduction

Atopic dermatitis, or eczema, is a common skin condition that leads to redness, inflammation and itching. It is often seen on the cheeks, arms, and legs. A family history of asthma or "hay fever" is a risk factor for this chronic skin condition.

Pathophysiology

The exact cause of atopic dermatitis is unknown. When an allergen trigger (internal or external) comes in contact with the body, the body triggers an immune response. This immune response results in inflammation of the skin, which can lead to redness and itching.

Assessment

Subjective and Objective Data

Patients with atopic dermatitis may present with dry, itchy skin. A rash or raised bumps might be seen; the raised bumps may leak and crust over if scratched. Due to frequent scratching, patients may have skin that is raw and sensitive.

Management

Topical corticosteroids react with receptor protein in the cytoplasm, which modifies inflammation and decreases itching. Topical steroids are available in different potencies. There are a number of nonsteroidal creams on the market for regular use, which may help to decrease the amount of steroids used. In more severe cases a number of systemic immune modulators are available and would typically be prescribed by a dermatologist or allergy specialist.

Non-pharmacological management includes keeping the clean, dry, and moisturized. Patients may also benefit from light therapy. Avoiding allergen triggers is also recommended.

Complications

Patients with allergic dermatitis may lead to a poor quality of sleep due to the increased need to scratch. Frequent scratching may result in broken skin, which could become infected.

Referrals

Referral to a dermatologist may be beneficial for patients with allergic dermatitis. An allergist or immunology referral may also be necessary.

Diagnosis: Anaphylaxis

ICD-10 T78.2: Anaphylactic shock, unspecified

Claudia Griffin, DNP, CPNP

Introduction

Anaphylaxis is a severe, life-threatening allergic reaction that happens suddenly and manifests itself in several systems. Anaphylaxis can impair breathing and cause the body to go into shock within seconds or minutes. The most common causative agents include bee stings, peanuts, medications, and latex.

Pathophysiology

The body's immune system reacts to the allergic trigger as an invader, which produces chemicals to cause an allergic response. Anaphylactic reactions can affect more than one body system and can be fatal if not treated immediately.

Assessment

Subjective and objective

A history of allergies, as well as asthma may increase the risk of developing anaphylaxis.

The following subjective and objective symptoms may occur with anaphylaxis within minutes of exposure to an allergic trigger:

- Fainting, light-headedness
- Difficulty breathing, shortness of breath, wheezing
- Hives, swelling of skin
- Rapid pulse

- Confusion
- Loss of consciousness

Pharmacologic Management

Treatment for anaphylaxis is the immediate injection of epinephrine, a sympathomimetic catecholamine. Epinephrine acts upon alpha and beta-andrenergic receptors, inducing vascular smooth muscle contraction and relaxes the bronchial smooth muscle, reversing bronchospasm. The patient should be transported to an emergency room for observation and follow-up.

Special Considerations

Patients with previous events of anaphylaxis are at an increased risk of future episodes. It is important to note future events will most likely be more severe than previous episodes. Persons with allergies should wear a medical alert necklace/bracelet and maintain a dose of epinephrine if they are at high risk.

Complications

Anaphylaxis is a life-threatening event, which can lead to death. Therefore, immediate injection of epinephrine must be provided.

Referrals

Following an anaphylactic event, patients should be transported to an emergency department for further treatment and observation. For patients with allergies, referrals to an immunologist or allergist is recommended.

Diagnosis: Autoimmune Disorders

Systemic Lupus Erythematous (SLE)

ICD-10 M32.9: Systemic lupus erythematosus, unspecified

Claudia Griffin, DNP, CPNP

Pathophysiology

Systemic Lupus Erythematous (SLE) is the most common type of lupus and causes widespread inflammation and tissue damage. SLE can affect tissues, organs, joints, skin, blood vessels, kidneys, and the brain. There is no cure and the cause is unknown. Symptoms can range from mild to life-threatening. Many people live with SLE for years before they are diagnosed, as the symptoms are similar to many other diseases.

Physical Assessment

Subjective Data

Patients with SLE may report feelings of fatigue, pain in their joints and sensitivity to the sun. Additionally, their fingers and toes may turn white/blue when cold or when under stressful situations.

Objective Data

Upon examination, the patient may have a fever, joint swelling, skin rashes, and other symptoms that affect lungs, heart, and kidneys. There may be a butterfly rash across the face that looks like a sunburn.

Laboratory/Diagnostics

There is no single test to diagnose SLE. A medical and family history should be obtained, as well as a complete physical examination performed. The antinuclear antibody (ANA) test may be positive for ANA in a person with SLE.

Criteria to diagnose lupus:

- Malar rash – a rash over the cheeks and nose, often in the shape of a butterfly
- Discoid rash – a rash that appears as red, raised, disk-shaped patches
- Photosensitivity – a reaction to sun or light that causes a skin rash to appear or get worse
- Oral ulcers – sores appearing in the mouth
- Arthritis – joint pain and swelling of two or more joints in which the bones around the joints do not become destroyed
- Serositis – inflammation of the lining around the lungs (pleuritis) or inflammation of the lining around the heart that causes chest pain which is worse with deep breathing (pericarditis)
- Kidney disorder – persistent protein or cellular casts in the urine
- Neurological disorder – seizures or psychosis
- Blood disorder – anemia (low red blood cell count), leukopenia (low white blood cell count), lymphopenia (low level of specific white blood cells), or thrombocytopenia (low platelet count)

- Immunologic disorder – anti-DNA or anti-Sm or positive antiphospholipid antibodies
- Abnormal antinuclear antibody (ANA)

Pharmacologic Management

Over the counter (OTC) non-steroidal anti-inflammatory drugs (NSAIDs) may be used to treat symptoms of pain. Corticosteroids such as prednisone can also help with swelling and pain. Antimalarials decrease autoantibody production and are effective in treating skin rashes, ulcers, and joint pain. Hydroxychloroquine (Plaquenil) and chloroquine (Aralen) are the most prescribed. These may take months to improve SLE symptoms. Other medications that may be used to treat SLE include anticoagulants and immunosuppressives.

Special Considerations

Pregnant women with SLE are considered high risk for miscarriage and should be educated on the importance of routine prenatal care during pregnancy to offer the best chance of a healthy pregnancy and baby. Antimalarial medications should be taken throughout pregnancy to avoid flare ups of lupus (Richman & Karakashian, 2018). It is recommended that women wait until they go six-months without a lupus flare up and the disease is latent before becoming pregnant (Bermas & Smith, 2018).

Referrals

Patients with SLE should be referred to a rheumatologist that specializes in lupus.

Diagnosis: HIV/AIDS

ICD-10 B20: Human immunodeficiency virus (HIV) disease

Claudia Griffin, DNP, CPNP

Pathophysiology

Human immunodeficiency virus, or HIV, attacks the body's immune system, targeting CD4 cells (Tcells). TCells work to fight infections and diseases. Since HIV destroys the TCells, it becomes difficult for the body to fight diseases and infections, which causes a weakened immune system. Due to the decreased immune system, the body is at risk for opportunistic infections or cancers. Once this happens, the body is considered in the end stage of HIV and considered to have acquired immunodeficiency syndrome (AIDS). The three stages of HIV include:

- Stage 1: Acute HIV infection – large amounts of virus is found in the blood and is highly contagious
- Stage 2: Clinical latency (HIV is not active)
- Stage 3: AIDS – high risk for opportunistic infections and severely decreased immune system

Assessment

Subjective and Objective Data

Signs of primary HIV infection may include fever and chills. As the virus progresses, the patient may report experiencing night sweats, being fatigued, as well as a loss of appetite. Additional symptoms may include abdominal pain or pain upon swallowing, swollen lymph nodes, as well as chronic diarrhea, ulcers, or a rash.

Laboratory/Diagnostic

The U.S Preventative Task Force (USPTF, 2019) recommends the following screening guidelines for HIV:

- Sexually active adolescents less than 15 years and older should be screened
- Screenings should be done on all patients ages 15- 65
- All pregnant women should be screened as routine testing

Diagnosis of HIV may be accomplished via use of antibody/antigen tests, which checks for the HIV antibody 2-4 weeks after exposure. Antibody screening tests (immunoassay or ELISA tests) and considered to be accurate and can diagnose within 2-8 weeks of being infected. The nucleic acid test (NAT) can be performed when high-risk individuals are displaying flu-like symptoms.

Pharmacologic Management

ART therapy (Antiretroviral Therapy) should be started as soon as a patient is diagnosed with HIV. The patient is to take the HIV regimen every day. Though ART therapy is not a cure for HIV, it can help patients live longer and decrease the possibility of transmission of HIV; the goal being that the virus would be undetected in the blood. It usually takes a patient 3-6 months before their viral load is undetectable.

Special Considerations

Pregnant women can pass HIV transplacental, during a vaginal birth, or through breastfeeding. HIV positive women are at an increased risk for pregnancy complications. HIV prenatal routine blood tests are recommended with the HIV testing by enzyme-linked immunosorbent assay (ELISA).

Complications

Patients with HIV are at an increased risk for opportunistic infections and cancer due to their decreased immune system.

Referrals

Patients with HIV may benefit from referral to an infectious disease specialist or an internist. A referral to a psychiatrist may be made to help patients cope with their diagnosis.

Chapter 11: Integumentary

Psoriasis Vulgaris

Contact Dermatitis

Urticaria

Cellulitis

Impetigo

Verrucae

Keratosis

Furuncle

Squamous Cell Carcinoma

Malignant Melanoma

Diagnosis: Psoriasis Vulgaris

ICD-10 L40.0: Psoriasis vulgaris

Alex Bahadori, DNP, MS, FNP-C

Pathophysiology

Psoriasis vulgaris (most common type of psoriasis) is a chronic inflammatory skin disease with a strong genetic predisposition and autoimmune traits. Environmental factors also appear to play a role. It is a chronic inflammatory disease that involves hyperproliferation of the keratinocytes in the epidermis, which leads to an increase in the epidermal cell turnover rate. Psoriasis typically affects the skin but may also affect the joints in up to 40% of patients.

Assessment

Subjective Data

Patients with psoriasis vulgaris may report itchy, painful skin, which is often exacerbated by extreme temperatures.

Objective Data

Upon examination, patients may present with well-demarcated, erythematous, plaques covered in silvery scales. The plaques often coalesce and cover large areas of skin. Common locations include the extensor surfaces of the limbs, scalp, and trunk.

Laboratory/Diagnostics

Diagnosis is usually determined by performing a thorough medical exam and patient history. A skin biopsy may be performed to confirm diagnosis and rule out other pathologies.

Pharmacologic Management

Mild to moderate psoriasis can be treated topically with a combination of glucocorticoids (i.e. triamcinolone), vitamin D analogues (i.e. calcipotriene), and sometimes phototherapy. Moderate to severe psoriasis may require systemic treatment. The presence of psoriasis arthritis is highly relevant in determining systemic treatment, and in these cases biologics (i.e. adalimumab) are usually prescribed (Rendon & Schakel, 2019).

Special Considerations

Topical corticosteroids should be limited in their application, and the selection of an appropriate steroid potency must be considered according to skin location. Less potent topical steroids should be prescribed in areas where the skin is sensitive and thin. These include the face, the back of the knees, inside of the elbows, the groin area, and the armpits.

Complications

Patients with psoriasis vulgaris may be at risk of:

- Psoriatic arthritis
- Eye Diseases
- Anxiety

- Depression
- Infection
- Obesity
- Cardiovascular disease
- Other autoimmune diseases

Referrals

Referrals include a dermatology specialist, as well as a rheumatology specialist.

Diagnosis: Urticaria

ICD-10 L50.9: Urticaria, unspecified

Alex Bahadori, DNP, MS, FNP-C

Pathophysiology

Urticaria involves intensely pruritic lesions with or without edema of the surrounding skin tissue. It is usually a self-limited, benign reaction, but can be chronic. Uncommonly, it may represent serious systemic disease or a life-threatening allergic reaction (Kanani, Betschel & Warrington, 2018). Urticaria is primarily caused by immunoglobulin E- and non–immunoglobulin E-mediated release of histamine and other inflammatory mediators from basophils and mast cells.

Assessment

Subjective Data

Patients with urticaria may report intensely pruritic lesions (hives) lasting for several hours. Individual lesions may come and go on other parts of the body.

Objective Data

Upon examination, well-circumscribed erythematous wheals ranging from several millimeters to several centimeters or larger in size may be noted. These wheals may occur with localized subcutaneous or interstitial non-pitting edema. The area is often warm to the touch.

Laboratory/Diagnostics

Diagnosis is typically determined by performing a thorough medical examination and patient history. Laboratory workup in the absence of indications of an underlying cause is not necessary. A skin biopsy may be performed to confirm diagnosis and rule out other pathologies. Allergy testing may also be performed but is not routinely indicated.

Pharmacologic Management

Second-generation (i.e. loratadine) or third generation H_1 antihistamines (i.e. levocetirizine) are the first line treatment for acute urticaria. In some cases, they may be titrated greater than the normal dose to control symptoms (Schaefer, 2017). First generation H_1 antihistamines (i.e. diphenhydramine) may provide immediate relief of symptoms; second and third generation antihistamines have longer onset times.

Special Considerations

It is critical to rule out anaphylaxis, which has findings or symptoms involving other body systems beyond the skin, such as the pulmonary (wheezing, stridor), cardiovascular (tachycardia, hypotension), gastrointestinal (diarrhea, vomiting, abdominal pain), or nervous system (dizziness).

Complications

Patients with chronic urticaria are risk for angioedema, anxiety, and depression.

Referrals

Referral to a dermatologist or an allergy specialist can be beneficial. To assist patients with feelings of depression or anxiety as a result of their condition, a referral to a psychiatrist might be considered.

Diagnosis: Cellulitis

ICD-10 L03.90: Cellulitis, unspecified

Dana Y. Preston, DNP, APRN, FNP-BC

Pathophysiology

Cellulitis results when cytokines and neutrophils respond to bacteria breaching the epidermis. This epidermal response includes the production of antimicrobial peptides and keratinocyte proliferation, all of which produce the characteristic examination findings of cellulitis. The predominant bacterial causes of cellulitis include Group A streptococcus, the most common, and *staphylococcus aureus*, less frequently.

Physical Assessment

Subjective Data

Patients with cellulitis may report areas of worsening erythematous skin that is warm and tender to palpation with associated swelling. There might be possible constitutional symptoms of generalized malaise, fatigue, and fevers. Additionally, patients might have painful regional lymphadenopathy, as well as a positive history of cellulitis and/or predisposing diagnoses such as diabetes mellitus, venous stasis, peripheral vascular disease, obesity, old age, chronic tinea pedis, and lymphedema.

Objective Data

Upon examination there may be the presence of spreading erythematous inflammation of the deep dermis and subcutaneous tissue (usually of the lower extremities and most often unilateral), edema, warmth, and tenderness. There may be skin microabrasions secondary to injuries, insect bites, pressure ulcers, or injection sites. If cellulitis is affecting the lower extremities, there may be fissuring, scaling, or macerations in the toe web spaces (secondary to tinea pedis). Patients may have a fever.

Pay careful consideration for the possible presence of predictors of lower extremity cellulitis, including asymmetry, leukocytosis, tachycardia, and advanced age (above 70). Beware of common cellulitis mimickers such as eczema, stasis dermatitis, stasis ulcers, gout, congestive heart failure, non-specific edema, lymphedema, lipodermatosclerosis, and deep venous thrombosis.

Laboratory/Diagnostics

Two of the four criteria (erythema, edema, warmth, or tenderness) are required to make the diagnosis of cellulitis, which is clinically based (Brown & Watson, 2019). Laboratory findings may include an elevated white blood cell count (WBC), elevated erythrocyte sedimentation rate, and elevated C-reactive protein. Blood cultures are unnecessary for typical cases of cellulitis.

Pharmacological Management

Antibiotic therapy is the first line treatment for cellulitis. Below is an overview of the various oral antibiotic choices (Table 11.1).

Table 11.1: First-Line Oral Treatment for Uncomplicated Nonpurulent Cellulitis

Streptococcal Coverage		
Drug	**Drug Class**	**Mechanism of Action**
Penicillin, Amoxicillin, Dicloxacillin Amoxicillin-Clavulanate Cephalexin	Penicillin beta-lactam antibiotics Penicillin beta-lactam antibiotic plus a beta-lactamase inhibitor Cephalosporin beta-lactam antibiotic	Bactericidal; beta-lactams act by binding to penicillin-binding proteins that inhibit a process called transpeptidation, leading to activation of autolytic enzymes in the bacterial cell wall; beta-lactamase inhibitors bind irreversibly to the catalytic site of an organism's penicillinase enzyme, which causes resistance to the original beta-lactam ring (Weber et al., 1984).
Clindamycin	Lincomycin antibiotic	Bacteriostatic; inhibits bacterial protein synthesis by binding to the 23S RNA of the 50S subunit of the ribosome (Pfizer, 2020)
Methicillin-Resistant Staphylococcus Aureus (MRSA) Coverage		
Drug	**Drug Class**	**Mechanism of Action**
Doxycycline	Tetracycline antibiotic	Bacteriostatic; binds to 30S and possibly 50S ribosomal subunit(s), inhibiting protein synthesis (Roberts, 1996)
Clindamycin	Lincomycin antibiotic	Bacteriostatic; inhibits bacterial protein synthesis by binding to the 23S RNA of the 50S subunit of the ribosome (Pfizer, 2020)
Sulfamethoxazole-Trimethoprim (SMX-TMP)	Sulfonamide antibiotic	Bactericidal; sulfamethoxazole competes with para-

		aminobenzoic acid (PABA), inhibiting folic acid synthesis and trimethoprim selectively inhibits dihydrofolate reductase, folate antagonist (Kemnic & Coleman, 2019).
Streptococcal and MRSA Coverage		
Clindamycin alone or the combination of either doxycycline or SMX-TMP with a beta-lactam such as penicillin, amoxicillin, or cephalexin.		

Nonpharmacological general treatment includes providing patient education on the following measures:

- Raise affected extremity as much as possible.
- Treat uncomplicated cellulitis with appropriate antibiotic for five days and extend for ten days if not improving.
- If lower extremity cellulitis, check interdigital toes spaces and treat if abnormal.

Special Considerations

Cellulitis is nearly always unilateral. Bilateral cellulitis is unusual as are findings that last over several months or pruritus, which suggests another condition (Blumberg et al., 2017). Evaluate the patient for purulent cellulitis which includes cellulitis with an abscess/carbuncle, or with drainage, or with exudate in the absence of a drainable abscess/carbuncle. Incise and drain the abscess/carbuncle and obtain a gram stain and culture of the purulent drainage. MRSA is an unusual cause of typical cellulitis and treatment for that organism is usually unnecessary. Coverage for MRSA may be prudent in cellulitis associated with penetrating trauma, especially from illicit drug use, purulent drainage, or with concomitant MRSA infection elsewhere (Stevens et al., 2014).

Complications

Patients with cellulitis are at risk for extensive tissue damage, gangrene, and bacteremia/sepsis. Additional complications include osteomyelitis, lymphadenitis, lymphangitis, endocarditis, bacterial meningitis, amputation and death.

Referrals

A referral to an infectious disease specialist may be needed for patients with recurrent cellulitis.

Diagnosis: Impetigo

ICD-10 L01.00: Impetigo, unspecified

Alex Bahadori, DNP, MS, FNP-C

Pathophysiology

Impetigo is a common bacterial infection of the superficial layers of the skin. Most infections are caused by gram-positive bacteria and are highly contagious. Common sources of infection include trauma, insect bites, eczema, surgery, burns, and varicella. It is very common for patients to auto inoculate other sites on the body once an impetigo lesion is present (Nardi & Schaefer, 2017).

Assessment

Subjective and Objective Data

Patients with impetigo may report feeling itchy and having pain at the sores. Upon examination, patients have a bullous (blistering) or non-bullous presentation. Non-bullous present with erythematous plaques and a yellow or honey color crust commonly on the face and extremities. Bullous impetigo presents with multiple flaccid bullae that contain a clear or yellow fluid. Ruptured bullae leave behind an erythematous base with scaling. Lesions most commonly occur on trunk or intertriginous areas of the body and do not form a honey colored crust. Fever or regional lymphadenopathy may occur with impetigo.

Laboratory/Diagnostics

Gathering a complete patient history and performing a physical examination are essential to diagnose impetigo. Bacterial cultures can be used for confirmation of diagnosis and should be obtained if a drug resistant bacterial infection is suspected. A skin biopsy may be considered if the case is not responding well to treatment, or to rule out other etiology.

Laboratory blood work is not routinely indicated for the diagnosis of impetigo. However, human immunodeficiency virus (HIV) testing should be considered when a previously healthy adult develops bullous impetigo

Pharmacologic Management

First line treatment includes topical antibiotics (i.e. mupirocin) alone or in conjunction with systemic antibiotics. Antibiotic coverage should cover both *S aureus* and *S pyogenes*. Impetigo is often self-limiting; however, antibiotics decrease the spread of lesions and duration of the illness. Also, antibiotic treatment decreases the chances of complications. Systemic antibiotics should be prescribed for bullous impetigo, non-bullous impetigo with five or more lesions, and suspected systemic infection. Cephalosporins (i.e. cephalexin) are commonly prescribed for systemic antibiotic therapy (Nardi & Schaefer, 2017).

Special Considerations

Approximately 5% of patients with impetigo will develop associated post-streptococcal glomerulonephritis. This typically occurs one to two weeks after a streptococcal infection. Patients may experience fever, hypertension, edema and hematuria. It is not clear whether or not systemic antibiotics reduce the chances of developing glomerulonephritis.

Complications

Complications of impetigo include renal failure/glomerulonephritis, septic arthritis, and scarlet fever. Patients may also be at risk for sepsis and staphylococcal scalded skin syndrome.

Referrals

A referral to a dermatology specialist or an infectious disease specialist may be necessary for patients with impetigo.

Diagnosis: Verruca Vulgaris (Common Warts)

ICD-10 B07.9: Viral wart, unspecified

Pamela Porter DNP, APRN, FNP-BC, CNS, PA-S

Pathophysiology

Verruca vulgaris, or the common wart, are benign epidermal lesions most commonly caused by human papillomavirus (HPV). Once an individual is infected, the virus causes a proliferation of epidermal cells at the site. They initially appear as flesh-colored papules and progress to a rougher texture, followed by hyperkeratotic growths with "black dots". These growths may have finger-like projections and are caused by thrombosed capillaries.

Over 30% of warts will resolve in 6-12 months without treatment but can spread to surrounding skin through autoinoculation. The verruca virus is transmitted by direct contact and can appear anytime throughout the lifespan; however, warts are more common in children and young adults. Additionally, individuals who are immunocompromised at increased risk of acquiring warts.

Physical Assessment

Subjective and Objective Data

Patients with warts may present with small, grainy bumps; mostly found on the fingers and hands. The number may vary and could present as a flesh-colored papule with a rough surface. There might also be a hyperkeratotic appearance with black dots from thrombosed capillaries.

Laboratory/Diagnostics

Diagnosis of warts is often done through examination and then are treated accordingly to type. In resistant cases, verrucae are biopsied to help identify the genotype.

Pharmacologic Management

Topical salicylic acid is often used to treat warts by removing the outer layer of the wart. Cryotherapy may also be used in conjunction to salicylic acid; side effects of cryotherapy can be pain and blistering at the affected site. At home, patients may use duct tape occlusion, or other over-the-counter remedies for warts.

Special Considerations

Most warts will resolve spontaneously over several years. Children and young adults may be at most risk for developing warts, as well as individuals with weakened immune systems.

Complications

Complications may include pain, inflammation, secondary infections, and scarring.

Referrals

Referral to dermatology is indicated if warts are resistant to conservative care.

Diagnosis: Keratosis Pilaris

ICD-10 L85.8: Keratosis pilaris, acquired

Sherri Richardson DNP, APRN-CNP

Pathophysiology

Keratosis pilaris is a disorder of the skin of unknown etiology. This disorder has been found to be an inheritable autosomal dominant disorder. There is some consideration the development occurs as a disorder of the follicles that can develop a horny plug, which occludes the hair follicle. When this process occurs, development of rough dry papules are formed causing a sandpaper texture. Locations of occurrence commonly seen are on the upper arms, thighs, and facial cheeks.

Physical Assessment

Subjective and Objective Data

Patients with keratosis pilaris may be asymptomatic. Upon examination, follicular pustules or small spiny keratotic papules may be seen. These can be pink or red but are mostly flesh colored.

Laboratory/Diagnostics

There are no diagnostic or laboratory data needed. Diagnosis is made by clinical findings.

Pharmacologic Management

The condition usually clears up on its own over time; however, first line treatment includes propylene glycol-glycerin-lactic acid mixtures. These serve to remove dead skin cells, hydrate the stratum corneum and control scaling.

Special Considerations

Topical corticosteroids should not be used in children less than three months of age. Prescribing to the aging adult with thinning skin should be approached with caution due to the side effects that can occur using topical corticosteroids.

Complications

Overuse of topical corticosteroids can cause thinning of the skin, hypopigmentation, contact dermatitis, telangiectasia, purpura, and striae. It is best to recommend a two week length of treatment to decrease the risk of side effects from topical corticosteroids.

Referrals

A referral to a dermatologist may be provided for patients with keratosis pilaris.

Diagnosis: Furuncle

ICD-10 L02.828: Furuncle, unspecified

Nicole Sinkler, DNP, MS, APRN, FNP-C

Pathophysiology

Furuncles, caused by staphylococcus aureus, are skin infections that are deeply seated underneath the skin and involve the entire hair follicle and nearby subcutaneous tissue. The most common sites are hairy regions on the body that are exposed to friction, irritation, and/or moisture such as the posterior neck, scalp, buttocks, axillae, and beards. Furuncles are often described as "lumps" and can be solitary or have several lesions that form a carbuncle, comprising adjoining hair follicles. Pain and tenderness are the presenting symptoms.

Physical Assessment

Subjective and Objective Data

Patients typically complain of pain and tenderness to the affected area. Solitary or multiple lesions may be present; the area, which gradually enlarges over time, is round or nodular-like and firm. The area can soften and become fluctuant with the spontaneous expulsion of pus and a core.

Laboratory/Diagnostics

A complete blood count (CBC) for white blood cell count is rarely required, but slight leukocytosis may be present. A culture of pus may be performed to determine the type of bacteria present and to rule out MRSA.

Pharmacologic Management

First line treatment is incision and drainage of the furuncle with systemic antimicrobial therapy. Sulfamethoxazole-trimethoprim (Bactrim DS), a combination of an antimicrobial and sulfonamide work together to inhibit enzyme systems involved in the bacterial synthesis of tetrahydrofolic acid (THF). SMX is a structural analog of para-aminobenzoic acid (PABA) and competes with PABA to inhibit the synthesis of dihydrofolic acid, an intermediate step in the formation of THF. SMX binds to dihydropteroate synthetase which catalyzes this reaction. TMP binds to bacterial dihydrofolate reductase (in preference to human dihydrofolate reductase), also preventing the formation of THF.

Special Considerations

The following factors increase the risk of developing furuncles:

- Diabetes mellitus- particular with insulin injection therapy
- Intravenous drug use
- Allergy injections
- HIV disease
- Hospitalized
- Prisons
- Military
- Sports teams
- Homelessness
- Three or more bouts of furunculosis within a 12-month period

Complications

Complications associated with furuncles include the potential for staphylococcal infection, which can lead to septicemia.

Referrals

Patients with repeated or frequent episodes may be referred to a dermatologist for follow-up.

Diagnosis: Squamous Cell Carcinoma

ICD-10 C44.02: Squamous cell carcinoma of skin, unspecified

Sherri Richardson DNP, APRN-CNP

Pathophysiology

Squamous cell carcinoma (SCC) is a form of non-melanoma skin cancer that can appear as a papule, plaque, or nodule in sun exposed areas. Like melanoma, this form of skin cancer can metastasize. SCC is usually not seen until middle adulthood and beyond, as it occurs as a result of cumulative damage of thermal injury to the epithelium skin from the mutation of the cellular DNA. The tumor develops from the proliferation of squamous cells, also called keratinocytes. The tumor develops when the damaged cells are unable to repair and regenerate, which leads to invasion to the dermal layers of the skin.

Risk factors include advancing age, a history of blistering sunburns, having fair skin, red or blonde hair, and hazel or blue eyes. Additional risk factors including living in the south and a history of solar radiation exposure during childhood, ultraviolet A treatment (PUVA), oral psoralen psoriasis treatment and or a history of other melanoma and non-melanoma skin cancers.

Physical Assessment

Subjective Data

Patients with a SCC may have a lesion that is tender/painful. They may report the lesion easily bleeds.

Objective Data

The location of a SCC varies and can present on the lower/upper extremities, head, neck, scalp, ears, lips, tongue, or the genitalia. The lesion is pink or red in color and is sharply demarcated. SCC can appear in small erosions, which can be crusted over or ulcerated.

Laboratory/Diagnostics

A shave biopsy with a histopathological evaluation should be used to confirm the diagnosis.

Pharmacologic Management

The gold standard is surgical excision of the lesion. Alternatively, radiation may be used. The use of pharmacological agents is only recommended if the neoplasm is superficial. 5-Fluorouracil cream, which is an anti-neoplastic, can be used. This drug will interfere with the DNA synthesis by inactivating the nucleotide thymidylate synthase that is responsible for DNA replication. The end result is apoptosis of high proliferating cells.

Imiquimod 5%, an immunomodulator, can also be used. This drug forms an RNA expression that stimulates the cytokine production that will activate apoptosis of the treated tissue.

Special Considerations

Treatments with 5-Fluoracil and Imiquimod for the management of SCC should be managed by a specialist such as a dermatologist or oncologist. Actinic keratosis (AK) can be a precursor to development of squamous cell carcinoma. Approximately 20% of AK can develop into SCC.

Complications

Untreated SCC has the risk of metastasizing to cartilage, bone, and the lymphatic system. Metastasis also affects solid organs such as the lungs and liver.

Referrals

Referral to a dermatologist, surgeon trained in Moh's surgery or an oncologist may be needed for a patient with SCC. Dermatology

Diagnosis: Malignant Melanoma

ICD-10 C90.0: Multiple melanoma

Sherri Richardson DNP, APRN-CNP

Pathophysiology

Melanoma is a form of skin cancer that can develop from melanocytes located at the epidermal level of the skin. Melanocytes absorb ultraviolet radiation and serve as a protection against mutations that can occur from the ultraviolet rays. When melanocytes degenerate, they can become neoplastic. Once they become neoplastic, then they are no longer constrained to the basal layer of the epidermis and then can migrate slowly either horizontally or vertically. When the degenerated melanocytes begin to migrate vertically toward the dermis, this serves as the pathway of metastasis. There are multiple risk factors that can contribute to the development of melanoma, including:

- Atypical moles
- >75-100 moles
- History and family history of non-melanoma skin cancer, history of blistering sunburns
- Congenital nevus
- Immunosuppression
- Freckling, fair skin
- Red or blonde hair

- Tanning bed use
- Solar radiation

Physical Assessment

Subjective and Objective Data

Patients may be asymptomatic. It is important to perform the ABCDE assessment to evaluate for asymmetry, border, color, diameter and evolving of moles. Table 11.1 demonstrates objective findings for the various types of melanomas.

Table 11.2: Malignant Melanoma Objective Findings

Type	Location	Color	Shape and Size
Superficial Spreading Melanoma	For men, on the trunk; women, on the legs	Flat or elevated can be multi-colored: brown, black, blue, red or white	Irregular Diameter >6mm
Nodular Melanoma	Trunk and legs	Brown to black	Irregular, raised plaque, dome shaped Diameter >6mm
Lentigo Maligna Melanoma	Head, neck, arms (sun damaged skin)	Brown or black Blue-black	Irregular, large macule 3-6 cm or raised nodule
Acral Lentiginous melanoma	Palms, soles phalanges, under nail plate	Brown or black	Irregular macule or papule

Laboratory/Diagnostics

A punch biopsy can be used for obtaining an initial diagnosis; however, the best technique is to perform a complete excisional biopsy to include all margins. This can be a preferred option for the areas that are cosmetically important. A special surgeon such as a Moh's surgeon will perform a complete excision. If the malignant melanoma has metastasized to the lymph nodes, then a sentinel node biopsy may be required to predict the risk of reoccurrence.

Adjuvant treatment may be recommended for a patient with advanced disease. These treatments can include Interferon, chemotherapy, and/or radiation. Sentinel lymph node biopsy may be performed for patients with a skin lesion that is greater than one millimeter in thickness due to the higher risk of metastasis. These treatments will need to be managed by a specialist.

Special Considerations

For malignant melanoma that is metastatic, it is important for a Dermatologist to perform a full skin assessment at regular intervals every four to six months for the first few years. Physical examination should include palpation of lymph nodes both regional and distal to site of melanoma.

Complications

Melanoma is classified into stages based on the Breslow thickness and Clark level of the neoplasm. For melanoma cases that are localized, there is a 99%, five-year survival rate. When regional involvement occurs, the survival rate percentage is 65%. If metastasis to distal sites occurs, the survival rate decreases to 25%. Note the survival rates are general statements, as there are multiple factors that can improve the patient's chance of survival such as age, overall health, and response to treatments.

Referrals

Patients with melanoma should be referred to a dermatologist for follow up and treatment. Additional referrals may include a Moh's surgeon or an oncologist.

Chapter 12: Reproductive

Cervical Cancer

Testicular Cancer

Prostate Cancer

Diagnosis: Mastalgia

ICD-10 N64.4: Mastodynia

Diana Meeks PhD, RN, MSN, CS, CNE, NE-BC, FNP

Pathophysiology

There are two types of breast pain, cyclical and noncyclical. The pathophysiology s dependent on the cause of the breast pain. Cyclical is most common in patients 20-30 years of age and is menstrual related in 2/3 of cases. Pain is related to hormonal stimulation during the luteal phase of ovulation. Noncyclical mastalgia, common in persons aged 40-50 years, occurs in 1/3 of cases. Pain occurs from the breast (mammary) or from somewhere else in the body, such as nearby muscles or joints.

Physical Assessment

Subjective and Objective Data

Symptomology is dependent on whether the pain is cyclical or noncyclical (see Table 12.1).

Table 12.1 : Subjective and Objective Data of Mastodynia

	Cyclical	Noncyclical
Subjective Data	• Pain is diffuse, bilateral, radiation to axilla • Pain can be dull and/or achy • Related to menstrual cycle or cyclic hormonal therapy • Pain decreases or ceases	• Pain is focal or diffuse • Pain is described as tight, burning, or sore and cam be unilateral or bilateral, intermittent • Not related to menstrual cycle • Pain is present all the time and is in only one specific

	with menses	location. • Medication history may identify a pharmacological cause
Objective Data	• Pain and/or tenderness upon palpation in both breasts Assess for asymmetry, masses, nipple discharge	• Focal pain or tenderness with palpation • Assess for asymmetry, masses, nipple discharge • If related to infection there may be erythema or edema

Laboratory/Diagnostics

A pregnancy test may be performed if the patient is not menopausal. Available imaging includes mammogram and ultrasound. Any palpated mass requires a diagnostic mammogram. Cyclic pain without a palpable mass does not require imaging due to low risk of cancer.

Pharmacologic Management

Cyclical mastalgia treatment will vary based on symptoms, age, general health, and the severity of the symptoms. Most mastalgia resolves without pharmacologic treatment. For cyclic mastalgia, a non-steroidal anti-inflammatory drug (NSAID) such as a topical diclofenac gel or patch, is the first line treatment for mild cases. The NSAIDs inhibit cyclooxygenase-1 and 2 enzymes (COX-1 and COX-2), which decreases prostaglandin precursor formation, resulting in analgesic, and anti-inflammatory effects. Symptoms with noncyclic mastalgia often resolve spontaneously once the cause is identified and successfully treated.

Nonpharmacological treatments include providing reassurance, and assessing bra fit for adequate support. Caffeine reduction, dietary modification and vitamin supplementation are often recommended; however, most clinical trials do not show evidence of their effectiveness.

Considerations

When breast pain occurs, many women are concerned it may be breast cancer. A thorough history and clinical evaluation is required. Overall, the presence or absence of pain does not determine malignancy.

Referrals

A referral to an obstetrics and gynecology (OB/GYN) or to a breast specialist may be necessary for a palpated mass and/or confirmed diagnostic imaging of a mass. An OB/GYN referral may also be needed for moderate to severe mastalgia.

Diagnosis: Fibrocystic Breast Disease

ICD-10 N60.1: Diffuse cystic mastopathy

Dana Y. Preston, DNP, APRN, FNP-BC

Pathophysiology

Changes in the mammary glandular tissue, determined by a predominance of estrogen stimulation and progesterone deficiency, result in hyperproliferation of connective tissue (fibrosis), which is followed by facultative epithelial proliferation.

Physical Assessment

Subjective Data

Mastalgia is the most common symptom of fibrocystic breast changes. Complaints can include a palpable solitary breast lump, or diffuse lumpiness, and nipple discharge.

Objective Data

Upon examination, the provider may note focal tenderness, palpable lump(s), or nodule(s), and nipple discharge. Nipple discharge is pathologic if spontaneous, serous, or bloody, and usually unilateral and single duct.

Laboratory/Diagnostics

For palpable lesions:

- Diagnostic mammogram- for palpable lesions in women >35 years old. A diagnostic mammogram in conjunction with an ultrasound can be used for evaluation of discrete palpable lesions in women over 35 years old.

- Ultrasound- appropriate for imaging in women < 35 years of age.
- core or fine needle aspirate biopsy- appropriate for evaluation of complex cysts containing both fluid and solid matter, and for solid lesions. Required to determine the presence or absence of malignancy.

For nipple discharge

- pathological discharge- a hemoccult card or urine dipstick to test for occult blood, diagnostic mammogram and galactography.
- serum prolactin level -Milky discharge (galactorrhea)

A screening mammogram is recommended for patients over 35 with physiologic discharge. In patients < under 35 with only physiologic discharge only reassurance is necessary.

Pharmacologic Management

Pharmacologic treatment options are demonstrated in Table 12.2

Non-pharmacological treatment includes providing patient education on the following:

- Practicing daily relaxation exercises: anxiety along with other psychological disorders have been found to be more frequent among women with mastalgia.
- Smoking cessation or reducing the number of cigarettes smoked daily (smoking was identified as being a factor associated with mastalgia).
- Wearing well-fitted, supportive bra for the relief of mastalgia.

- Caffeine reduction or elimination to alleviate breast pain has not been sufficiently studied; however, many practitioners recommend that patients restrict their caffeine intake based on their clinical experience.

Table 12.2: First-Line Options for the Treatment of Cystic Mastalgia

Name	Drug Class	Mechanism of Action
Aspirin, Ibuprofen (oral or topical)	Nonsteroidal anti-inflammatories	Inhibits the activity of the cyclooxygenase (COX) enzyme; anti-inflammatory actions thought to be due to inhibition of COX-2.
Evening Primrose Oil (EPO)	Herbal supplement	Improves deficiencies in gamma-linolenic acid (GLA), an essential fatty acid, and restores the saturated/unsaturated fatty acid balance and decreases sensitivity to steroidal hormones; researchers propose that deficiencies in prostaglandin E and GLA, its precursor, increase breast sensitivity during the luteal phase of the menstrual cycle.
Vitamin B6	Vitamin supplement/ Antioxidant, co-factor agent	Enhances the therapeutic efficacy of other drugs and may be used in combination with hormonal drugs or as a safe alternative to hormonal therapies; has the same therapeutic effect as EPO and has a lower cost and more availability.
Progesterone, Progestogens, Progestins	Hormonal supplement	Progesterone therapy improves the estradiol/progesterone (E2/P) ratio; with local therapy for at least six months, mastalgia and average size and cyst number significantly decreased and disappeared.

Special Considerations

Some special considerations associated with fibrocystic breast disease include:

- Some studies have shown that low-dose oral contraceptives (20 μg ethinyl estradiol) were effective in reducing the severity and duration of cyclic breast discomfort.

- Reducing the estrogen dosage in post-menopausal women's hormonal replacement therapy or adding an androgen to the estrogen replacement therapy appears to reduce breast pain.
- Vitamin E is the most commonly used and studied vitamin to use as treatment for cyclic mastalgia and is considered ineffective
- Metformin has been suggested to reduce the excessive cell proliferation, promoting fibrocystic changes in the breast, caused by associated hormones.
- Tamoxifen (or raloxifene) can be offered preventatively to patients with benign breast lesions imparting an increased risk of breast cancer.

Complications

The benign lesions of fibrocystic breast disease are not associated with an increased malignancy risk. However, the benign lesions are associated with an up to 50% risk of developing breast cancer under certain histopathological and clinical circumstances.

Referrals

Referral to a surgeon is warranted for pathological nipple discharge and for cysts which repetitively, despite frequent fine needle aspiration, have an intra-cystic solid appearance on ultrasound or have atypical cells present upon cytopathological evaluation.

Diagnosis: Candidiasis

ICD-10 B37.9: Candidiasis, unspecified

Nathalie Grant, EdD, APRN, ADM-BC

Pathophysiology

Candida is a strain of fungus that can cause a skin infection in many different areas of the body. *Candida albicans* normally lives on the skin, in the mucous membrane, on the skin the mouth, throat, gut, and vagina, and penis without causing any problems. The exact pathophysiology is unknown. One cause is due to changes in the immune system, *Candida* can cause infections with increased growth and change to a pathogen with antibiotic use.

Candidiasis, Oral (Thrush)

Thrush is the most common fungal infection of the oral cavity; it is uncommon in healthy adults. Oral candidiasis is most common infections among newborns, older adults, denture wearers, and the immunocompromised, including those with HIV (Human Immunodeficiency Virus) infection/AIDS, cancer, diabetes. Antibiotics or corticosteroids, including inhaled corticosteroids can promote overgrowth.

Vaginal Candidiasis

Candidal vulvovaginitis is caused by inflammatory changes in the vaginal and vulvar epithelium secondary to infection with *Candida* species, most commonly candida albicans.

Balanitis

C. Albicans is the most common pathogen causing balanitis in men. In uncircumcised males, the moist and warm space beneath the foreskin promotes candida growth

Cutaneous candidiasis

In cutaneous candidiasis, the skin is infected with *candida* fungi. Most often found where two skin areas rub together. Most often it occurs in warm, moist, creased areas such as the armpits and groin.

Physical Assessment

Subjective and Objective Data

Both subjective and objective data findings depend on the type of candidiasis.

Table 12.3: Subjective and Objective Data Findings of Candidiasis

Diagnosis	Subjective	Objective
Oral Candidiasis	Cotton like feeling in mouth, loss of taste, dysphagia, odynophagia	White plaques are present on the buccal mucosa and the undersurface of the tongue and represent thrush. When wiped off, the plaques leave red erosive areas.
Vulvovaginitis	Dysuria, itching , burning	Inflammation of perineal area, white discharge, swelling or irritation
Balanitis	Burning, itching, painful sexual intercourse	Redness, swelling, papules, thick lumpy discharge, inability to retract the foreskin, foul odor.
Cutaneous Candidiasis	Itching, pain, soreness	Rash, cracks in the skin, erythema, maceration

Diagnostic/Laboratory

For oral candidiasis, a histologic examination is performed on a glass slide stained with Gram or potassium hydroxide stain.

With vaginal candidiasis, the following tests may be performed: wet mount, whiff testing, and pH testing., the vaginal PH is < 5, hyphae can be seen on microscopic exam

Pharmacologic Management

For an uncomplicated adult with oral thrush, clotrimazole may be prescribed via 10 mg troches 5 times daily, for 7-14 days miconazole 50 mg buccal tablet applied to the mucosal surface (canine fossa) daily for 7–14 days. With severe/resistant infections, fluconazole, 100–200 mg by mouth daily, for 7–14 days may be prescribed. Long-term prophylactic therapy with fluconazole 100-200 mg by mouth 3 times weekly is recommended for immunosuppressed patients (e.g., those with cancer or AIDS), due to high rates of recurrence.

For uncomplicated vulvovaginitis, Fluconazole 150 mg by mouth for one dose may be prescribed. With complicated vulvovaginitis,
Fluconazole, 150 mg by mouth every 72 hours for a total of 2-3 doses may be provided if symptoms persist. For those unresponsive to oral azoles, a boric acid gelatin capsule, 600 mg daily per vagina for 14 days may be prescribed. With recurring vulvovaginitis, Nystatin 100,000 units via intravaginal suppositories may be given daily for 10-14 days, followed by fluconazole 150 mg by mouth weekly for 6 months. Finally, with balanitis, clotrimazole cream 1% topical application twice daily for 10 days may be prescribed.

Special Considerations

Amphotericin B is the treatment of choice for invasive candidiasis in pregnant women. Fluconazole, itraconazole, posaconazole, and isavuconazole should be avoided in pregnant women, especially those in the first trimester. Voriconazole is contraindicated during pregnancy because of fetal abnormalities observed in animals. Flucytosine is contraindicated during pregnancy.

Complications

Potential complications of oral candidiasis include dysphagia or respiratory distress, bronchopulmonary candidiasis, and systemic infection.

Referral

Referrals include an immunologist or infectious disease if immunocompromise is suspected.

Diagnosis: Chlamydia

ICD-10 A74.9: Chlamydial infection

Shanna Chapman, DNP, APRN, FNP-C, FAANP

Pathophysiology

Chlamydia is a sexually transmitted infection caused by the bacteria *C. trachomatis*. It is acquired through oral, anal, or vaginal intercourse in both men and women. Women can develop infections in the throat, cervix, or anus; while men can develop infections in the throat, penis, or anus. Infants can acquire the infection through vaginal childbirth, resulting in conjunctivitis with or without pneumonia. Newborns typically start showing symptoms at five to seven days of age.

Physical Assessment

Subjective Data

It is quite common for both men and women to not experience any symptoms. Female symptoms include strong vaginal odor with discharge, pain with intercourse, and dysuria. Men can be asymptomatic or may experience penile discharge, dysuria, burning or pain at the opening of the penis and testes swelling. Infection of the anus typically results in itching, pain around the anus, discharge, or bleeding.

Infection of the throat may cause symptoms or sore throat, painless lesions in the mouth, tonsillitis, exudative tonsillitis, and lesions similar to cold sores around the mouth. Infection of the eye causes typical conjunctivitis symptoms of redness, itching, and drainage.

Objective Data

A full examination should be completed. Women should have a pelvic exam while men should have a penile and testicular examination. Both should have a rectal examination. Women will often experience pain during the pelvic examination due to the inflammation of the cervix. It is normal to visualize discharge, erythema, and irritation.

Men should have a full penile and testicular examination. Men may have a normal assessment; however, some men may have purulent drainage out of the penis head or papules/petechiae on the head of the penis. The head of the penis may be tender to palpate. The testes may be swollen and may or may not be tender to palpate.

If the rectum has become infected, it will often be erythematous, have purulent drainage, and may have small ulcers. If the throat is infected, both male and female patients will have an erythematous pharynx, exudative or nonexudative tonsillitis, and can have small sores. There may be lesions around the mouth that resemble herpes simplex virus (HSV) sores. Eye infections demonstrate pus drainage, redness, and erythema.

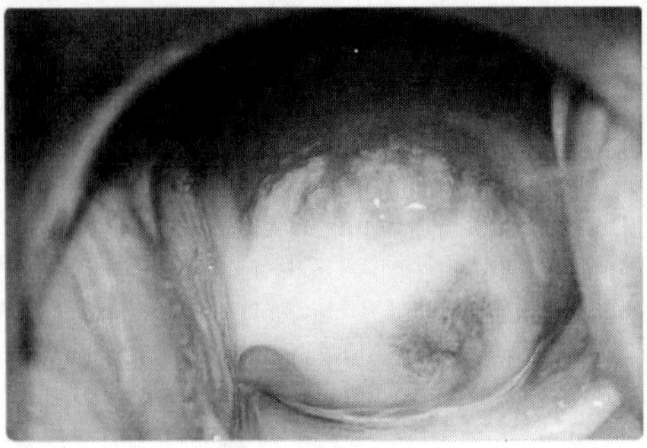

Cervicitis

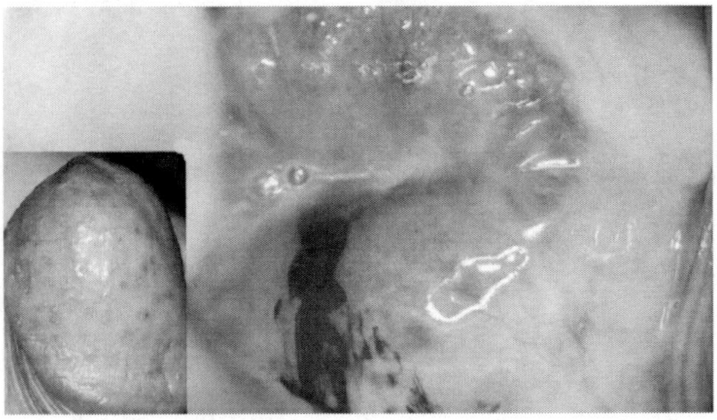

Early Chlamydial Infection of Cervix, Insert Pic of Penile Chlamydial Infection (Healthline.com)

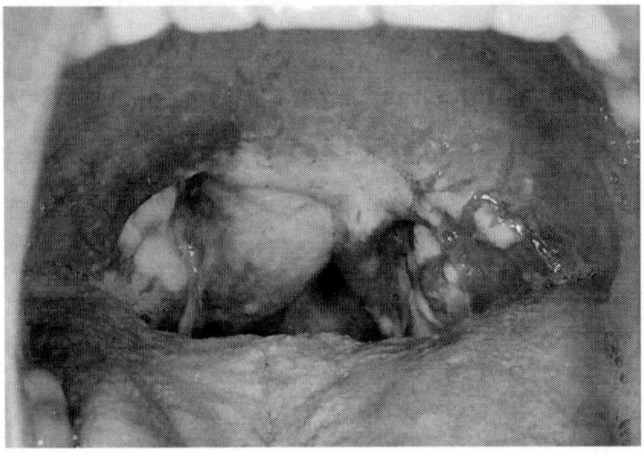

Exudative tonsillitis with Chlamydial infection

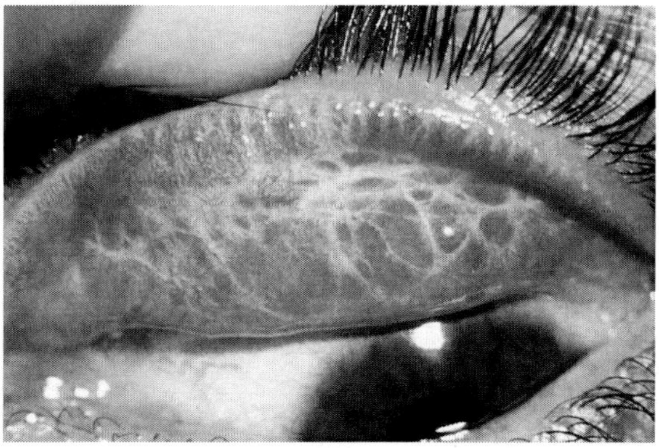

Conjunctivitis due to *C. Trachomatis*

Laboratory/Diagnostics

Women should have an endocervical swab completed while having a pelvic examination. A NAAT (Nucleic acid amplification test) urinalysis can be conducted. Men should have either a penile swab or a NAAT urinalysis for *C. trachomatis*. If rectal, eye, anus, or throat infection is suspected, a swab needs to be completed and tested.

Pharmacologic Management

The first line treatment for chlamydia is Azithromycin, 1gram, for one dose. As a macrolide antibiotic, Azithromycin inhibits protein bacterial synthesis and translation.

One alternative treatment is Amoxicillin, 500mg, by mouth three times a day for seven days. As a penicillin class of antibiotic, amoxicillin treats gram positive and negative bacteria by inhibiting cellular wall biosynthesis that results in the death of the bacteria.

An additional alternative treatment is Erythromycin, 500mg twice daily for seven days. As a macrolide antibiotic, Erythromycin works to inhibit protein synthesis.

Special Considerations

Patients with chlamydia should also be tested for HIV, syphilis, trichomonas, and gonorrhea due to the high incidence of co-infections. Chlamydia is often asymptomatic, which can result in complications such as pelvic inflammatory disease, ectopic pregnancy, and female infertility.

Azithromycin is excreted in breast milk and has a Pregnancy Category of B, which indicates that either no risk or minimal risk is noted for the neonate. Patients with chlamydia should be advised to not have intercourse for at least seven days and until all partners are treated.

Complications

Asymptomatic patients with chlamydia can progress without treatment, which can then lead to complications including pelvic inflammatory disease, infertility, and ectopic Pregnancy.

Female patients that are pregnant are at an elevated risk for spontaneous abortion or preterm labor. Pregnant patients also need to be rescreened during the third trimester to prevent infant chlamydial infections. While prescribing, remember that doxycycline is contraindicated in pregnancy.

Referrals

Referrals to specialists are not needed.

Diagnosis: Trichomoniasis

ICD-10 A59.9: Trichomoniasis, unspecified

Shanna Chapman, DNP, APRN, FNP-C, FAANP

Pathophysiology

The *Trichomonas vaginalis* protozoa have four flagella on the anterior portion of the protozoa that propels it forward and one posterior flagella. Infection from the protozoa occurs when it excretes cytotoxic substance that destroys epithelial cells. The incubation period is 5-28 days. The protozoa reside in men's external genitalia, urethra, bladder, prostate, and anus. In females, the parasite lives in the urethra, bladder, cervix, Bartholin Glands, Skene's Glands, and anus. There are some reports of lateral transmission in newborns. There is a lack of information known about this condition or how it is transferred.

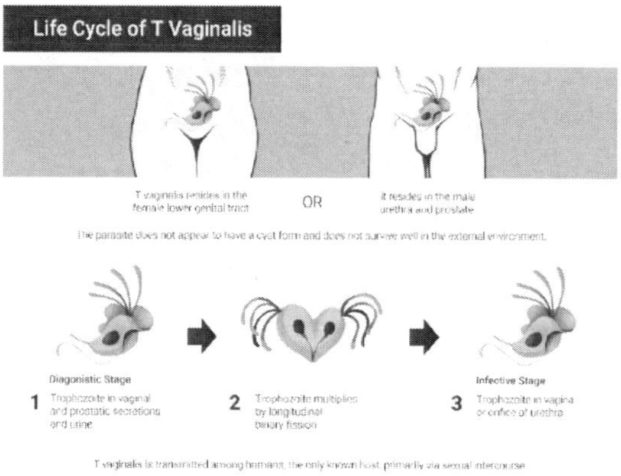

Photo courtesy of CDC.org

Physical Assessment

Subjective and Objective Data

Patients are usually asymptomatic; approximately 25% of patients will exhibit symptoms. Females may report dysuria, painful intercourse, vaginal discharge, a fishy odor, or have itching or swelling of their genitals. Upon examination, colpitis mascularis (Strawberry cervix) from punctuate hemorrhage may be present in half of the cases, as well as foul odor and an elevated pH of 4.5.

Males may experience dysuria, painful ejaculation, discharge from the penis, or itching and irritation outside the penis. Upon examination, inflammation of the urethra may be noted, as well as discharge, balanoposthitis, prostatitis, cystitis, or epididymo-orchitis.

	Female	Male
Symptoms	Dysuria Painful intercourse Erythema of Genitals Vaginal Discharge Fishy Odor Itching of Genitals	Dysuria, Painful ejaculation, Discharge from penis Itching or Irritation inside the penis
Assessment	Colpitis mascularis (strawberry cervix) Genital edema/erythema Foul odorous discharge Elevated pH >4.5 Vaginal leukocytosis	Dysuria Urethritis Inflammation of Urethra Discharge Balanoposthitis Prostatitis Cystitis Epididymo-orchitis

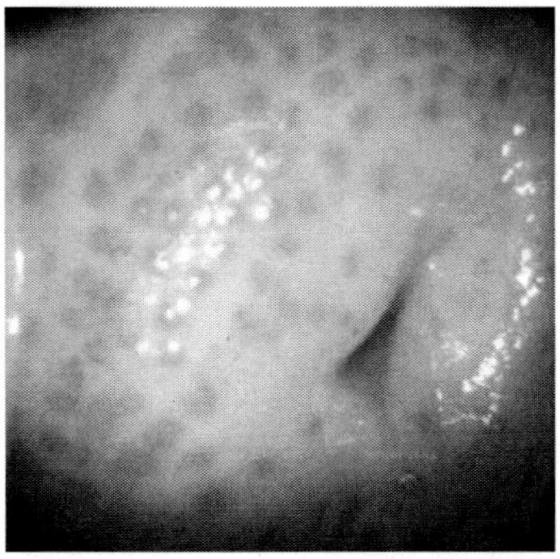

Strawberry Cervix present in *T. vaginalis* (CDC.org)

Laboratory/Diagnostics

NAAT (Nucleic acid amplification test) urine testing is the most reliable test in male patients; however, it is not as reliable in females. The preferred testing in female patients is an endocervical or vaginal swab. A wet mount and PCR (Polymerase Chain Reaction), which is less sensitive, can also diagnose Trichomonas.

Pharmacologic Management

The first line treatment is Metronidazole, an nitroimidazole, which works by inhibiting cellular synthesis by disrupting the DNA of microbial cells. Metronidazole 2 gm po one time dose.

Tinidazole, also a nitroimidazole, may be used as an alternative treatment. Tinidazole has an anti-protozoal effect, which is caused by the free nitro radical that is generated. Tinidazole 2 gm po one time dose.

Special Considerations

Infection during pregnancy can cause spontaneous abortion or pre-term labor. Babies born with low birth weight have been attributed to patients with T. vaginalis infection. Patients with T. vaginalis should be screened for HIV, as they are often co-infections. Women in their first trimester should be screened for T. vaginalis to prevent vertical transmission to the fetus. Patients with trichomoniasis should be educated to not have any further sexual intercourse until all partners are treated.

Complications

Patients can have recurrent or resistant infections of T. vaginalis. Therefore, it is important to determine if the patient is having a resistant, recurrent infection or if the patient is becoming re-infected.

Referrals

No referral is needed for patients with trichomoniasis.

Diagnosis: Syphilis

ICD-10 A53.9 Syphilis, unspecified

Cathleen Crowley-Koschnitzki DNP, CNM, WHNP-BC, FNP-C, PMHNP-BC

Pathophysiology

Syphilis is a sexually transmitted infection caused by the bacterial spirochete *Treponema pallidum.* This bacterial is transmitted through sexual contact, transplacentally to a fetus in utero, through blood products and breaks in skin. *T. pallidum* enters mucous membranes via direct contact and can enter the lymphatics and blood stream. Incubation time is 10- 90 days post exposure.

Physical assessment

Subjective Dat

Client symptoms vary based on the stage of infection.

Stage 1- chancre. A painless genital lesion which heals within a week. Often not noticed by client.

Stage 2: overall body rash (2-10 weeks post exposure). Clients may present with reports of sore throat, fever, anorexia, stiff neck, or rash. The rash can be generalized or limited to palms of hands and soles of feet.

Stage 3 (latent): asymptomatic. This phase can last for years.

Stage 4 (tertiary): progression of latent syphilis that did not resolve causing degenerative changes. Neurological system lesions can result in cognitive changes and vision and hearing changes. Neurosyphilis can result in dementia, stroke, and paresis.

Objective Data

exam findings are related to the disease stage

Stage 1: Chancre noted to genitalia. Localized painless lymphadenopathy

Stage 2: erythematous maculopapular nonpruritic rash, can be all over body or localized to pals of hands and soles of feet. possible patch alopecia.

Latent phase: can last for years. granulomas form which causes organ damage

Tertiary: cognitive changes, CVA (Cerebrovascular Accident),

Laboratory/Diagnostics

It is important to note that syphilis testing remains reactive for life. Tests include:

VDRL- not sensitive in early syphilis

RPR- used for diagnosis in the primary stage

FTA-ABS- first test to become positive in early syphilis

T. pallidum particle agglutination test- test if RPR or VDRL is positive, confirms infection

Lumbar puncture- cerebral spinal fluid analysis will identify presence of *T. pallidum*

CT/MRI can assess complications

Pharmacologic Management

Pharmacoloic management differs based on stage of disease

Primary, secondary, and latent stages:

Penicillin G benzathine, a penicillin antibiotic, interferes with bacterial cell wall synthesis during active replication, causes cell wall death and bactericidal activity.

Dose: 2.4 million units intramuscularly X 1.

Tertiary: Penicillin G benzathine, 2.4 million units intramuscularly weekly for three weeks

Neurosyphilis: Penicillin G procaine, 2.4 million units intramuscularly once daily for 10 to 14 days and Probenecid, 500 mg orally four times daily for 10 to 14 day

Special Considerations

Syphilis in pregnancy can cause miscarriage, stillbirth, or congenital syphilis. All positive syphilis cases should be tested for HIV.

Repeat testing is necessary- Successful treatment of primary and secondary syphilis will have a fourfold decline in RPR/VDRL titer over the next three to six months.

Referrals

A neurology referral is recommended if cognitive changes are noted.

Diagnosis: Gonorrhea

ICD-10: A54.9 Gonococcus, gonococcal (disease) (infection)

ICD 10 code will vary depending on location

Cathleen Crowley-Koschnitzki DNP, CNM, WHNP-BC, FNP-C, PMHNP-BC

Pathophysiology

Neisseria gonorrhoeae is gram negative diplococcal bacterial organism that infects mucous membranes via sexual transmission and during childbirth. *N. gonorrhoeae* pili (hair like projections) allow the bacterium to attach to mucosa or the cervix, urethra, and conjunctiva. Gonococcal organisms can genetically mutate, making them resistant to the body defense mechanisms and medications.

Physical assessment

Subjective Data

Pharyngeal gonorrheal infection can be asymptomatic. Some cases of genital infection are asymptomatic. Women can present with complaints of dysuria, genital pruritis, purulent vaginal discharge. Men can present with complaints of dysuria and copious purulent penile discharge.

Objective Data

Physical exam findings will vary depending on the location of the infection.

- Pharynx: erythema or exudate, cervical lymphadenopathy
- Speculum exam: cervicitis may be noted 5-10 days post exposure.
- Purulent discharge may be noted in males and females.

Laboratory/Diagnostics

Female specimens should be obtained from the endocervix, male specimens from the urethra

- Urethral Gram stain- identify gram negative intracellular diplococci
- Culture and sensitivity: identification of *N. gonorrhoeae* and appropriate treatment.
- Pharyngeal culture for coinfection, if suspected

A CT or MRI can assess complications if necessary

Pharmacological management:

Treatment is based on antibiotic sensitivity due to genetic mutation causing antibiotic resistance.

First line treatment:

Ceftriaxone (Rocephin), 250 mg IM in a single dose, plus

Azithromycin (Zithromax), 1 g orally in a single dose, or doxycycline, 100 mg orally twice per day for 7 days.

Fluoroquinolones should not be used to treat gonorrhea due to antibiotic resistance .

Special considerations

Patients who test positive for gonorrhea should also be tested for syphilis, chlamydia, HIV (Human Immunodeficiency Virus), (Herpes Simplex Virus) and hepatitis C as coinfection is common.

Sex partners of the last 60 days should be offered treatment.

Retesting for gonococcal reinfection is recommended three to six months post treatment, regardless of partner treatment.

Complications

Untreated gonorrhea can cause pelvic inflammatory disease in women with risk of infertility. Neonatal gonococcal infections from exposure to infected cervical secretions during birth can cause sepsis, conjunctivitis, meningitis, and arthritis. Gonococcal conjunctivitis can cause blindness. Gonococcal blood infections can cause arthritis, myocarditis, or meningitis.

Referrals

Gynecology referral is recommended for pelvic inflammatory disease symptoms.

Diagnosis: Herpes Simplex Virus (HSV) Type 1 and Type 2

ICD-10 B00.9 Herpesviral infection, unspecified.

Shanna Chapman, DNP, APRN, FNP-C, FAANP

Pathophysiology

Herpes Simplex Type 1 (HSV-1) and 2 (HSV-2) are both viruses that are contracted through direct contact with an active lesion or the body fluid of an infected person. The virus invades mucosal membranes and replicates.
During initial infection, viral DNA travel via axons to the sensory ganglion of the spinal cord where it persists for life. Asymptomatic viral shedding commonly occurs on 10% to 20% of all days and occurs most often during the first-year post infection. ICD 10 codoes are specific to area of infection.

In HSV-1, the trigeminal nerve is most often the nerve involved while in HSV-2, the sacral nerve root typically is involved. Once infected, the virus lays dormant in the nerve ganglia until reactivated. HSV-1 has an affinity for the oral mucosa while HSV-2 has an affinity for genitalia mucosa. However, a patient may experience HSV-2 on their oral mucosa and HSV-1 on the genitalia. This is becoming more and more common with oral sex practices.

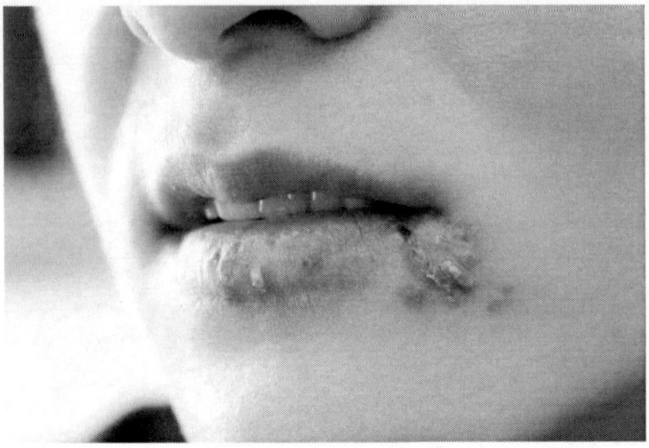

Pic #1: HSV 1 of the Oral Mucosa (Healthline.com)

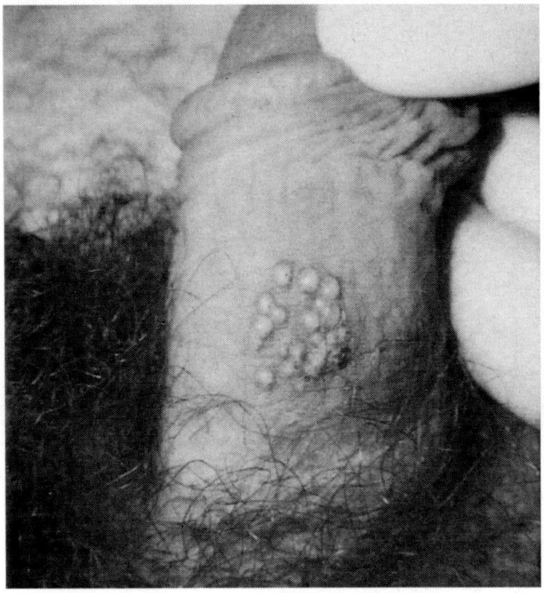

Pic #2: HSV 2 on a Male Penis (Healthline.com)

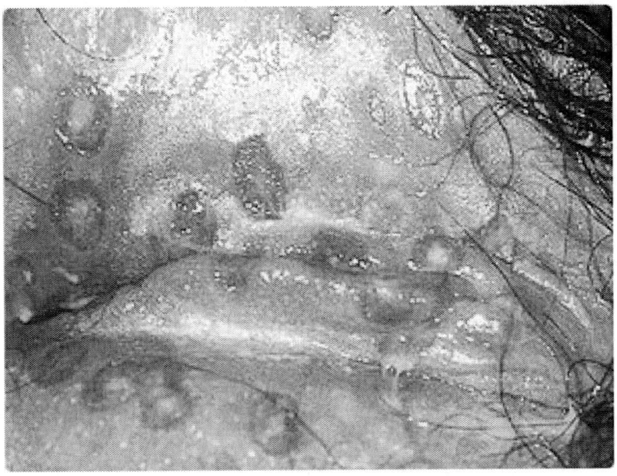

Pic #3 HSV 2 on a Female Labia (Healthline.com)

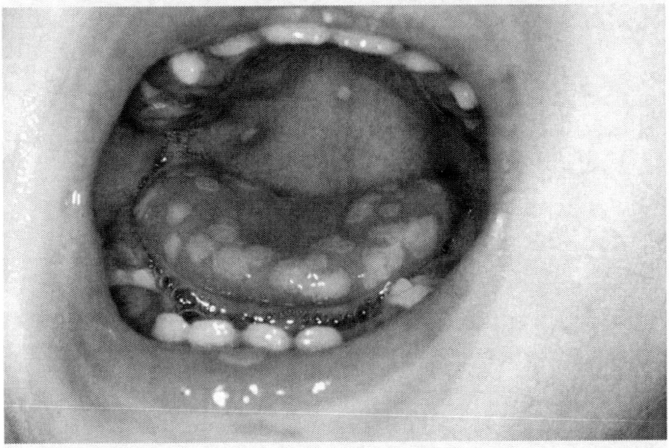

Pic #4 Herpetic Gingivostomatitis of a Child (Healthline.com)

Physical Assessment

Subjective Data

The chief complaint can vary on whether this is a primary or subsequent outbreak (see Table 12.4).

Table 12.4: HSV Subjective Data

	Primary outbreak	Subsequent outbreaks
Prodrome	May report pain, tingling, burning, or itching for hours or days prior to the appearance of the lesions.	
Physical complaints	May report malaise, fever, or adenopathy Patients may also report few or no symptoms. 65-90% of HSV + patients are unaware of the infection.	May report milder symptoms. Lesions last 6-12 days
Lesions	Visible outbreak: Reports painful fluid filled lesions at site of infection. May have vesicles that have opened, ulcerated, and reformed. Lesions can last up to 2 weeks	Reports painful fluid filled lesions at site of infection. May have vesicles that have opened, ulcerated, and reformed. Lesions last 6-12 days

Objective Data

Upon examination, presence of a single or cluster of vesicles or crusted lesions (or both) on an erythematous base noted at site of infection, usually orolabial or genital. Fever and adenopathy may be noted near the affected site.

Laboratory/Diagnostics

If active lesions are present, a viral culture may be ordered, as well as a polymerase chain reaction test. If no lesions are present, but the patient has suggestive symptoms, a Western Blot or an ELISA may be necessary. Otherwise, routine testing is not recommended.

Pharmacologic Management

The first line treatment is the same for HSV-1 and HSV-2 and is suppression treatment for the reduction of symptom severity, recurrence, and transmission. Patients can also be offered episodic outbreak treatment.

Antiviral medications such as Acyclovir (Zovirax) and Valacyclovir (Valtrex) can be prescribed. These nucleo-side analogues inhibit DNA synthesis and viral replication by competing with deoxyguanosine triphosphate for viral DNA polymerase and being incorporated into viral DNA.

Special Considerations

There is no cure for herpes. Antiviral medications are used prophylactically or to shorten outbreaks. Pregnant women with a known HSV history are treated prophylactically at 36 weeks of pregnancy until delivery. Newborn transmission can occur if the mother is not diagnosed and effectively treated prior to delivery. Women with active genital lesions should deliver via Cesarean section to decrease the risk of transmission.

All nucleosides are safe in pregnancy and breastfeeding. Partner testing for HSV infected persons requires testing a two-week to six-month window post exposure. Serial testing may be required if the first test is negative.

Complications

Complications of HSV include acute urinary retention, disseminated herpes, aseptic meningitis, hepatitis, neonatal infection, and pelvic inflammatory disease (PID). HSV infected persons have a three times higher incidence of contracting human immunodeficiency virus (HIV), as the open lesions can facilitate HIV transmission during sexual contact.

Referrals

Referrals are not necessary for uncomplicated HSV.

Diagnosis: Pelvic Inflammatory Disease

ICD-10 N73.9: Female pelvic inflammatory disease, unspecified

Shanna Chapman, DNP, APRN, FNP-C, FAANP

Pathophysiology

Pelvic inflammatory disease (PID) is a complex condition. It begins when bacteria introduced into the vagina ascends through the cervix to the upper genital tract. Common bacteria are from sexually transmitted infections such as chlamydia and gonorrhea. Without adequate treatment, it is quite common to develop complications such as infertility, ectopic pregnancy, tubo-ovarian abscess, and chronic pelvic pain.

Physical Assessment

Subjective Data

PID is often not recognized by women or their healthcare providers. Therefore, early detection and treatment are key to avoiding complications. Patients may report abdominal and pelvic pain, vaginal discharge and/or bleeding, irregular menstrual bleeding, dysuria and frequency of urine, painful coitus, as well as cervical motion tenderness.

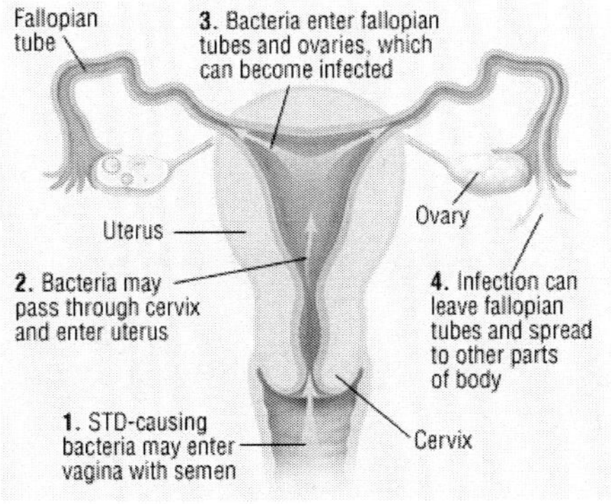

Healthline.com

Objective Data

Upon examination, patients with PID may exhibit one or more of the following:

- Fever of 101° F or greater
- Cervical mucopurulent drainage
- Cervical friability
- uterine and adnexal tenderness

Laboratory/Diagnostics

- Presence of abundant white blood cells (WBC) in vaginal discharge
- Elevated CRP and ESR (Erythrocyte Sedimentation Rates)
- urine NAAT (Nucleic acid amplification test)- positive chlamydia or gonorrhea

An endometrial biopsy may be used for specific diagnostic testing. A transvaginal ultrasound or MRI (Magnetic Resonance Imaging) of the pelvis may demonstrate thickened, fluid filled tubes with or without free fluid. Laparoscopic findings may be consistent with findings of PID.

Pharmacologic Management

The treatment plan should include antibiotics that treat *C. trachomatis* and *Neisseria gonorrhoeae*. First-line treatment includes Ceftriaxone 250 mg intramuscularly (one time), Doxycycline 100 mg twice a day by mouth for 10 days, as well as Metronidazole 500 mg by mouth, twice a day for 14 days.

Ceftriaxone works by inhibiting bacterial cell wall synthesis; Doxycycline inhibits bacteria synthesis by binding to the 30S ribosomal subunit; and Metronidazole inhibits cellular synthesis by disrupting the DNA of microbial cells.

Special Considerations

Pregnancy testing should be ordered for all female clients of reproductive age. Patients are recommended to abstain from sexual intercourse until all treatment is completed and PID is resolved. All sexual partners in the prior sixty days need to be treated and the patient should be retested in three months. Additionally, the patient should be tested for human immunodeficiency virus (HIV), as well as sexual partners.

Complications

Without early intervention, the patient has a high chance of experiencing complications such as infertility, ectopic pregnancy, and abscess.

Referrals

A referral to a gynecologist is necessary if there is no improvement within 72 hours, or if there is a high probability of hospitalization and laparoscopic intervention.

Diagnosis: Premenstrual Syndrome (PMS) and Premenstrual Dysphoric Disorder (PMDD)

ICD-10 N94.3: Premenstrual tension syndrome

ICD-10 F32.81: Premenstrual dysphoric disorder

Tracy Stogner DNP, APRN, PMHCNS-BC

Pathophysiology

There is still limited understanding as to the cause of Premenstrual syndrome (PMS) or Premenstrual dysphoric disorder (PMDD). Hormones are thought to play a role in both PMS and PMDD, particularly estrogen and progesterone and their impact during the week leading up to menstruation. Some women with PMDD may be more sensitive to the hormonal influences of serotonergic functioning, particularly estrogen. Other potential biological factors include a genetic component as well as well as a Central Nervous System sensitivity to reproductive hormones.

Physical Assessment

Subjective Data

Symptoms associated with PMS usually range from mild to moderate and include breast tenderness, fatigue and loss of concentration and mood swings. More severe symptoms of mood swings associated with the menstrual cycle are referred to as PMDD.

At least 5 of the following symptoms must be present the week right before the onset of menses and then symptoms are alleviated and end when menses begins.

PMDD must include at least 2 of the following symptoms to meet DSM V criteria

One or more of the following symptoms need to be present:

1. Marked affective lability (e.g., mood swings, feeling suddenly sad or tearful, or increased sensitivity to rejection)
2. Marked irritability or anger or increased interpersonal conflicts
3. Markedly depressed mood, feelings of hopelessness, or self-deprecating thoughts
4. Marked anxiety, tension, and/or feelings of being keyed up or on edge

In addition, one or more of the following symptoms must be present and when combined with the above symptoms, there must be at least 5 symptoms present in order to meet the criterion for a PMDD diagnosis.

- Reports of decreased concentration
- Decrease in interest in previous activities
- Complaints of lack of energy, fatigue and change in appetite.
- Sleep patterns changes- either insomnia or increased somnolence.
- Reports of a sense of being overwhelmed.
- Physical symptoms can include, bloating, breast tenderness and joint and muscle pain

Objective Data

There are no real physical characteristics associated with PMS or PMDD, mood lability and a tearful or depressed affect may be noted.

Laboratory/Diagnostics

There are no specific lab results used to diagnose PMDD. The lab tests listed below are important in order to rule out other types of disorders that can present with similar symptoms.

- TSH, T4- hyperthyroidism and hypothyroidism, depressive type symptoms
- CBC- anemia or leukemia

Pharmacologic Management

First line treatment for PMS includes providing supportive therapy or counseling to cope with symptoms. Vitamin B12 has also been shown to be helpful.

First line treatment for PMDD includes selective serotonin reuptake inhibitors (SSRI) and Serotonin-norepinephrine reuptake inhibitors (SNRI). Supportive therapy and counseling can be provided to learn to cope with the symptoms has also shown some benefit.

Cognitive behavioral therapy (CBT) has been shown to be successful in patients with PMDD. Some of the common SSRI drugs that have been used in the treatment of PMDD are fluoxetine, paroxetine, citalopram and escitalopram. These medications can become effective in the treatment of symptoms related to PMDD within days which is different than onset of action in depression. These drugs are often given in lower doses than what is used to treat MDD and is given only during the luteal phase of a women's menstrual cycle which is from ovulation to menstruation.

Special Considerations

PMS and PMDD only affect women and adolescents of childbearing age. SSRIs can increase suicidal ideation (SI) in adolescents and young adults. Include this information in education and assess for SI at each follow up visit.

Complications

A thorough psychiatric evaluation may be warranted to evaluate for depression or additional mood disorders. The use of an SSRI or SNRI in bipolar depression can activate mania. Serotonin syndrome may also occur.

Referrals

Patients with PMS or PMDD can be referred for counseling. A psychiatric mental health specialist may be needed if symptoms do not resolve and/or symptoms extend longer than the luteal phase

Diagnosis: Menstrual Irregularities

ICD-10 N92.6: Irregular menstruation, unspecified

Candice Phillips, PhD, RN, APRN, CNM, CNE

Pathophysiology

Menses cycles demonstrate consistent patterns in individual women following ovulation unless significant health changes occur that impact the hypertrophic pulmonary osteoarthropathy (HPOA). For example, menstrual irregularities can often occur around menarche and menopause due to anovulation and inadequate follicular development. Menstrual cycle disorders also result from conditions that affect the hypothalamus, pituitary gland, ovaries, uterus, cervix, or vagina.

The etiology of menstrual irregularities include:

- Organ/Systemic illness: thyroid disease, blood dyscrasias, adrenal imbalance, von Willebrand's disease, liver disease, kidney disease, leukemia, clotting disorders, abnormal hormone secretion
- Pelvic malignancy: ovary, uterus, vagina, bladder, rectum, nodes
- Ovarian functional change (perimenopause)
- Uterine polyps, prolapse, tumors, leiomyomata, or trauma
- Endometrial polyps, leiomyomata, hyperplasia, structural abnormalities, or endometriosis
- Adenomyosis
- Vaginal tumors or trauma

- Cervical lesions, polyps, leiomyomata, carcinoma, or trauma
- Ectopic Pregnancy/Abortion/Placental Accidents
- Sexually Transmitted Infections (STI), Pelvic Inflammatory Disease (PID)
- Urethral prolapse
- Stress, excessive exercise

Physical Assessment

Subjective Data

Subjective symptoms for menstrual irregularities may include midcycle bleeding or variation in normal menstrual flow. Spotting or a sudden onset of heavy bleeding may occur, as well as passing blood clots larger than a quarter. Fatigue or shortness of breath may be present. Menstruation may be longer than seven days with cycle intervals less than 21 days; or more than 38 days but less than 90 days.

Objective Data

Vital signs may be abnormal or abnormal. Objective findings for menstrual irregularities may include one or more soaked sanitary pads or tampons every hour for several consecutive hours. Additionally, prolonged or excessive uterine bleeding of more than 80 mL may occur. Upon a bimanual examination, the patient may demonstrate tenderness on palpation; the uterus size may be normal or abnormal.

Laboratory/Diagnostics

Laboratory diagnostics for menstrual irregularities may include:

- Complete blood count (CBC) to assess for anemia

- Bleeding and clotting time, if indicated
- Serum Pregnancy test, if indicated
- Urinalysis
- Wet mount to assess for a sexually transmitted infection (STI) or bacterial vaginosis
- Thyroid studies to assess for HPOA axis pathophysiology
- von Willebrand's testing, if indicated
- Hormone levels such as luteinizing hormone (LH), follicle-stimulating hormone (FSH), prolactin, gonadotropin-releasing hormone (GnRH), serum estradiol

Pharmacologic Management

The first-line treatment for menstrual irregularities involving light flow and/or irregular bleeding entails observation for two or three cycles with a menstrual diary to determine an effective treatment plan. Pharmacologic management is demonstrated in Table 12.5. The first-line treatment for menstrual irregularities involving heavy bleeding include a physician consultation or referral.

Table 12.5: Pharmacological Management of Menstrual Irregularities

Name	Class	Mechanism of Action
Oral Progestin: Numerous Generic and Brand Names Camila, Errin, Heather, Jolivette, Micronor, Norethindrone, Ovrette	Steroid Hormone Synthetic Progesterone only oral contraceptive	Suppression of the midcycle surge of luteinizing hormone (LH); inhibition of the release of gonadotropin-releasing hormone (GnRH) and pre-ovulatory LH surge, preventing follicular maturation and ovulation; thinning of the endometrial lining
Numerous Generic and Brand Names Alesse, Brevicon, Loestrin, Modicon, Wera, Balziva, Briellyn, Gildagia, Philith, Zenchent	Steroid Hormone Monophasic combined estrogen-progestin oral contraceptive	Ovulation suppression through inhibition of gonadotropin-releasing hormone (GnRH), luteinizing hormone (LH), follicle-stimulating hormone (FSH) and the mid-cycle LH surge; thinning of the endometrial lining
Meclofenamate Sodium (Meclomen)	Nonsteroidal anti-inflammatory drug (NSAID)	Inhibition of prostaglandin synthesis

Special Considerations

A consultation or referral may be necessary for women with a positive human chorionic gonadotropin (hCG) if bleeding persists, as well as for women who miss more than three menstrual periods (either consecutively or over the course of a year), and those with post-menopausal bleeding. Consider low-dose contraceptives for three cycles or supplemental estrogen for heavy bleeding with Depo-Provera. Consider an endometrial biopsy for postmenopausal women or for women of any age if bleeding persists without known etiology.

Complications

Complications of menstrual irregularities include anemia, severe hemorrhage, shock, and systemic illness symptoms.

Referrals

Patients with menstrual irregularities may be referred to obstetrics and gynecology (OB/GYN) or a hematologist.

Diagnosis: Dysmenorrhea

ICD-10 N94.4 Primary dysmenorrhea

N94.5 Secondary dysmenorrhea

N94.6 Dysmenorrhea, unspecified

Linda Wilson, DNP, FNP-C

Pathophysiology

The pathophysiology of dysmenorrhea is not fully understood. It is thought to be initiated by the release of prostaglandins in the menstrual fluid, which creates uterine contractions and pain. Prostaglandins are controlled by progesterone, when progesterone levels decrease prostaglandin levels increase. Vasopressin may play a role increasing uterine pain by increasing contractility. Vasoconstriction and ischemia cause inflammation and stimulation of pain fibers pain one to two days before menses starts.

Physical Assessment

The primary evaluation goal is a detailed history of the onset, duration of pain and a negative physical exam to rule out any additional pathology.

Subjective Data

The patient presents with complaints of lower abdominal pain, which may include radiation to the back and thighs. Pain is most significant the first eight to 72 hours of menses. Pain can be severe enough that absenteeism from school, work, and daily activities may occur. Additional symptoms can include nausea, vomiting, diarrhea, fatigue, and sleep deprivation.

Objective Data

The physical exam is usually normal. A pelvic exam is not considered necessary at the time of initial presentation.

Laboratory/Diagnostics

There are no specific laboratory testing or diagnostics for initial diagnosis of dysmenorrhea.

If symptoms do not improve in three-six months with conservative treatment, a pelvic exam and ultrasound should be considered.

STD (sexually transmitted diseases) testing should be included at that time.

Pharmacologic Management

First line treatment of dysmenorrhea are analgesics, specifically nonsteroidal anti-inflammatories. NSAIDS (Non-steroidal anti-inflammatory drugs) inhibits prostaglandin synthesis and produce analgesic, anti-inflammatory effects and should be taken one to two days before menses onset. Ibuprofen 400mg to 600mg every four to six hours or naproxen sodium 500mg every 12 hours.

If the patient does not achieve relief with NSAIDS then a secondary treatment option is low dose oral contraceptives (OCPs). OCPs can be initiated cyclically or continuously, taking only active pills. Suppression of ovulation is associated with decreased menstrual pain.

Special considerations

Primary dysmenorrhea usually starts at menarche or shortly after. An increase in age and childbearing tend to eliminate symptoms. Primary dysmenorrhea occurs without gynecological disease.

Secondary dysmenorrhea may have pathological origins of endometriosis, adenomyosis, fibroids or pelvic inflammatory disease. Secondary tends to occur greater than two years after menses begins.

Complications

There are no significant complications with primary dysmenorrhea. The treatment is supportive.

Referrals

Moderate to severe dysmenorrhea that interferes with lifestyle and is nonresponsive to treatment should be referred to gynecology.

Diagnosis: Amenorrhea

ICD-10:N 91.0 Primary amenorrhea

N91.1 Secondary amenorrhea

N91.2 Amenorrhea, unspecified

Pamela Porter DNP, APRN, FNP-BC, CNS, PA-S

Pathophysiology

Numerous etiologies can be at the core of amenorrhea, but three physiologic causes need to be ruled out initially in all childbearing ages; physiological causes include pregnancy, lactation, and menopause. Amenorrhea is categorized as primary or secondary.

Primary amenorrhea

Pregnancy

Hypergonadotropic/ hypogonadism

Eugonadism (imperforate hymen, transverse vaginal septum are reversible)

Secondary amenorrhea

Ovarian disease (PCOS)

Hypothalamic dysfunction (eating disorder, exercise, stress congenital GnRH (gonadotropin releasing hormone) deficiency)

Pituitary diseases (hyperprolactinemia, empty sell syndrome, Sheahan's syndrome, s/p radiation)

Asherman's syndrome

Drug induced

Congenital adrenal hyperplasia, Cushing's, thyroid disorders

Exercise, stress, or weight loss induced

Table 12.6: Causes of Amenorrhea

	Common Cause	**Pathophysiology**
Normal Physiologic processes	Pregnancy	Sustained High Estrogen & progesterone
	Menopause	Lack of estrogen
Uterine disorders	Disorders of development	Excessive androgen exposure
	Congenital abnormalities	e.g., imperforate hymen
	Asherman's Syndrome	Endometrial adhesions following curettage
Ovarian disorders	Gonadal dysgenesis	Deletion of genetic material X chromosome
	Premature ovarian failure	Lack of viable follicles
	Polycystic ovary syndrome	Altered intraovarian hormone balance
Disorders of the Hypothalamus or pituitary	Stress, athletes in training, underweight- anorexia	Altered GnRH pulses

Physical Assessment

Subjective Data

Clients will report lack of menarche or cessation of menses. Additional complaints, which vary on pathophysiology, can include lack of female physical maturation, infertility, constipation,

Objective Data

physical exam findings will vary based on pathology as noted in Table 12.7

Table 12.7: Pathology and Exam findings in Amenorrhea

Pathology	Physical exam findings
Anatomical/functional	Transverse vaginal septum Imperforate hymen Perirectal fullness Progressive cyclic pelvic/ abdominal pain
Pituitary	Galactorrhea Pituitary adenoma- N/V and vision changes
Hypothyroidism	Weight gain 10-20 pounds Cold intolerance Hair loss Dry skin hypotension bradycardia
PCOS	Masculine features Hirsutism acne Obesity 60-80 %
Androgen insensitivity	breast development present Absent pubis, axillary hair Retained testes (groin or inguinal) noted on imaging
Mullerian agenesis	breast development present Pubic & axillary hair present Absent uterus and upper vagina Ovaries present Possible renal and vertebral anomalies
Gonadal dysgenesis	breast development present No dysmorphic features
Turner Syndrome	Short stature Epicanthic folds Low-set ears High arched palate Webbing of the neck Otitis media Square chest Absent breast development

Laboratory/ Diagnostics

Laboratory testing and diagnostics will vary based on the pathology.

Normal Physiologic processes- Serum hCG; Serum FSH (follicle stimulating hormone) if menopause suspected

Uterine disorders- Pelvic ultrasonography or MRI to assess anatomy, estrogen-progesterone trial, visualization of endometrium

Ovarian disorders- Genetic testing Karyotype- done when the uterus is absent, or Turners syndrome is suspected. Ultrasound for follicles, check gonadotropin levels.

Disorders of the Hypothalamus or pituitary- Serum TSH, T4, PRL, gonadotropins

Pharmacological management

Treatment of amenorrhea is determined by the etiology.

Table 12.8: Amenorrhea Treatment

Disorders	**First-line treatment**	
Normal Physiologic processes	Medroxyprogesterone to promote withdrawal bleeding. Inhibits pituitary gonadotropin release, blocking follicular maturation and ovulation, transforms proliferative into secretory endometrium	Provera 5-10 mg for 5-10 days
hypogonadism	An oral contraceptive, either combined or intermittent or continuous progesterone is prescribed to prevent endometrial hyperplasia	OCP: Multiple choices
	Vitamin D3- stimulates intestinal Ca and PO4 absorption; stimulates bone mineralization and prevents osteoporosis	Vitamin D3 Cholecalciferol 800 units PO qd
PCOS (polycystic ovarian syndrome)	Oral Contraception- suppresses LH (Luteinizing Hormone) and FSH, inhibiting ovulation; alters cervical mucus and endometrium.	OCP: Multiple choices
	Insulin-sensitizing agents, Biguanides, reduce insulin resistance and improve ovulatory function.	Insulin-sensitizing agents Metformin 500 mg tid or 850-1000 mg PO bid

	Androgen antagonists/ aldosterone receptor antagonists- antagonizes aldosterone-specific mineralocorticoid receptors. Prescribed for acne and hirsutism	Spironolactone 50-200mg qd

Special considerations

Untreated amenorrhea can lead to infertility.

Other considerations are related to pathophysiology of the cause.

Complications

Complications of amenorrhea included osteoporosis, endometrial hyperplasia, uterine cancer and infertility.

Referrals

A referral to Gynecology is recommended

Diagnosis: Polycystic Ovarian Syndrome

ICD-10 E28.2: Polycystic ovarian syndrome

Tiney Ray PhD, DNP, FNP-BC

Pathophysiology

Polycystic ovarian syndrome (PCOS) is an endocrine disorder classified as a syndrome where women have an abnormality in the metabolism of androgens and estrogen that affects fertility and menstrual cycle. In PCOS, the ovaries are usually bilaterally enlarged and contain multiple follicles.

Physical Assessment

Subjective Data

The most common symptoms of PCOS include menstrual dysfunction, and hirsutism, infertility, obesity, and metabolic syndrome. Diabetes and obstructive sleep apnea may also be reported.

Objective Data

Upon examination, virilization signs may be noted, as well as acanthosis nigricans, hypertension and enlarged ovaries.

Laboratory/Diagnostics

For patients with suspected PCOS, the following testing may be used:

- Serum HCG for all women of childbearing age
- Thyroid function tests
- Prolactin level
- Testosterone levels
- Cosyntropin stimulation test
- Serum 17-hydroxyprogesterone (17-OHPG) level
- Urinary free cortisol (UFC) and creatinine levels
- Low-dose dexamethasone suppression test
- Serum insulin-like growth factor (IGF)–1 level
- Androstenedione level
- FSH and LH levels
- GnRH (gonadotropin releasing hormone) stimulation testing
- Glucose level
- Insulin level

Imaging tests may include:

- Transvaginal ultrasound to assess anatomy
- Pelvic CT (Computed Tomography) scan or MRI (Magnetic Resonance Imaging) to visualize the adrenals and ovaries

Pharmacologic Management

Lifestyle modifications are considered the first-line treatment for women with PCOS. Women are encouraged to lose weight through diet and exercise. Pharmacologic treatments are reserved to address anovulation, hirsutism, and menstrual irregularities- of an oral contraceptive to regulate menses. Ethinyl estradiol and progesterone, contraceptives, may suppress LH and FSH from the pituitary gland by decreasing the amount of GnRH.

Special Considerations

PCOS is difficult to diagnose in adolescents due to the similarity of the clinical and biochemical manifestations along with irregular menstrual cycle and the normal pubertal development. Therefore, diagnosis should be deferred at least two years following menarche.

Complications

Patients with PCOS are at an increased risk for endometrial hyperplasia and carcinoma due to the chronic anovulation.

Referrals

A referral to a gynecologist or reproductive endocrinologist may be needed if the female patient has difficulty conceiving or is having difficulty regulating their menstrual cycle.

Diagnosis: Uterine Fibroids

ICD-10 D25.9: Leiomyoma of uterus, unspecified

Tiney Ray PhD, DNP, FNP-BC

Pathophysiology

Uterine fibroids (leiomyomas) are benign monoclonal tumors which arise from the smooth muscle cells of the myometrium most commonly during childbearing years. Uterine fibroids rely on estrogen for growth and can increase in size and number as estrogen increases which can occur during pregnancy, oral contraceptive use, and insulin resistance. Uterine fibroids can range in size from seedling which are undetectable by the human eye to bulky masses that can distort and enlarge the uterus. Uterine fibroids shrink when estrogen levels decline such as during menopause or with the use of a progesterone only oral contraceptive.

Physical Assessment

Subjective Data

Patients with uterine fibroids may report symptoms including:

- Menorrhagia
- Blood clots associated with menses
- Dysmenorrhea (pelvic or back pain)
- Urinary symptoms
- Dyspareunia
- Mittelschmerz
- Reproductive problems (preterm labor / miscarriage/ infertility)
- Fatigue

Objective Data

The patient may exhibit heavy menstrual bleeding and have a feeling of hardness in their lower abdomen or pelvic area. Pelvic examination may note lesions, as well as anemia.

Laboratory/Diagnostics

For suspected uterine fibroids, a complete blood count (CBC) can be ordered to assess for anemia related to menorrhagia Pelvic ultrasound or endovaginal scanning may be used to evaluate nonspecific pelvic pain and anatomical abnormalities

Pharmacologic Management

First line treatment is using conservative measures to control the symptoms. Asymptomatic women, those with small or slow-growing fibroids, or those with larger fibroids who want to preserve their fertility can benefit from pharmacologic management such as non-steroidal anti-inflammatory drugs (Ibuprofen, meloxicam, Aleve, Celecoxib, Naprosyn). These drugs inhibit the cyclooxygenase enzyme and lower the production of pro-inflammatory prostaglandins, which can decrease dysmenorrhea and menorrhagia.

Tranexamic acid, an antifibrinolytic agent can be used. This drug inhibits fibrinolysis by forming a reversible complex that displaces plasminogen from fibrin and inhibits plasmin proteolytic activity, reducing the menstrual blood. Finally, a progesterone-only oral contraception may be prescribed, which serves to repress the estrogenic stimulated growth of the endometrium; this class of medications consequently decreases blood loss during menstruation

Special considerations

The prevalence of fibroids increases with maternal age and is higher in black women than in white or Hispanic women. Women with larger fibroids who decline medical intervention require annual sonograms to monitor the progression of the fibroids.

Complications

Uterine fibroids can lead to infertility. Severe pelvic pain and fever in women with a history of fibroids can suggest necrosis of the fibroid tumor

Referrals

A referral to a gynecologist may be necessary if there is a noted pelvic mass. A surgical myomectomy, removal of myometrium including leiomyoma or hysterectomy, is not appropriate for women in childbearing years. Interventional radiology can treat uterine artery embolization, which blocks blood flow to the uterine body.

Diagnosis: Ovarian Cysts

ICD-10 N83.29: Unspecified ovarian cysts

Tiney Ray PhD, DNP, FNP-BC

Pathophysiology

The exact pathophysiology of the ovarian cyst is unclear. An ovarian cyst is a sac filled with fluid material found in the ovary. These cysts can occur in females at any stage of life, from the neonatal period to post menopause. ovarian cysts are often divided into two categories, ovarian cystic neoplasms, and functional ovarian cysts.

Physical Assessment

Subjective Data

Patients with ovarian cysts may be asymptomatic. Some patients are symptomatic due to the cyst type and size. Subjective complaints can include:

- Pain in the lower abdomen
- Menstrual irregularities
- Urinary symptoms (larger cysts)

- Dyspareunia
- Pain during bowel movements (Grabosch, 2018).

Objective Data

The pelvic examination may reveal unilateral or bilateral tenderness. The cyst may be palpated during exam.

Laboratory/Diagnostics:

A pregnancy test (urine) may be used to assess for pregnancy or tubal pregnancy. A urinalysis can help to rule out an infection, while endocervical swabs can rule out a sexual transmitted disease. Finally, a transvaginal sonogram may be used to assess the anatomy.

Pharmacologic Management

Non-steroidal anti-inflammatory drugs such as ibuprofen, meloxicam, Aleve, celecoxib, and Naprosyn may be beneficial. These drugs inhibit the cyclooxygenase enzyme cyclooxygenase and lower the production of pro-inflammatory prostaglandins, which have been shown to improve dysmenorrhea and menorrhagia.

Special Considerations

Risk factors for an ovarian cyst include the need for infertility treatment, the use of tamoxifen, pregnancy, tubal ligations, cigarette smoking, hypothyroidism, and maternal gonadotropins. In the postmenopausal women with new ovarian growths, there should be a high suspicion of cancer.

Complications

Ovarian cysts larger than 4 cm in diameter have over a 10% chance of causing ovarian torsion. Though rare, a spontaneous rupture of a dermoid cyst can cause peritonitis, which warrants an emergency surgery.

Referrals

Patients with severe abdominal pain should be referred to an emergency department.

Diagnosis: Endometriosis

ICD-10: N80.9: Endometriosis, unspecified

Tiney Ray PhD, DNP, FNP-BC

Pathophysiology

Endometriosis is an inflammatory condition in which endometrial tissues are found in extrauterine locations. The endometrial lining can grow on various parts of the female reproductive track, including fallopian tubes, ovaries, cul-de-sac (the space behind the uterus) and abdominal organs including the peritoneum, bladder, ureters, and rectum. Endometrial tissue bleeding during the menstrual cycle can adhesions.

Physical Assessment

Subjective and Objective Data

Complaints may include menorrhagia, menstrual blood clots, dysmenorrhea (pelvic or back pain), dyspareunia, infertility and painful micturition or defecation. Tenderness may be noted, which is related to the site involved.

Laboratory/Diagnostics

A laparoscopy-tissue biopsy may be used to confirm the diagnosis of endometriosis.

Pharmacologic Management

Treatment depends on the extent of the disease, the patient symptoms, and whether the patient desires fertility. Endometriosis can be treated with medication, surgery, or both. When pain is the primary problem, medication usually is tried first. Pain relievers such as ibuprofen, meloxicam, Aleve, celecoxib, and Naprosyn may be used. These non-steroidal anti-inflammatory drugs (NSAID) can inhibit the cyclooxygenase enzyme, which then lowers the production of pro-inflammatory prostaglandins; this has been shown to improve dysmenorrhea and menorrhagia.

Special Considerations

For pediatric patients, early assessment of any patient with moderate to severe dysmenorrhea requires aggressive treatment to conserve future fertility. Surgical options include laparoscopic surgery to remove lesions, relieve pain, and improve fertility; a hysterectomy may be necessary for unresolved pain in women not seeking fertility.

Complications

Complications of endometriosis include infertility, ovarian cysts, and adhesion of organs. Additionally, urinary and bowel complications may occur.

Referrals

Referrals include an obstetrician/gynecologist (OB/GYN) or specialists in reproductive endocrinology, urology, and colorectal surgery. A referral to gynecologic oncology may also be necessary.

Diagnosis: Infertility

ICD-10: N97.9: Female infertility, unspecified

ICD-10: N46.9: Male infertility, unspecified

Tiney Ray PhD, DNP, FNP-BC

Pathophysiology

Infertility is the inability to conceive after one full year or more of unprotected sexual intercourse. Pathophysiology differs according to the cause which can include abnormal sperm production, reproductive tract abnormalities, physical or chemical agents, endocrine disorders/ nerve damage, sexual transmitted disease, frequency of intercourse, overall health, lifestyle, and mental health state.

Physical Assessment

Subjective and Objective Data

Persons with an inability to conceive after one full year or more of unprotected sex may be infertile. A physical and pelvic examination should be performed initially to determine if there are any obvious causes of infertility.

Laboratory/Diagnostics

Testing includes semen analysis, cervical swabs and cultures to test for a sexually transmitted infection (STI), complete blood count (CBC), endometrial biopsy, and hormone testing such as prolactin, progesterone, and testosterone levels.

Pharmacologic Management

Infertility treatment depends on the age of the couple, the cause and length of the infertility and their personal preferences. Treatment may include changing lifestyle factors, medications to improve sperm count and fertility medications to stimulate ovulation, sperm retrieval or surgery to restore fertility

Special Considerations

Infertility treatment can be an exhausting option and it can have significant effects on the couple's relationship. Additionally, infertility treatment is costly and may lead to financial debt.

Complications

Potential complications depend on the choice of treatment. Bleeding or infection may occur with invasive treatment. Multiple pregnancy is a common complication of infertility treatment. Ovarian hyperstimulation syndrome may occur from some fertility medications, which can cause edema of the ovaries; this is extremely painful and is considered a medical emergency.

Referrals

Patients/couples may be referred to an infertility specialist for treatment.

Diagnosis: Breast Cancer

ICD-10 C50.919: Malignant neoplasm of unspecified site of unspecified female breast

LaTonya Carroll, DNP, FNP-C, CPNP-PC

Pathophysiology

The genes whose function to suppress tumor genes are BRCA1 and BRCA2. If the genes mutate, the progression of the cell cycle can occur as well as limiting DNA repair. Mutation can affect other tissues; cyclin D1 is in estrogen/progesterone and cell cycle progression when mutations involve c-myc expression.

Physical Assessment

Subjective Data

Breast cancer can be symptomatic or asymptomatic. Symptoms may include pain in the breast or axilla, heaviness, swelling, thickening, redness, or dimpling of the skin. Nipple discharge, often bloody, erosion or retraction could also be reported, as well as a lump in the axilla or supraclavicular area.

Objective Data

Upon examination, the breast will have an asymmetrical appearance. Additional findings include a breast mass, breast dimpling, nipple discharge, axillary lymphadenopathy, skin thickening or discoloration, retraction or scaling of the nipple.

Laboratory/Diagnostics

A mammogram can detect an irregular mass, clustered microcalcifications, and linear branching calcifications. A breast ultrasound may also be used, which can visualize a hypoechoic mass, an irregular mass with internal calcification, and enlarged axillary lymph nodes. Additionally, a breast MRI can enhance areas of significant architectural distortion.

A breast biopsy will be needed to make a definitive diagnosis of breast cancer. Hormone receptor testing may be positive or negative; the HER2 receptor test may also be positive or negative in someone with breast cancer.

Pharmacologic Management

Management is based on the location and staging of the cancer (0, I, II or IIIA [T3N1M0]). Raloxifine, a selective estrogen receptor modulator (SERM), as well as Tamoxifen, an antineoplastic agent, estrogen receptor antagonist, and SERM may be used.

For the post-menopausal women, Raloxifine acts to select binding activating estrogenic pathways in some tissues and antagonizing estrogenic pathways to block some estrogen effects in the breast and uterine tissues. In the bone it acts like an estrogen agonist to prevent bone loss, which increases bone mineral density and decreases fracture incidence.

Tamoxifen competitively binds to estrogen receptors on tumors and other tissue targets, decreasing DNA synthesis and inhibiting estrogen effects; potent antiestrogenic properties compete with estrogen for binding sites in the breast and other tissues.

Special Considerations

In pregnancy treatment for breast cancer is dependent upon what trimester the woman is in. A mastectomy or breast conservation are preferred in pregnancy due to radiation being contraindicated. Chemotherapy can be given during pregnancy in the second and third trimesters; however, trastuzumab is contraindicated. Radiation can be considered after delivery, but not while a woman is breast feeding.

Complications

Complications include chemotherapy-related nausea and/or vomiting; drug-related vasomotor symptoms; neutropenia/neutropenic fever; chemotherapy-related ovarian failure; lymphedema; chemotherapy-related leukemia; tamoxifen-related

DVT; tamoxifen-related pulmonary embolus; endocrine therapy-induced vascular disease; tamoxifen endometrial cancer.

Referrals

Patients with breast cancer should be referred to gynecological oncology.

Diagnosis: Ovarian Cancer

ICD-10 C56.9: Malignant neoplasm of unspecified ovary

Gloria Okoh, PhD, FNP-C

Pathophysiology

The three most common types of ovarian cancers are Epithelial (most common), Germ-cell, and Stromal. The pathophysiology of each differs. Epithelial ovarian cancer type 1 originates in the ovary. Epithelial ovarian cancer type 2 originates in the fallopian tube and is linked to genetic mutations. Germ cell ovarian cancer are histologically similar to germ cell tumors in the testes of men. Stromal ovarian cancer develops from the sex cord, stromal cord or both and is the least common ovarian cancer.

Physical Assessment

Subjective Data

Symptoms are vague and non-specific and can include abdominal bloating, abdominal pain, urinary frequency, and changes in bowel habits.

Objective Data

Abdominal or pelvic bimanual examination commonly identifies an adnexal mass. Ascites may be detected.

Laboratory/Diagnostics:

Serum CA125 level (MUC16; cancer antigen 125)- used for diagnosis and evaluation of treatment response

- Over 80% of ovarian malignancies express elevated levels of CA125
    - Elevated levels are more often detected in advanced or recurrent disease
    - The following are considered positive results:
        - Level above 50 units/mL in premenopausal women
        - Level above 40 units/mL in premenopausal women using oral contraceptives
        - Level above 30 units/mL in postmenopausal women
- Serum HE4 level (WFDC2; human epididymal protein 4)
    - Tumor marker secreted and overexpressed by serous and endometrioid epithelial ovarian cancer

- Serum HE4 level has a very high negative predictive value (about 99%), indicating that almost all patients with negative test results will have benign ovarian pathology
- Combination of serum HE4 and CA125 levels has higher sensitivity and specificity than either test used alone

Imaging

- Transvaginal ultrasonography with color Doppler is the preferred modality; some centers perform additional transabdominal scan
    - Major ultrasonographic characteristics suggesting malignancy include:
        - Irregularly shaped solid tumor
        - Tumor with multiple (more than 4) papillary structures
        - Irregularly shaped solid, multiloculated tumor more than 10 cm in largest dimension
        - Tumor that demonstrates very strong flow on color Doppler
        - Ascites
- MRI of abdomen/pelvis

- Usually indicated to assess for local metastasis after initial ultrasonographic evaluation; may help if diagnosis is unclear based on ultrasonographic findings alone
  - More specific for diagnosis of malignancy than ultrasonography; may reduce false-positive findings
  - Superior to CT at detecting local metastasis to bladder, vagina, rectum, and pelvis
- Findings suggestive of malignancy include presence of vegetations in cystic masses and ascites

- CT of abdomen/pelvis
  - Usually not useful for diagnosis but may be used to detect local metastases after initial ultrasonography
  - CT can be helpful for assessing disease in lymph nodes and upper abdomen

Diagnosis is confirmed by histopathologic examination of surgical specimen

- Surgical removal of the complete ovary or ovaries, rather than tissue biopsy, is recommended to determine whether ovarian cancer is present
- Aspiration biopsy of an ovarian mass is contraindicated if malignancy is suspected owing to risk of peritoneal contamination

Pharmacologic management

First line treatment: Goal is eradication of tumors and long-term disease free

Surgery: total abdominal hysterectomy with bilateral salpingo-oophorectomy and comprehensive surgical staging. Followed by comprehensive chemotherapy.

Pathological staging and Chemotherapy treatment is noted below:

Stages I A, B or C: Observe or Fertility sparing therapy for selected patients Platinum-based chemotherapy Regimen OR, Paclitaxel and carboplatin IV chemotherapy regimen.

Stage II-IV: Complete surgery as indicated by the tumor and Platinum-based Chemotherapy Regimen

Special considerations

Ovarian Cancer is the most common lethal of all the gynecological cancers, often diagnosed in advanced staged due to the vague symptoms. About 70% of ovarian cancer are at stages III and IV at time of diagnosis.

Elderly patients 70 or older may not tolerate combination chemotherapy regimens. Alternative regimens may be appropriate for elderly patients with stage I through stage IV epithelial ovarian cancer, including: Carboplatin every 3 weeks Paclitaxel plus carboplatin every 3 weeks Paclitaxel plus carboplatin weekly for 18 weeks.

Complications

Complications associated with ovarian cancer include metastasis to peritoneal cavity, ascites, intestinal or ureteric obstruction, premature menopause secondary to oophorectomy, tumor recurrence and chemotherapy complications.

Referrals

- genetic counselor for breast, ovarian, and colorectal cancer risk evaluation
- gynecologic oncologist for clinically suspicious lesions and for comprehensive staging and surgical treatment
- medical oncologist for management of systemic chemotherapy
- reproductive endocrinologist for consultation regarding fertility-preservation procedures

Diagnosis: Uterine Cancer

ICD-10 C55: Malignant neoplasm of uterus, part unspecified

Gloria Okoh, PhD, FNP-C

Pathophysiology

Endometrial cancer is usually preceded by endometrial hyperplasia. Endometrial carcinoma is commonly classified into 2 types. Type I tumors are usually estrogen-responsive and low-grade. Endometrioid adenocarcinoma is the most common histology. Type II tumors are usually high-grade (eg, serous or clear cell histology).

Physical Assessment

Subjective Data

Reproductive age women may present with reports of missed periods, heavy or irregular menstruation. Pelvic or bladder pain and painful intercourse. Post-menopausal women can present with reports of vaginal spotting or bleeding. Other symptoms may include painful micturition, dyspareunia, vaginal discharge, odor, and pelvic pain.

Objective Data

The physical examination may be unremarkable. Other possible exam findings include enlarged uterus. A pelvic mass may be palpated in advanced stages.

Laboratory/Diagnostics:

Human chorionic gonadotropin (hCG) to rule out pregnancy

Endometrial biopsy-Positive histologic findings is confirmatory

Cancer antigen 125 (CA-125) serum levels can be elevated

Transvaginal ultrasound and endometrial biopsy with hysteroscopy- assess anatomy

Dilation and curettage required if biopsy is negative in patients with persistent symptoms.

Treatment

Surgical options include total hysterectomy, bilateral salpingo-opherectomy, pelvic and para-aortic lymph-denectomy. In medically inoperative or patients with complications such as morbid obesity or cardiopulmonary disease, treatment includes chemotherapy and radiation followed with surgical resection and surgical staging. Treatment option for surgical stages include:

Stage I: Observe, Vaginal radiation therapy and or chemotherapy.

Stage II: Radiation

Stage III: Chemotherapy and or radiation

Stage IV: Chemotherapy and or radiation.

Complications

Complications of uterine cancer can include anemia related to vaginal bleeding, infertility, premature onset of menopause, metastasis to surrounding organs, radiation vaginitis, radiation cystitis and infection secondary to chemotherapy.

Referrals:

Refer to Gynecology is suspicion of uterine cancer. The gynecologist will coordinate with oncology.

Diagnosis: Cervical Cancer

ICD-10 C53.9: Malignant neoplasm of cervix uteri, unspecified

LaTonya Carroll, DNP, FNP-C, CPNP-PC

Pathophysiology

Changes to the cervical epithelial tissue consists of dysplasia early in the disease process, which starts out mild and then becomes progressively severe. The dysplasia typically occurs with the squamous epithelial cells of the external cervical os of the cervix (the transformation zone) at the junction of the columnar cells.

The neoplasia of the cervical intraepithelial is graded from I to III depended on the dysplasia severity and the degree of the cell differentiation. Carcinoma in situ, which is where many disorganized, undifferentiated, abnormal cells are present (severe dysplasia) in seen in grade III. The timeline from mild dysplasia to carcinoma in situ can take up to 10 years.

Physical Assessment

Subjective Data

Common symptoms include postcoital bleeding, intermenstrual or postmenopausal bleeding and/ or vaginal discharge. Less common symptoms: painful sex, low back with radiation down the posterior leg, lower extremity edema, vesicovaginal and rectovaginal fistula, and urinary symptoms.

Objective Data

The pelvic exam is typically normal with microinvasive disease. Additional findings include exophytic, endophytic, polypoid, papillary, ulcerative, or necrotic lesions; watery, purulent, or bloody discharge and lymphadenopathy of the supraclavicular or inguinal lymph nodes. In advanced disease there may be ascites, and decreased breath sounds, which would indicate metastases.

Laboratory/Diagnostics

A vaginal or speculum examination should be performed, which may demonstrate a cervical mass or bleeding. Cervical screening for precancerous and cancerous cells can be accomplished via a Papanicolaou test. Human papillomavirus (HPV) testing is recommended for pap smear findings of atypical squamous cells of undetermined significance (ASCUS). A colposcopy can assess for abnormal vascularity, white changes with acetic acid, or obvious exophytic lesions. Finally, a biopsy can confirm cervical cancer histologically and identify the subtype.

Management

Cervical cancer is treated through surgery, chemotherapy, and radiation. The treatment plan is based on staging.

Special Considerations

During pregnancy, there should be a multidisciplinary approach. Chemotherapy can be given during the second and third trimesters; however, surgery should be avoided. Radiation is an absolute contraindication in pregnancy.

ASC-US patients who are HPV-positive should be referred for colposcopy.

Complications

Patients with cervical cancer are at risk for the following:

- Loss of ovarian function
- Hemorrhage
- Pelvic infection
- Bladder dysfunction
- Sexual dysfunction
- Ureteral obstruction with renal failure
- Bowel obstruction
- Pulmonary embolism
- Lower extremity lymphedema

Referrals

Once a diagnosis is confirmed, multidisciplinary management will occur with various disciplines including primary care, gynecology, and gynecological oncology.

Diagnosis: Testicular Cancer

ICD-10: C62.90 Malignant neoplasm of unspecified testis, unspecified

Joel Regalado, DNP, ACNP-BC, CCRN-CMC, PCCN

Pathophysiology

Germ cell tumors (GCT) account for 90% of testicular cancers. The main type of GCTs are seminomas and non-seminomas. Seminomas tend to grow and spread more slowly than non-seminomas. The main two subtypes that usually occur in men between 25 and 45 years old. Spermatocytic seminoma, a rare slow growing germ cell tumor, occurs more commonly in men over 50 years of age.

Non-seminomas tend to occur among late teens and early 30s. Non-seminomas are classified into four (4) types: **Embryonal carcinoma** are tumors that look like tissues of early embryos. Embryonal carcinomas increased level of AFP and hCG. **Yolk sac carcinoma** is termed as the cells are similar to early human embryo. This is the most common type of testicular cancer in children but rare in adults. **Choriocarcinoma** spreads aggressively to other parts of the body including the lungs, bones, and brain. This tumor increases the level of hCG. **Teratoma** are tumors that look like the three layers of the embryo (endoderm, mesoderm, and ectoderm). Teratomas do not increase AFP or hCG levels.

Physical Assessment

Subjective and Objective Data

Patients with testicular cancer commonly present with testicular discomfort, as well as a feeling of heaviness. They may also complain of gynecomastia or breast soreness (with certain types of germ cell tumors, hCG levels rise).

With metastatic disease, symptoms vary depending on the metastatic site and can include:

- Neck mass in supraclavicular lymph node metastasis
- Cough and dyspnea in lung metastasis
- Anorexia, nausea, vomiting in retro duodenal metastasis
- Bone pain in skeletal metastasis
- Lower extremity swelling in iliac or caval venous obstruction or thrombosis

Laboratory/Diagnostics

A scrotal ultrasound can distinguish intrinsic from extrinsic testicular lesions with a high degree of accuracy. Additionally, serum tumor markers (AFP, beta-hCG, lactate dehydrogenase can be beneficial in the diagnosis of testicular cancer. A computed tomography (CT) scan may be needed for suspicion of metastasis. If brain metastasis is suspected, a magnetic resonance imaging (MRI) test may be needed.

Biopsy is not recommended due to the risk of spreading the cancer. Finally, a positron emission tomography (PET) scan is useful post treatment to evaluate residual masses.

The staging system most often used for testicular cancer is the American Joint Committee on Cancer (AJCC) TNM system, which is based on 4 key pieces of information. The system considers the extent of the disease based upon primary tumor (T), lymph node involvement (N), presence of metastasis (M) and the serum (S) blood level of tumor markers.

Treatment Options

Management is based on tumor markers and imaging results and should be made in a multidisciplinary setting involving specialists such as urology, medical oncology, radiation oncology, pathology, and radiology. Treatment may include a radical inguinal orchiectomy and retroperitoneal lymph node dissection.

Chemotherapy administered in cycles lasting approximately three to four weeks is also used. Chemotherapy agents include cisplatin, etoposide, bleomycin, ifosfamide, paclitaxel and vinblastine. Due to high dose chemotherapy, which can mitigate suppression of bone marrow, a stem cell transplant may be necessary.

Complications

Complications of testicular cancer include infertility, as well as retrograde ejaculation after retroperitoneal lymphadenectomy. Men diagnosed with testicular cancer should be given the option for semen cryopreservation prior to initiating therapy. A baseline sperm count and banking should be performed to avoid radiation exposure.

Referrals

Patients with testicular cancer may be referred to a urologist, medical oncologist, radiation oncologist, as well as a pathologist.

Diagnosis: Prostate Cancer

ICD-10 C 61 Malignant neoplasm of prostate

Joel Regalado, DNP, ACNP-BC, CCRN-CMC, PCCN

Pathophysiology

Prostate adenocarcinoma results from a genetic mutation in the luminal or basal cells resulting in uncontrolled cell division. The two gene mutations have been linked specifically to prostate cancer are breast cancer gene 1 and 2, also known as BRCA1 and BRCA2. Once the mutation occurs, the affected cells begin to grow and replicate, forming a tumor. Prostate cancer is a slow process compared to other types of cancer.

Physical Assessment

Subjective and Objective Data

Most patients may present with nonspecific subjective and objective urinary symptoms including

- urgency
- frequency
- nocturia
- incontinence
- abnormal bladder sensation
- hematuria
- low stream
- intermittency
- hesitancy
- terminal dribble
- dysuria

- Digital Rectal Exam - may detect nodules, induration, or asymmetry

Symptoms of metastatic disease include pain secondary to osseous metastases, although many remains asymptomatic despite extensive spread.

Laboratory/Diagnostics

- Serum PSA (Prostate Specific Antigen) –not specific for malignancy. Can be elevate in benign conditions. Refer to PSA testing guidelines for appropriate ordering and counseling for this test. (See special considerations)

- Prostate Imaging - transrectal ultrasound, computed tomography (CT), and magnetic resonance imaging (MRI) to image the prostate can be useful when treatment choice is dependent on total prostate volume.

Treatment Options

For prostate adenocarcinoma, active surveillance is warranted when the tumor is confined to the prostate - including routine tumor marker measure and imaging to confirm that tumor is not progressive.

If there is tumor progression options may include:

- radical prostatectomy with pelvic lymph node dissection
- radiation therapy
- brachytherapy
- orchiectomy – removing the testes removes the source of testosterone and can shrink or stop the growth of cancer
- androgen deprivation therapy (ADT) or hormone therapy
    - luteinizing hormone - releasing hormone (LHRH) agonist or GnRH (gonadotropin releasing hormone) are drugs that lower the amount of testosterone. Medications available in the US are Lupron, Zoladex, Triptorelin and Histrelin.
    - LNRH Antagonist - can lower testosterone level quickly without the effect of tumor flare. Available on the market is Firmagon.

- Chemotherapy – can be taken orally or intravenously if prostate cancer has spread and hormone therapy is ineffective. Available chemotherapeutic agents are Taxotere, Jevtana, Novantrone, and Emcyt
- Immunotherapy – use to stimulate the immune system to recognize and destroy cancer cells. Provenge is a vaccine that boosts the immune system to destroy prostate cancer cells.

Special considerations

The severity of the symptoms can be quantitated using the American Urological Association (AUA) symptoms score/International Prostate Symptom Score (IPSS). The AUA symptom score and the IPSS use the same questions and scale.

There is no specific numerical PSA threshold that accurately determines the presence of prostate cancer. As such, the AUA in their published guideline for early detection of prostate cancer does not recommend PSA screening in men under 40 years old because of low prevalence in this age group. Men between 40-54 years should be evaluated based on risk factors such as African American race and those with family history of metastatic cancer. The greatest benefit of screening is between 55-69 but should be a shared decision making between the patient and provider. A routine screening interval of two years or more may be preferred over annual screening in those men who have taken part in shared decision-making and decided on screening. A routine PSA screening is not recommended for men over 70 years old or any man with less than 10-15 years life expectancy. Similarly, a prostate biopsy is not warranted if patient has significant comorbidities that limit life expectancy.

Complications

Complications associated with prostate cancer include renal stones, hydronephrosis, obstructive uropathy and renal failure

Referrals

Urology, Nephrology and Oncology as indicated.

Chapter 13: Perinatal Disorders

Spontaneous Abortion

Hyperemesis Gravidarum

Ectopic Pregnancy

Gestational Diabetes

Iron Deficiency Anemia

PUPPS

Preeclampsia/Eclampsia

Preterm Labor

Incompetent Cervix

Diagnosis: Spontaneous Abortion

ICD-10 O03: Complete or unspecified spontaneous abortion without complication

Amanda Marshall DNP, APRN, WHNP-BC

Pathophysiology

Early pregnancy loss occurs in the first trimester of pregnancy and is identified by an empty gestation sac or absent activity of the fetal heart. Approximately half of cases are related to fetal chromosome abnormalities.

Physical Assessment

Subjective Data

Patients may report vaginal bleeding, passage of clots or products of conception. Cramping can be present or absent. The last menstrual period (LMP) greater than 28 days may also be reported.

Objective Data

The blood pressure and pulse may be affected dependent on blood loss. The pelvic examination may reveal vaginal bleeding or products of conception noted in the vagina or cervix. Bright red or pink blood indicates active bleeding, while dark red or brown blood indicates earlier bleeding. Cervical motion tenderness or adnexal pain may indicate an ectopic pregnancy.

Laboratory/Diagnostics

Vaginal bleeding may occur in 25% of women. The presence and location of a live fetus must be verified prior to any treatment. Vaginal ultrasound is used to assess for the presence of an intrauterine fetus and cardiac activity. Serum β-hCG levels should be run; quantitative hCG levels should double every 48 hours with viable pregnancy. If the hCG level is > 3000 miu/ml, a gestational sac should be noted on an ultrasound. Type and screen to assess for blood type and Rh factor may be necessary, as well as a complete blood count (CBC) to monitor for hemodynamic changes and/or anemia from blood loss

Pharmacologic Management

First line treatment is to allow the miscarriage to occur naturally without interventions. Expectant management is limited to the first trimester and lasts up to eight weeks.

For incomplete abortions or terminations, Misoprostol 800 micrograms can be provided initially with a repeat dose, if needed. Misoprostol is a prostaglandin E1 analogue, which can induce uterine contractions. It is important to confirm complete expulsion with a follow-up ultrasound or serum β-hCG levels.

Special Considerations

Incomplete abortions or terminations require medical and/or surgical management. Educate expectant management patients on when to seek medical attention related to blood loss, pain, and infection, along with the possibility of needing surgical intervention. Negative Rh blood type requires Rho (d) immunoglobulin with any pregnancy bleeding to prevent Rh positive antibody formation.

Complications

Complications of a spontaneous abortion include hemorrhage, hemodynamic instability, and infection.

infection

Referrals

A referral to obstetrics and gynecology (OB/GYN) is warranted for patients with complications or for management of threatened, incomplete or missed abortions. The patient may be referred to the emergency department for active bleeding with hemodynamic instability. Finally, it may be beneficial to refer patients to support groups for pregnancy loss.

Diagnosis: Hyperemesis Gravidarum (HEG)

ICD-10 O21.1: Hyperemesis gravidarum with metabolic disturbance

Amanda Marshall DNP, APRN, WHNP-BC

Pathophysiology

Hyperemesis gravidarum (HEG) refers to intractable nausea and vomiting resulting in dehydration, weight loss and ketonuria. HEG begins in the first trimester and affects 2-3% of pregnant women. Symptoms start at approximately 3-5 weeks of gestation and most cases resolve by 20 weeks gestation.

The pathophysiology of HEG is unknown. Suspected contributing factors include rising human chorionic gonadotropin (hCG), estrogen and progesterone levels.

Physical Assessment

Subjective and Objective Data

Patients may report severe nausea, vomiting, weight loss, fatigue, and excessive salivation (ptyalism). Upon examination, patients may exhibit vomiting, weight loss of greater than 5% of pre-pregnancy weight, dehydration, and ptyalism.

Laboratory/Diagnostics

Laboratory data includes a urinalysis, which will demonstrate positive ketones and an increased urine specific gravity. Patients may have an increased blood urea nitrogen (BUN), abnormal levels of sodium and potassium, increased liver enzymes, abnormal thyroid, and parathyroid levels (decreased TSH, elevated T4), and an increased hematocrit.

Pharmacologic Management

First line treatment for HEG is Zofran (Ondansetron), which is an antiemetic. Routes include oral tablet, Subcutaneous (SQ) pump, liquid, quick dissolve film, or intravenous (IV). Dosage is 4-8 mg every 6-8 hours.

Special Considerations

Mild nausea and vomiting symptoms can be treated with ginger, pyridoxine, antihistamines, and metoclopramide Electrolyte imbalances are corrected with IV fluids and enteral or total parenteral nutrition is given for sustained weight loss. Vitamin supplements such as thiamine are recommended to prevent Wernicke's encephalopathy. Evaluation consists of serial weights, heart rate, orthostatic blood pressure, urine ketones, electrolytes, and obstetric ultrasound If severe nausea onset occurs after nine weeks other medical conditions should be considered.

Complications

Complications of HEG include malnutrition, esophageal tears, gastric ulcers, esophageal bleeding, kidney and liver damage, gallbladder disease, depression, anxiety, temporomandibular joint disorders, dental caries, diabetes, difficulty with weight management, motion sickness, preterm labor, low birthweight, and preeclampsia. HEG can lead to severe complications such as Wernicke's encephalopathy, peripheral neuropathy, and central pontine myelinolysis, and acute tubular necrosis

Referrals

Referrals for HEG include an obstetrician for management, as well as a dietician. Referral to a social worker or support group may be needed, as well as a mental health specialist to treat anxiety and depression.

Diagnosis: Ectopic Pregnancy

ICD-10 O00.9: Ectopic pregnancy, unspecified

Amanda Marshall DNP, APRN, WHNP-BC

Pathophysiology

Ectopic pregnancy occurs because of abnormalities in fallopian tube anatomy or function. Causes of fallopian tube dysfunction can include infections, surgeries, or medications that can cause scaring of the reproductive tract. Potential causes include in vitro fertilization, endometriosis, prior ectopic pregnancy, endometriosis, in utero DES exposure, appendectomy, pelvic surgery, tubal sterilization, intrauterine device (IUD), and malformation of the fallopian tubes. Common sexually transmitted infections that cause scarring include Chlamydia and Pelvic Inflammatory Disease. Surgeries include past cesarean sections. Cigarette smoking can cause decrease mobility in the fallopian tube. The fertilized ovum implants in the epithelium, the embryo or fetus can be absent.

Physical Assessment

Subjective Data

Patients may present with complaints of pain, either generalized or unilateral; continuous or intermittent; sharp or cramping, abdominal or pelvic location. Dizziness can be present, or shoulder pain. Shoulder pain or urge to defecate could indicate internal bleeding from the fallopian tube or posterior cul-de sac. Vaginal bleeding may or may not be present.

Objective Data

Upon examination, findings may include pallor, tachycardia, hypotension, and infection. Speculum examination may demonstrate vaginal bleeding or spotting; bluish coloration of the cervix, which normally appears in pregnancy; bulging cul-de-sac, which occurs with hemoperitoneum in rupture. Bimanual examination may demonstrate abdominal tenderness, cervical motion tenderness, and mild uterine enlargement may be noted. Adnexal mass may be palpated depending on gestational age.

Laboratory/Diagnostics

For patients with an ectopic pregnancy, a urine hCG will be positive. A transvaginal ultrasound may show the location of the gestation, which must be verified prior to any treatment. With serum β-hCG levels, quantitative hCG levels should double every 48 hours with viable pregnancy. Levels will decrease or fail to double as expected. If the hCG level is > 3000 miu/ml, a gestational sac should be noted on ultrasound. A serum progesterone level of < 5 ng/ml will indicate nonliving intrauterine pregnancy or ectopic pregnancy. Levels > 25 ng/ml will rule out ectopic pregnancy. Type and screen may be used to assess for blood type and Rh factor. Additionally, a complete blood count (CBC) is needed to monitor for hemodynamic changes and/or anemia from blood loss

Management

Management is determined by the level of activity of the ectopic gestation.

It is important to determine if Expectant, Medical, or Surgical management is appropriate. For expectant (very inactive ectopic gestation), low and plateauing hCG <1500 will often resolve without intervention. With medical (less active), early, unruptured ectopic pregnancies with B-hCG levels less than 3000 mIU/mL, gestational sac less than 3.5 cm or absent and no fetal cardiac activity on ultrasound examination.

Asymptomatic, hemodynamically stable women with no hepatic or renal disease and no evidence of leukopenia or thrombocytopenia can be treated with methotrexate, which is a folic acid antagonist. Methotrexate interferes with cellular multiplications and DNA synthesis. Post methotrexate evaluation includes:

- Day 4: Repeat hCG titer and assess symptoms
- Day 7: Repeat hCG titer
- If hCG titer does not decrease by at least 15%, a second dose of Methotrexate is indicated
- If hCG titer decreases by at least 15% on the seventh day, continue to monitor hCG weekly, until undetectable.

Special Considerations

Negative Rh blood type requires Rho (d) immunoglobulin with any pregnancy bleeding to prevent Rh positive antibody formation. Women should abstain from sexual activity for at least 3 months following Methotrexate therapy, due to the potential teratogenic effects. Women may experience increased abdominal pain, 5 to 10 days following Methotrexate therapy, which would require further evaluation to rule out tubal abortion and rupture.

Complications

Parity and history of ectopic pregnancy increase the risk of rupture. A ruptured ectopic pregnancy can cause acute, excessive bleeding and be life threatening. Sudden death, caused by internal hemorrhage and infection can result from a misdiagnosis, which occurs in 12% of cases.

Referrals

Immediate referral to an Emergency Department with OB/GYN services is necessary for a positive hCG, abdominal pain, and vaginal bleeding, hemodynamic failure, hemoperitoneum, high hCG levels, pain, and syncope require surgical management. Support groups can help assist with grief from the pregnancy loss and fears about future pregnancies

Diagnosis: Gestational Diabetes Mellitus (GDM)

ICD-10 O24.419: Gestational diabetes mellitus in pregnancy, unspecified control

Amanda Marshall DNP, APRN, WHNP-BC

Pathophysiology

Gestational diabetes mellitus (GDM) is an abnormal metabolic adaption to pregnancy, a transient insulin resistance beginning in the second trimester of pregnancy because of physiologic changes in placental hormones. An increase in estrogen, progesterone, cortisol, leptin, placental lactinogen and placental growth hormone cause result in insulin resistance. The glucose is transplacentally transported to the fetus, causing macrosomia.

Physical Assessment

Subjective Data

Patients may be asymptomatic or present with reports of polyuria, polydipsia, weight loss, fatigue, nausea/vomiting, or blurred vision.

Objective data

Upon examination, patients may have abnormal glucose values, elevated blood pressure, or candida vaginitis.

Laboratory/Diagnostics

Test blood glucose levels at 24-28 weeks gestation for all pregnant women one-hour Oral Glucose Tolerance Test (OGTT) with 50-gram glucose solution. If the one-hour plasma glucose is >140 mg/dl, the patient will complete a three-hour fasting OGTT with 100-gram glucose solution. Two or more elevated glucose levels on the three-hour confirms a diagnosis of GDM.

Management

Nonpharmacologic management includes a standard diabetic diet, moderate intensity exercise, and self-monitoring blood glucose (SMBG) up to four times daily, prandial, and pre-prandial.

If dietary management ineffective, Metformin, an antidiabetic agent biguanide (previously Category B) may be used. Metformin decreases hepatic glucose production and intestinal absorption of glucose. Increases insulin sensitivity by increasing peripheral glucose uptake and utilization.

Special Considerations

Monitor maternal weight, blood pressure, and fundal height. Additionally, monitor fetal well-being with ultrasounds and non-stress tests. Provide education and emotional support for the diagnosis and self-monitoring of blood glucose levels (SMBG). Review SMBG record at each prenatal visit, monitor for compliance, and adjust insulin dosage/frequency as needed.

Complications

Maternal risks include hypertensive disorders, perineal lacerations, c-section due to infant macrosomia, and risk of Type 2 diabetes. Fetal risks include macrosomia, birth trauma, and shoulder dystocia. Neonatal risks include hypoglycemia, hyperbilirubinemia, polycythemia, hypocalcemia, thrombocytopenia, and respiratory distress syndrome (RDS).

Referrals

Referral to obstetrics and gynecology (OB/GYN) is needed if insulin is required. Additional referrals may include a certified diabetic educator, as well as a maternal fetal medicine specialist.

Diagnosis: Iron Deficiency Anemia (IDA) of Pregnancy

ICD-10 O99.109: Anemia complicating pregnancy, unspecified trimester

Amanda Marshall DNP, APRN, WHNP-BC

Pathophysiology

Physiologic anemia occurs during pregnancy, due to hemodilution, an increased volume of maternal plasma and red blood cells, or inadequate dietary iron intake. As the blood volume increases and the placenta and fetus grow, so do the requirements for iron. A hemoglobin < 11 in the first and third trimesters or a hemoglobin < 10.5g/dl in the second trimester meets criteria for IDA of pregnancy.

Physical Assessment

Subjective and Objective Data

Patients with iron deficiency anemia (IDA) may report fatigue, pica (craving strange substances such as ice), headache, decreased appetite.

Objective Data

Upon examination, patients may exhibit pallor, tachycarida, icterus.

Laboratory/Diagnostics

A complete blood count (CBC) is beneficial to assess hemoglobin (Hgb) and hematocrit levels. A Hgb may be <11 in the first and third trimester or <10.5 in the second trimester. Serum ferritin levels may be < than 15mcg/L.

Pharmacologic Management

First line treatment is a multivitamin containing 16-20 mg of elemental iron, such as ferrous sulfate. Ferrous sulfate replaces iron and allows transportation of oxygen via hemoglobin.

Special Considerations

Other sources of iron include prenatal vitamins and food such as meats, fruits, vegetables, bread, and grain products. IDA in pregnancy increases the risk of infant neurodevelopment impairment, low birth weight, premature birth, and maternal mortality. Patients may require parenteral iron or blood transfusion if severe anemia is present.

Complications

Complications of IDA may include perinatal and postpartum depression, preterm labor, intrauterine growth restriction, and hemorrhage.

Referral

A referral to a dietician may be needed to assist with patient education.

Diagnosis: Pruritic Urticarial Papules and Plaques of Pregnancy (PUPPPs)

ICD-10 O26.86: Pruritic urticarial papules and plaques of pregnancy (PUPPP)

Amanda Marshall DNP, APRN, WHNP-BC

Pathophysiology

Pruritic Urticarial Papules and Plaques of Pregnancy (PUPPPs), also known as polymorphic eruption of pregnancy, is thought to result from the physiologic changes of pregnancy; however, the exact cause is unknown. Theories include skin changes occur in response to fetal antigens or as a response to connective tissue damage from skin stretching.

Physical Assessment

Subjective and Objective Data

Patients with PUPPP may present with pruritis, or a rash in the third trimester of pregnancy. Urticarial erythematous papules and plaques with striae involvement may be present. PUPPP will typically begin on the lower abdomen in the striae gravidarum around 36 weeks gestation.

Laboratory/Diagnostics

Patients may need a punch biopsy to rule out herpes gestationis.

Pharmacologic Management

First line treatment for PUPPPs is the use of a topical or systemic corticosteroid such as prednisone. Reserve oral corticosteroids for severe cases. Prednisone decreases inflammation by suppressing migration of polymorphonuclear leukocytes and reversing increased capillary permeability.

Special Considerations

PUPPPs will resolve 1-3 weeks after delivery, so if it is tolerable, no treatment is needed. Oral antihistamines, like diphenhydramine, can be used to relieve pruritis.

Complications

There are no fetal or maternal effects associated with PUPPP.

Referral

Referral to a dermatologist is recommended if first line treatment fails.

Diagnosis: Preeclampsia/Eclampsia

ICD-10: O14.90: Unspecified pre-eclampsia, unspecified trimester

Amanda Marshall DNP, APRN, WHNP-BC

Pathophysiology

The specific etiology is not clear. Placental implantation factors are thought to be the cause behind the endothelia dysfunction, vasoconstriction and poor blood flow to the kidneys and other organs.

Physical Assessment

Subjective and Objective Data

Patients may report headaches, visual disturbances, right upper quadrant or epigastric pain, increased swelling, and sudden weight gain.

Objective Data

Upon examination, patients may have a systolic blood pressure of ≥140, diastolic blood pressure ≥90, or both. Pitting edema of lower extremities or generalized edema may be present, as well as epigastric pain.

Laboratory/Diagnostics

A 24-hour urine will demonstrate proteinuria is >300 mg. A urinalysis: ≥0.3 protein/creatinine ratio. With severe preeclampsia, platelets may be <100 in a complete blood count (CBC). Serum creatinine will be >1.1 mg per dL or doubling.

Pharmacologic Management

First line treatment is based on severity Labetalol (beta-blocker) and/or Hydralazine (vasodilator) may be given intravenously (IV). When IV access is not available, immediate-release oral nifedipine (calcium channel blocker) may be used. Magnesium Sulfate is used for the prevention and treatment of seizures. Low dose aspirin (81 mg daily) is recommended as prophylaxis for at risk women.

Special Considerations

Increased fetal monitoring and surveillance is necessary through the remainder of pregnancy. The onset of seizures warrants immediate delivery of fetus. The condition is cured through delivery of the fetus; however, risk remains through six weeks postpartum. Schedule a blood pressure check within 7-10 days after birth and review postpartum preeclampsia precautions. Postpartum patients discharged on antihypertensives should follow-up with their obstetric providers within 72 hours.

Complications

Provide postpartum patient education regarding the increased risk for cardiovascular disease and stroke.

Referrals

Patients should be referred immediately to an Emergency Department if they have signs of increased headache or swelling, as well as if there is new onset seizure activity in a pregnant patient.

Diagnosis: Preterm Labor (PTL)

ICD-10 O60.00: Preterm labor without delivery, unspecified

ICD-10 O60.10X0: Preterm labor with preterm delivery, unspecified

Amanda Marshall DNP, APRN, WHNP-BC

Pathophysiology

Pathological causes of preterm labor (PTL) include inflammation, pathologic distention of the uterus, decidual hemorrhage, and activation of the hypothalamic-pituitary-adrenal axis in the mother or fetus.

Physical Assessment

Subjective Data

It is important to gather a thorough history and identify risk factors for PTL. Patients may report cramps, painful or painless contractions, a change in vaginal discharge, low dull backache, pelvic pressure.

Objective Data

Upon examination, there may be cervical dilation, effacement, or both or 2cm on initial exam. Determine the cervical length and look for rupture of membranes. Regular contractions occurring every 10 minutes or more often with a 30 second duration may indicate PTL. Use the Bishop score to assess risk of preterm birth.

Laboratory/Diagnostics

Perform a sterile speculum exam to obtain a fetal fibronectin sample. A negative result decreases probability of PTL 87%. Speculum examination can test vaginal fluid for pH and ferning. A transvaginal ultrasound showing cervical length <25mm is considered short. External fetal monitoring may be used to assess contractions and fetal heart rate.

Pharmacologic Management

First line treatment for PTL is the use of tocolytic therapy by an obstetrician or perinatologist, on an intrapartum unit, with the goal of extending pregnancy and administering prenatal corticosteroids. Magnesium sulfate is a tocolytic, which inhibits uterine contractions by decreasing acetylcholine in motor nerve terminals.

Special Considerations

Antenatal corticosteroid administration accelerates fetal lung development. Advise pelvic rest with symptoms of PTL, which restricts sexual intercourse, heavy lifting, orgasm, and douching. Bedrest has not been proven to prevent PTL. For patients with a history of preterm birth, administer 17 α-hydroxyprogesterone caproate weekly beginning at 16-18weeks' gestation until term. Cervical cerclage may be placed after 24 weeks in women with or short cervical length or cervical incompetency.

Complications

Preterm birth alone is the largest cause of cerebral palsy and increases the risk of developmental delays

Referrals

PTL should be managed an obstetrician or perinatologist.

Diagnosis: Incompetent Cervix

ICD-10 N88.3: Incompetence of cervix uteri

Amanda Marshall DNP, APRN, WHNP-BC

Pathophysiology

The cause of incompetent cervix is unknown. It is associated with abnormal cervical development, as well as previous cervical trauma.

Physical Assessment

Subjective Data

Patients with incompetent cervix may report a a feeling of pelvic fullness or pressure. These patients may have a history of miscarriage or preterm delivery.

Objective Data

With a cervicaldigital or ultrasound examination, cervical dilation more than 3 mm and cervical length less than 2.5 cm indicates incompetent cervix.

Laboratory/Diagnostics

A transvaginal ultrasound can be used and may demonstrate funneling of the cervical canal, and cervical length less than 2.5 cm.

Pharmacologic Management

There is no pharmacologic treatment. First line treatment is cervical cerclage (prophylactic or therapeutic). Cerclage is offered prior to fetal viability with a cervical length of less than 2.5 cm and intact membranes to prevent further cervical dilation and preterm delivery. The sutures are removed after 37 weeks of gestation.

Special Considerations

Transvaginal ultrasound may be used every 2 weeks to check cervical length and funneling. For patients with a history of cervical incompetence, prophylactic cerclage may be provided at 2-14 weeks of gestation.

Complications

Complications include pregnancy loss, preterm rupture of membranes, preterm delivery, and infection. There is a risk of rupture of membranes if cerclage placed after 23 weeks.

Referrals

Patients may be referred to an obstetrician or maternal fetal medicine specialist.

Chapter 14: Mental Health

Unipolar Depression

Bipolar Depression

Anxiety

Panic

Substance Abuse

Diagnosis: Mood Disorders

ICD-10 F30-F39: Mood (affective) disorders

Cathleen Crowley-Koschnitzki DNP, CNM, WHNP-BC, FNP-C, PMHNP-BC

Pathophysiology

The underlying pathophysiology of depression is not clearly understood. Neurobiological circuits are responsible for mood, a dysfunction results in a mood change. According to the MAO hypothesis, depression, or any mood disorder which includes depression, mania and hypomania is the result of the imbalance of dysfunction of the monoamine transmitter system. Involved neurotransmitters include serotonin, norepinephrine, and dopamine. In mania, neuroimaging has shown increased activity in the amygdala, which is associated with emotions.

Physical Assessment

Subjective and Objective Data

Clients may present with depression symptoms listed below (see Table 30), which are similar in both unipolar and bipolar depression. Previous history should include assessment for previous times of hypomania or mania in all patients presenting with depression symptoms.

Table 14.1 : Mood Disorder Subjective and Objective Data

	Unipolar Depression	**Bipolar Depression**
Subjective Data	Clients may present with complaints of daily low or sad mood, fatigue, decreased interest in	Depression symptoms are consistent in unipolar and bipolar depression.

	previously pleasurable activities, weight changes (loss or gain), sleep changes (insomnia or hypersomnia), agitation, feelings of guilt, feelings of worthlessness, difficulty concentrating, or suicidal thoughts.	**Depression:** Clients may present with complaints of daily low or sad mood, fatigue, decreased interest in previously pleasurable activities, weight changes (loss or gain), sleep changes (insomnia or hypersomnia), agitation, feelings of guilt, feelings of worthlessness, difficulty concentrating, or suicidal thoughts. **Mania:** Decreased need for sleep, euphoria, hypersexuality, impulsive behaviors leading to relationship discord, occupational problems, or legal problems. An obsession with religion, politics, finance as well as grandiose delusions may be noted. **Hypomania:** Elevated mood, decreased need for sleep, very productive period lasting a minimum of 4 days. Absence of psychotic symptoms. No relationship issues or legal implications due to behavior.

Objective Data	Flat affect, weight changes (loss or gain). Low affect.	**Depression:** Flat affect, weight changes (loss or gain) Hypomania- no symptoms may be present. **Mania:** Hyperactive and/or hyperverbal-pressured speech, flight or ideas, inability to stop talking or stay seated may be noted.

Pharmacological Management

For unipolar depression, first line treatment includes selective serotonin reuptake inhibitor (SSRI) and Serotonin-norepinephrine reuptake inhibitors (SNRI). Escitalopram is the best tolerated SSRI with the fewest drug interactions. SSRIs inhibit reuptake of serotonin in the central nervous system which increases available serotonin in the synaptic cleft.

In bipolar depression, treatment can be initiated with mood stabilizers such as Lithium if the client is presenting in a state of mania. Lithium is a natural element thought to alter sodium transport across nerve and muscle cell membranes.

Special Considerations

Women experience depression twice as frequently as men. Depression symptoms such as fatigue and insomnia also present as symptoms of other diagnoses, particularly anemias and thyroid abnormalities. Depression is common in chronic diagnoses.

Lithium is considered neuroprotective and is also used to decrease suicidal ideation.

Complications

Inaccurate diagnosis and treatment of bipolar patients with antidepressants can activate a manic episode. Treatment compliance may be difficult in bipolar disorder, clients report mania feels good. Clients with mood disorders have increased risk for suicide. Women attempt suicide twice as often as men, but men are more likely to succeed because men choose more lethal means. Manic clients can be a danger to themselves or others when psychotic. Lithium has a small therapeutic window; lithium levels are monitored to prevent toxicity.

Referrals

Primary care providers can treat depression. If bipolar disorder is suspected initiate treatment and refer to psychiatry for management.

Diagnosis: Anxiety

ICD-10 F41.9: Anxiety disorder, unspecified

Cathleen Crowley-Koschnitzki DNP, CNM, WHNP-BC, FNP-C, PMHNP-BC

Introduction

Anxiety disorders are the most prevalent psychiatric illness, affecting 10-30% of the population. The Diagnostic and Statistical Manual of Mental Disorders (DSM) defines anxiety as anticipation of future threat and differentiates anxiety disorders by thought content and situation.

Pathophysiology

Anxiety occurs in response to a sense of threat, releasing norepinephrine. Norepinephrine increases alertness and can activate the sympathetic nervous system, resulting in the common physical signs of anxiety. Response to the perceived threat also occurs in the limbic system, specifically the amygdala. The amygdala compares the current threat with memories of previous perceived threats to determine the fear response. In perceived threat, the amygdala responds with neurotransmission to the hypothalamus, activating the hypothalamic-pituitary-adrenal (HPA) axis which results in cortisol release.

Physical Assessment

Subjective Data

Clients may report feelings of distress when separating from others (separation anxiety), inability to speak in certain social situations (selective mutism), excessive worry (general anxiety disorder), fear of certain objects, locations or situations (specific phobia), heart racing, sweating, gastrointestinal upset in social situations (social anxiety), inability to leave home or avoidance of certain locations that cause increased worry or fear (agoraphobia). Muscle tension, headaches, sleep disorders, nightmares and difficulty with concentration are also reported.

A through medication history should be included taking note of medications which can mimic anxiety symptoms. Medications which can mimic anxiety include antidepressants, antipsychotics, stimulants, antihypertensive, decongestants, bronchodilators, caffeine, St John's Wort, Yohimbe, and antihistamines. Illicit substances which mimic anxiety can include cocaine, methamphetamine, cannabis, ecstasy, and lysergic acid diethylamide.

Objective Data

Acute discomfort may be noted during the examination, as well as fidgeting, tense body posture and hypervigilance. Affect may be affected; flat affect, irritability, or anger may be present. Speech rate and rhythm may be affected with loud or pressured speech. Notable thought content and processes include obsessive thoughts, perseveration. Impaired concentration, insight and judgement may be noted.

Laboratory/Diagnostics

It is important to rule out physical diagnoses which present with anxiety symptoms and identify substance abuse. The following laboratory testing may be used:

- Urine drug screen- CNS stimulant or cannabis intoxication or withdrawal from CNS depressants (alcohol and barbiturates) are associated with increased anxiety or panic
- TSH, T4- hyperthyroidism and hypothyroidism
- CBC- anemia
- Evaluate for cardiorespiratory disorders such as asthma, chronic lung diseases, arrhythmias, coronary artery disease as appropriate

Pharmacologic Management

Pharmacological treatment is specific to anxiety diagnosis and diagnosis is based on DSM criteria. First line treatment includes selective serotonin reuptake inhibitors (SSRI) and Serotonin-norepinephrine reuptake inhibitors (SNRI) Escitalopram is the best tolerated SSRI with the fewest drug interactions. SSRIs inhibit reuptake of serotonin in the central nervous system which increases available serotonin in the synaptic cleft.

Special Considerations

Not all SSRIs are the same. Each SSRI has additional properties due to specific neurotransmitter targeting. Some SSRIs are better for atypical depression, meaning they treat hypersomnia, low energy, and low mood. These medications can be activating which may increase feelings of anxiety and panic. SSRIs which are better for atypical depression include fluoxetine and sertraline.

Selective mutism and separation anxiety are most common in children.

SSRIs can increase suicidal ideation (SI) in children, adolescents, and young adults. Include this information in education and assess for SI at each follow up visit. Most SSRIs are not associated with birth defects and can be used in early pregnancy. The one exception is Paxil which has been associated with increased incidence malformations including cardiac malformations. SSRIs have been associated with third trimester and neonatal complications such as respiratory distress, transient newborn irritability and increased maternal bleeding at delivery.

Complications

Anxiety can be a complication of a chronic illness such as diabetes, cardiovascular disease, thyroid disorders, and substance abuse Anxiety often occurs comorbidly with depression.

Referrals

Anxiety can be treated successfully in primary care. Referral to mental health may be required for inadequate symptom reduction. Additionally, referral to specialists may be required if physical diagnoses that mimic depression require specialist evaluation.

Diagnosis: Panic disorder

ICD-10 F41.0: Panic disorder (episodic paroxysmal anxiety)

Cathleen Crowley-Koschnitzki DNP, CNM, WHNP-BC, FNP-C, PMHNP-BC

Pathophysiology

Panic etiology is not known. What is known is that persons prone to panic are sensitive to pH alterations in the brain, specially the amygdala.

Physical Assessment

Subjective Data

Clients can report one or more of the follow symptoms: palpitations, sweating, trembling/shaking, shortness of breath, sensation of smothering. Choking sensation, chest discomfort, nausea, feeling dizzy, lightheaded, numbness or tingling, fear of losing control, fear of dying. Client reports persistent worry that another panic attack will occur and/or reports behavioral changes or activity restriction in hopes of avoiding a future panic attack.

Objective Data

Unless examined during a panic attack, there is no objective data. Depending on severity, objective data noted during an attack can include tachycardia, sweating, trembling/shaking, shortness of breath and vomiting.

Laboratory/Diagnostics

Laboratory tests should include testing for physical diagnoses that present with symptoms of panic and identify substance abuse. The following testing may be used:

- Urine drug screen- CNS stimulant or cannabis intoxication or withdrawal from CNS depressants (alcohol and barbiturates) are associated with panic attacks.
- TSH, T4- thyroid disorders can present with similar symptoms
- Evaluate for respiratory disorders such as asthma and chronic lung diseases as appropriate
- Holter monitor if arrhythmia is suspected

Pharmacologic Management

SSRIs (Selective Serotonin Reuptake Inhibitors) are first line treatment for panic disorder. Paroxetine and sertraline are both FDA (Food and Drug Administration) approved for the treatment of panic disorder. SSRIs inhibit reuptake of serotonin in the central nervous system which increases available serotonin in the synaptic cleft.

Benzodiazepines (BZO) are used as adjunct or augmentation to SSRIS and are not first line treatment for panic disorders. SSRIs can take 4 or more weeks to obtain efficacy, BZOs can be used temporarily for immediate symptom relief if necessary, in person's without history of drug dependence. BZO are used for the shortest period of time at the lowest dose for symptom relief. Long term BZ use, four weeks or more, can lead to physical and psychological dependence. Additional caution should be used when considering prescribing BZ) to the elderly due to risk of adverse events.

Special Considerations

Panic attacks can occur as part of any mental health disorder, substance use and certain medical diagnoses such as cardiovascular, respiratory and gastrointestinal disorders. Panic attacks can be differentiated from times of increased anxiety (anxiety attack) by the absence of a trigger, symptom peak within 10 minutes of onset and resolution within 30 minutes.

Panic attacks rarely have full remission and can occur episodically throughout the lifetime. Up to 80% of persons with panic disorder will respond to SSRIs, cognitive behavioral therapy (CBT) or a combination of the two. CBT will reinforce that the symptoms are not fatal and provide coping skills to use in panic episodes relaxation techniques and cognitive restructuring.

Panic disorder is associated with infant low birth weight. Age of onset is typically late adolescence or early adulthood with a median age of 20-24. Panic attacks rarely present for the first time in the elderly. Evaluate for physical cause.

Complications

Panic disorder can lead to agoraphobia due to the fear of embarrassment or loss of control. Severe cases can lead to individuals becoming housebound. Clients are at increased risk for cardiovascular disease. Those with known coronary artery disease can experience a myocardial infarction during a panic attack.

Referrals

Referrals include a therapist for Cognitive Behavioral Therapy. Panic disorder may require referral to specialty practices if further workup is required for physical diagnoses

Diagnosis: Substance Use Disorders

ICD-10 F10-F19: Mental and behavioral disorders due to psychoactive

Patricia D Bailey, PhD, MSN, CNP, CNE, CME

Pathophysiology

Opioid receptors are located within both the central and peripheral nervous system. Opioids activate specific neurotransmitter receptors (mu, kappa, delta) that couple G proteins. G proteins are molecular intermediaries that initiate the intracellular communication process. Activation of endogenous mu opioid receptors results in the prototypic opioid effects of reward, withdrawal, and analgesia. Activation of mu receptors in the central nervous system results in responses such as respiratory depression, analgesia, euphoria, and miosis. Stimulation of peripheral mu opioid receptors, in smooth muscle of the bronchi and intestines, results in cough suppression and opioid-induced constipation.

Physical Assessment

Subjective Data

Clients may report the following symptoms: anxiety, increased cravings, nausea, muscle aches in the lower back and legs, muscle cramps, intestinal cramps, and diarrhea. Opioid use causes irregular periods and erectile dysfunction.

If reported or suspected, a substance history is required. Substance use history should address what substances the patient is currently using or have used in the past, last date of use, dose, frequency of consumption, amount consumed, route of administration, prior opioid treatment history, age at first use, as well as losses as a consequence of use.

Objective Data

Several findings on physical examination should raise the consideration of opioid dependence. Findings include constricted pupils, drowsiness or frequent nodding. Intranasal users may have nasal septal erosion or perforation. Injection drug users often have needle marks or track marks in the antecubital fossae or forearms. Some also inject in other locations, including veins in the neck, legs, groin, and axilla. There are some users who also inject subcutaneously into the upper arm, thigh or buttock.

Early signs and symptoms of withdrawal include anxiety, increased cravings, nausea, muscle aches in the lower back and legs, muscle cramps, intestinal cramps, and diarrhea. Worsening withdrawal acute discomforts can include- rhinorrhea, lacrimation, vomiting, piloerection, or sweating. A dysphoric mood may also be noted. Withdrawal symptoms peak in 12 hours and can last for 3 to 4 days. It typically takes a maximum of 7 days for the withdrawal to run its course.

Laboratory/Diagnostics

If the patient has been using heroin or abusing prescription opioids by snorting or injecting, obtain the following basic labs:

- Urine drug screen- identify substance(s)
- drug use is associated with sexually transmitted and blood borne infections

- HIV
- Hepatitis A, B, and C
- Liver function tests- assess for liver function
- Complete blood count- assess for infection
- Tuberculosis testing- a potential coexisting infection

Pharmacologic Management

Treatment of addiction involves facilitating the initial transition from frequent use of the reinforcer into sobriety by the process known as detoxification. After detoxification, the treatment focus is on maintaining sobriety.

Medications useful for opioid withdrawal discomfort symptoms include clonidine (multiple symptoms including anxiety), prochlorperazine (nausea), loperamide (diarrhea), ibuprofen (aches), and trazodone (insomnia).
Agents used for treatment for ongoing opioid dependence include buprenorphine/naloxone, methadone, and Vivitrol.

With opioids such as buprenorphine (Sublocade, Subutex) and buprenorphine/naloxone (Suboxone, Zubsolv), the patient must be in early withdrawal. Buprenorphine is a partial agonist with high-affinity binding to the mu-opioid receptors. Due to its partial agonist effect, withdrawal symptoms are milder and less uncomfortable for the patient. Once in the body, buprenorphine is broken down by the cytochrome CYP 34A enzymes to an active metabolite (norbuprenorphine). The average half-life of buprenorphine is about 38 hours.

Methadone has been used for decades as maintenance treatment for opioid dependence. Methadone is a full mu-agonist with a long half-life. It has pharmacologic actions similar morphine and is active by oral and parenteral routes of administration. Methadone may mimic endogenous opioids, enkephalins, and endorphins and affect the release of other neurotransmitters—acetylcholine, norepinephrine, and dopamine.

Naltrexone, an opioid, is long acting and available in oral or injectable form. The injectable form of naltrexone is known as Vivitrol. If patients try to use an opioid within four weeks of a Vivitrol injection, they will not feel a high. Naltrexone is only helpful for patients who have discontinued opioid completely and are highly motivated to continue abstinence. Before initial of oral Naltrexone or an injection with Vivitrol, the person must abstain from opioid for at least seven days. Patients should carry ID card or bracelet to alert medical personnel in emergency.

Naltrexone is an opioid antagonist with high affinity for the mu opioid receptor. Naltrexone competes and binds to opiate receptors. If binds successfully, naltrexone displaces opioid drugs from these receptors thereby antagonizing most of the effects of opiates, including respiratory depression, miosis, euphoria, and drug craving.

Sobriety Maintenance

The medications discussed below will focus on options that can be used to maintain sobriety after the detoxification of other important substance use disorders including alcohol.

Alcohol Use Disorder

Alcohol use disorder is potentially deadly. Inpatient detoxification initially or if patient has a history of prior complicated withdrawals. Once the patient is detoxified off alcohol, the following medication assisted treatments can be considered:

- Acamprosate acts by opposing glutamate. Contraindicated in CrCl < 30ml/min; No hepatic adjustment needed. Should be initiated after withdrawal when abstinence has been achieved; Diarrhea most common side effect; monitor for depression and suicidality. Other side effects include syncope, palpitations, edema, insomnia, anxiety, depression, weakness, nausea, vomiting, and constipation.
- Disulfiram introduces an element of positive punishment to drinking by making the person fell sick if takes a drink while on this medication (blocks metabolism of ethanol). No renal adjustment needed. However, use cause with hepatic cirrhosis of insufficiency; Can cause severe Disulfiram-Alcohol reaction (flushing, nausea, hypotension). This medication is contraindicated in severe myocardial disease, coronary occlusion, psychosis, EtOH use or Metronidazole use. The patient will need to be abstinent from alcohol or

alcohol containing products (cough syrup, mouthwash, cologne) for > 12 hours. A metallic taste is a common side effect. Monitor for hepatotoxicity. Possible side effects include drowsiness, headache, fatigue, psychosis, rash, dermatitis, metallic aftertaste, impotence, hepatitis, polyneuritis, peripheral neuropathy, and optic neuritis.

- Naltrexone (Vivitrol) blocks the ability of alcohol to activate opioid receptors which reduces the pleasurable sensation the individual gets from drinking. Available in tablet form or a monthly intramuscular (IM injection). Contraindicated in opiate use or positive urine drug screen; must be opioid free for 7 days minimally. Monitor for signs and symptoms of depression, suicidality, and hepatotoxicity. Patients should carry an ID card or bracelet to alert medical personnel in emergency. Common side effects include nausea, vomiting, decreased appetite, dizziness, dysphoria, anxiety, insomnia, nervousness, headache, low energy. Abdominal cramping, and arthralgia. With IM injection, common side effects include injection site reactions-pain, tenderness, pruritis, induration, swelling, erythema, or bruising.

Nicotine/Tobacco Use Disorder

Nicotine and tobacco are considered the most addictive substances. No impatient detoxification needed. Effective treatment strategies include nicotine replacement therapy (patches, gums, and lozenges); nicotinic receptor partial agonist (varenicline), the antidepressant bupropion. Smoking cessation can be a long process with multiple attempts before complete cessation is achieved. For this reason, psychosocial treatments are also helpful in providing support in teaching the individual how to cope effectively with cravings.

- Nicotine Products (gum, patch, lozenges, actuation nasal spray) must be used as directed; no more than 24 pieces of gum per day and no more than 20 lozenges per 24 hours. Renal or hepatic adjustment is needed. Possible side effects with gum or lozenge include tachycardia, headache, nausea, vomiting, dyspepsia, acid reflux, excessive salivation, belching, increased appetite, mouth/throat soreness, jaw muscle ache, and hiccups. Possible side effects with patch include insomnia, abnormal dreams, pruritis, cough and pharyngitis (Rastegar & Fingerhood, 2015; Stahl, 2017).
- Varenicline (Chantix) is a partial agonist at alpha4-beta2 ($\alpha 4\beta 2$) neuronal nicotinic acetylcholine receptors (nAChRs). Produces modest levels of mesolimbic dopamine thus reducing or diminishing nicotine cravings and withdrawal symptoms. Additional benefit of occupying nicotine receptors sites therefore reducing reward of nicotine upon patient relapse of nicotine use. Possible side effects include nausea, vomiting, constipation, weight gain, insomnia, abnormal dreams, headache (Rastegar & Fingerhood, 2015; Stahl, 2017).
- Bupropion (Zyban) is an antidepressant. Common adverse effects include agitation, dry mouth, insomnia, headache, nausea, constipation, weight loss or gain, tremor, hypertension (Stahl, 2017).

- Hallucinogens are a group of agents that act at serotonin synapses in the reward system. D-lysergic acid diethylamide (LSD), psilocybin (mushrooms, shrooms), dimethyltryptamine (DMT); mescaline (peyote), 2,5-dimethoxy-4-methylamphetamine (DOM); mescaline, 3,4-methylenedioxymethamphetamine (MDMA) and '*Foxy*' (5-methoxy-diisopropyltryptamine). Treatment options include cognitive behavioral therapy and motivational interviewing therapy. Since these substances can produce a psychotic state, an antianxiety or antipsychotic medication may be needed to decrease agitation and stabilize blood pressure (Rastegar & Fingerhood, 2015; Miller, 2018; Stahl, 2017).

Cannabis Use Disorder

There is no specific pharmacological treatment for cannabis use disorder. Nonpharmacological treatment options include cognitive behavioral therapy and motivational interviewing therapy. N-Acetylcysteine (NAC) is an over the counter prodrug that has been tested in adolescents for cannabis cessation. If withdrawal from cannabis induces a state of anxiety or psychosis, an antianxiety or antipsychotic medication may be administered to control symptoms

Special Considerations

Screening, counseling and medication assisted treatment (MAT) appears to be modestly effective in reducing subsequent drug use. Clients within MAT develop tolerance and physical dependence following repeated use. In addition, there is a high potential for abuse and drug diversion. Close observation is required in the first few hours after initiation of any long-term treatment. Pregnant women being treated for opioid addiction should be treated with methadone or monotherapy buprenorphine (Subutex). Always work closely with the OB/GYN provider and consider their recommendations as part of the overall treatment program. Treatment with monotherapy buprenorphine (Subutex) is an option for pregnant women to avoid naltrexone exposure.

Detoxification with Buprenorphine followed by drug-free therapy or naltrexone is the treatment of choice for adolescents because of their short addiction histories. If opioid maintenance is needed after detoxification, Naltrexone is a valuable therapeutic adjunct after detoxification. Geriatric clients typically have reduced metabolism and absorption rates. Caution should be exercised during buprenorphine induction due metabolism, absorption, body composition and the possibility of medication interactions.

Complications

A heart murmur may indicate subacute bacterial endocarditis. Hepatic enlargement may indicate acute hepatitis whereas a small, hard liver may indicate chronic hepatitis B or C virus. Clients develop a physical dependence to MAT medications and should not be discontinued abruptly. Medications should be continued in an inpatient setting if the client is hospitalized for any reason.

Referrals

Referral to an addiction specialist may be necessary for the treatment of addiction disorders requires specialized training. Only specially trained providers should treat opioid addiction disorders. Intensive detox is needed for patients with more severe addictions and those with comorbid medical or psychiatric disorder. Pregnant women presenting for treatment of opioid addiction may need to be referred to specialized services in methadone maintenance treatment programs.

Diagnosis: Sleep and Sleep Disorders

ICD 10 G47.9 Sleep disorder, unspecified

Kelly Holben, DNP, APRN, FNP-BC, PMHNP-BC

Pathophysiology

The neurobiology of sleep occurs in the hypothalamus-pituitary-adrenal (HPA) axis, cortex, cerebrum, sympathetic nervous system, and amygdala. The circadian rhythm is stamped on the hypothalamus-pituitary-adrenal (HPA) axis, and the lowest concentration is near midnight or nadir, cortisone levels will start to increase approximately 2-3 hours after the start of sleep and continue to increase into the waking hours with a peak around 0900, the decrease in cortisol will be potentiated by sleep and the cycle starts over.

Sleep-wake cycle changes occur in response to increased and sustained stress. An increase in stress hormones in response to stress affects the genes and neuroplasticity. This neurobiological change from stress can be permanent.

Stress and the disruption of sleep will cause a rise in a patient's hemoglobin A1C (HbA1C). Diabetes can worsen depression, thus further interrupting sleep. For those that do not have diabetes, the elevated HbA1C can lead to misdiagnosis.

OSA is most often associated with obesity, or anatomical factors such large neck size, enlarged tonsils and adenoids or the tongue which blocks the airway. Central sleep apnea can result from hypoxia and lowered PaCO2. There are multiple etiologies for the loss of drive to breathe during sleep.

Physical Assessment

Subjective Data

When assessing for sleep disorders, a comprehensive history and physical examination is indicated. The patient may have reports of difficulty falling asleep or staying asleep. Sleep interruptions can vary, some root causes include worry, frequent urination, or snoring. Partner may report the patient stops breathing or struggles for air at times while sleeping. Patient may report waking up gasping during the night and not sure why. Daytime sleepiness or headache when waking. Client may report that involuntary legs movements keep them awake.

The history may help to identify the cause, such as shift work, the use of alcohol or illicit substance use. Medications can contribute to sleep disorders; a complete medication is necessary.

Objective Data

Increases in weight, BMI or waist circumference may indicate obesity, a contributing factor of OSA. There may be infraorbital darkening, mouth breathing, nasal atrophy, septal deviation, turbinate hypertrophy, collapsing of nasal alae on inspiration, a contributing factor of OSA; enlarged tonsils can contribute to obstruction.

Laboratory/Diagnostics

A complete blood count (CBC) can be used to assess for secondary polycythemia, a marker of low oxygen levels and a contributing factor of OSA. Thyroid function panel can identify hyperthyroidism, which affects sleep. A urine drug screen can identify if illicit substances are associated with insomnia

Sleep study options include nocturnal polysomnography. The multiple sleep latency test (MSLT) is used for hypersomnia. Actigraphy is a noninvasive watch like device used to assess circadian rhythm. The maintenance of wakefulness test (MWT) is also used in the evaluation of hypersomnia giving and the objective information on the ability of the patient to stay awake (Shelgikar, & Chervin, 2013).

The following objective tools can assist with assessing sleep disorder presence and severity. National Sleep Foundation's Sleepiness Test, Pediatric Sleep Questionnaire (PSQ), Pittsburg Sleep Quality questionnaire (PSQI) Insomnia Severity Index, Epworth Sleepiness Scale, STOP BANG Screening Questionnaire for OSA, and the National Sleep Foundation's Sleep Diary

Depression and anxiety- the PHQ9 and the GAD 7 can identify mental help issues contributing to sleep disorders.

Pharmacologic Management

Cognitive behavioral therapy is considered the first-line treatment for insomnia. Melatonin, 3-5 milligrams by mouth at bedtime may induce sleep by binding to the melatonin MT1 and MT2 receptors.

Benzodiazepines are not recommended for treatment of sleep disorders. If used, short term duration is recommended due to known physical dependence. Benzodiazepines should not be used in the elderly, pregnancy, or those with OSA and COPD.

Special Considerations

Elderly are at an elevated risk of adverse effects from sedation, agitation, wandering, balance issues, and impaired ability to do activities of daily living such as driving due to age related metabolism changes. With pregnant patients, it is important to determine the cause of insomnia prior to initiating treatment. Benzodiazepines are not indicated for insomnia due to risk for mother and fetus.

For pediatric patients, the first line recommendation is to treat any underlying psychological cause (anxiety) or medical cause (OSA) with therapy. Antihistamines diphenhydramine and hydroxyzine are FDA approved for short term use.

Complications

Screening for alcohol use is indicated prior to starting benzodiazepines or the z-drugs. OSA-Adverse reactions are varied depending on the drug of choice.

Referrals

Referral to an eye, ear, nose, and throat (EENT) specialist may be needed for evaluation of structural obstruction such as deviated nasal septum or tonsillar hypertrophy. A bariatric specialist can assist with weight loss if the BMI and neck circumference are contributing factors for OSA. Additionally, a psychiatric specialist can treat depression, anxiety or prescribe antipsychotics or long-term benzodiazepines for sleep.

Chapter 15: Obesity

Diagnosis: Obesity

ICD-10 E66.9: Obesity, unspecified

ICD-10 E66.01: Morbid obesity

Angela Golden DNP, FNP-C, FAANP

Pathophysiology

An overview of the pathophysiology of obesity as we know it today is presented here. Obesity is a neuroendocrine disorder. The pathophysiology is an intertwining of genetic, inflammatory, endocrinologic, and neurologic components. Genetics determines the persons capacity for fat mass, but the environment is the key that "turns on" the genetic possibility. There are two separate interconnected processes that are the core of obesity, an increase in amount of adiposity and the biological defense of the increased adiposity. Adipocyte tissue increases through hypertrophy and hyperplasia. Hypertrophy occurs first and when an area has become saturated with triglycerides then hyperplasia occurs. The next step after hypertrophy and hyperplasia is the ectopic fat deposition in organs like liver, muscles, kidneys and in the heart. Additionally, as adipocytes remodel and enlarge there is an increase in macrophages and other immune cells. The immune cells secrete cytokines that create a low-grade inflammation. Sick adipose tissue also secretes inflammatory factors leading to insulin and leptin resistance.

Endocrine Disease

Demonstrating the endocrine nature of the disease of obesity is shown through the metabolic dysfunction. This includes over or underproduction of adipokines and cytokines, impairments in hormonal conversion, or the bodies abnormal response to hormones.

There are many hormones involved in energy homeostasis, one hunger hormone, ghrelin, and numerous hormones for satiety with leptin leading the pack. Obesity then is a disease with the hormonal homeostatic system of energy metabolism broken.

Leptin is the hormone that signals satiety. It also modulates the function of the HPA axis and the systemic sympathetic/adrenomedullary system. Adipocytes are the major source of leptin. The feedback mechanism demonstrates the endocrine function of obesity. When there is excess energy, leptin triggers a release of melanocortin. This in turn goes on to activate melanocortin-4-receptor (MC4R), a protein encoded by the MC4R gene. MC4R suppresses food intake and stimulates energy expenditure. At the same time leptin suppresses AgRP/NPY which are suppressers of MC4R.

Figure X: Insulin response

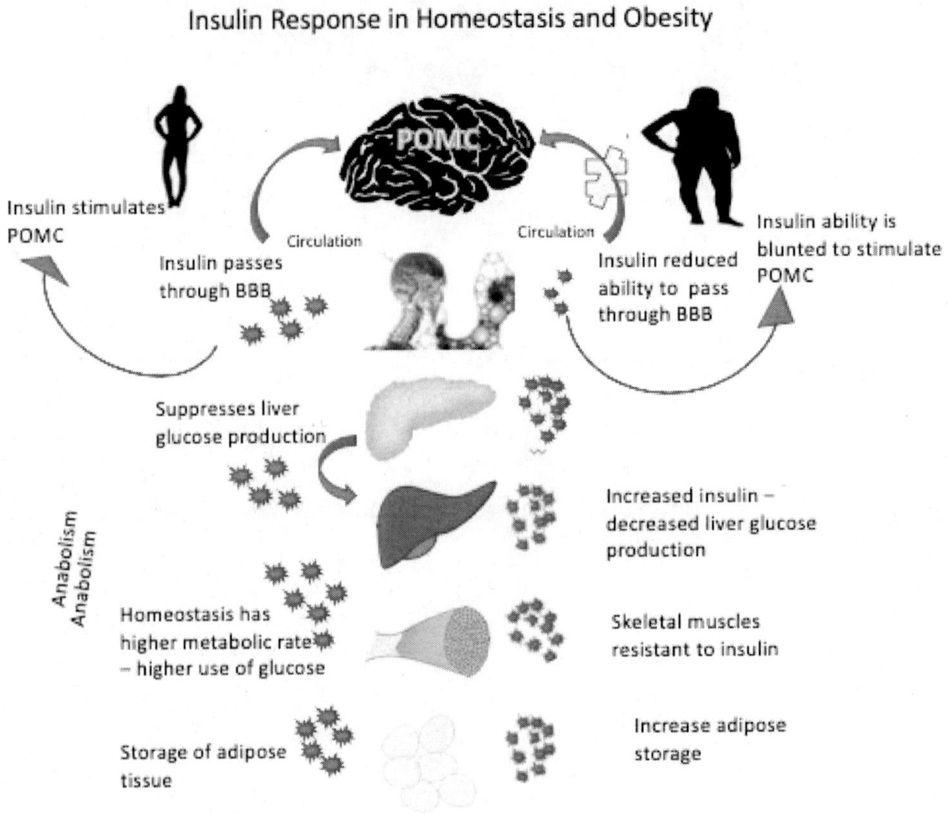

Insulins plays a role in obesity. In adipose tissue insulin promotes the uptake of fatty acids and the conversion to store triglycerides. This promotes a buildup of stored energy. Obesity is known to be a primary primary cause of insulin resistance (likely due to the proinflammatory aspect of obesity). In patients with visceral adiposity, higher concentrations of basal insulin are found and there is a higher secretion of insulin in response to a standard meal.

A change in insulin clearance occurs in the liver due to the increased concentration of free fatty acids from adipose tissue (see figure insulin response in homeostasis and obesity).

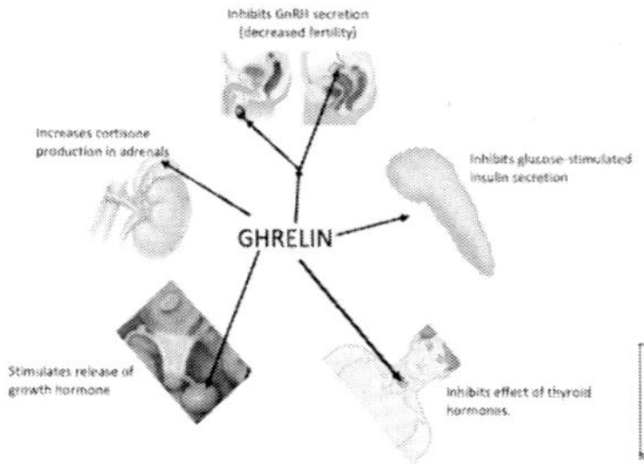

Figure X: Ghrelin impact

Ghrelin is the only known circulating hormone with strong orexigenic activity. Ghrelin is produced by the stomach and is a signal for eating. Its receptors are widespread almost everywhere in the body, but specifically in the hypothalamus and many endocrine organs including hypothalamus, pituitary, thyroid, parathyroid, pancreas, adrenal glands, placenta, and male and female gonads (see Figure Ghrelin impact). Ghrelin regulates multiple aspects of eating including food reward, stress induced feeding, motivation, and with learning and memory responses associated with eating.

Table 15.1: Additional Hormones Impacting Hunger and Homeostasis of Energy

Other Hormones	
ASP	• Stimulates glucose uptake, inhibits lipase, increases efficiency of triglyceride storage and synthesis
Amylin	• Plays a role in both acute satiation and long-term control of eating. The effect of amylin is centrally mediated in the hindbrain.
Adiponectin	• Primarily produced by adipose tissue with receptors in the liver and muscle. • Helps regulate insulin sensitivity and oxidation of fatty acids • Suppresses hepatic glucose production • Stimulates thermogenesis impacting weight homeostasis. Powerful anti-inflammatory agent and has antifibrotic actions in the liver

Table 15.2: Peptides Impacting Hunger and Homeostasis of Energy

Peptides - Peptides are derived from CART and POMC and are expressed in central and peripheral neurons that work on eating behaviors.	• CART is coexpressed with POMC in arcuate nucleus and is linked to satiety. These are stimulated by leptin
CART – cocaine and amphetamine regulated transcript	• Occurs with food consumption, inhibits food intake, role in reward mechanism of food
POMC - proopiomelanocortin	• Precursor to melanocortin. Occurs with food consumption, inhibits food intake, role in reward mechanism of food
Orexins	• Impact satiety thru the vagal receptors. • Have been found in the intestines, pancreas, adrenal glands, reproductive system and adipose tissue. • Found in many endocrine tissues including pituitary, thyroid, parathyroid, adrenals, testes, ovaries, and the pancreatic islets. Central orexins are found originating in the medulla with an impact on the HPA and affecting the SNS. • Impact hypothalamus for sleep and energy homeostasis beyond the impact on eating.
Neuropeptide Y (NPY)	• Found in the brain • Strong control of eating in the hypothalamus Encouraging an increase in food intake while decreasing energy expenditure by reducing thermogenesis • Also a mediator for food rewards.
Peptide YY (PYY)	• Secreted by the distal gut in response to a protein rich meal. Slows gastric emptying and reduces secretions from the pancreas and gallbladder. • Satiety peptide.

	• In obesity PYY secretion is blunted creating a reduced feeling of satiety.
Adrenomedullin	• Expressed in gastrointestinal tissues including liver, pancreas, stomach, duodenum, small intestines, colon, and pancreas. Inhibits gastric and intestinal emptying. • Stabilizes that gut barrier. • Satiety
Cholecystokinin	• Considered a brain/gut peptide • Found in intestinal endocrine cells and neurons • Regulates gastric acid secretion, gastric emptying, gallbladder contraction, and exocrine pancreatic secretion • Important in the communication of food intake
GLP-1	• Produced in the small intestine and a small set of neurons in the hindbrain • Inhibits eating • Peripherally receptors found in the pancreatic islets and the entire G.I. tract. • Centrally receptors are found in hypothalamus, amygdala, and in mesolimbic reward system allowing for the control of food intake and the regulation of energy balance.

Brain Disease

The brain is integral in the homeostatic system of energy. With obesity there is a chronic inflammation of the hypothalamic– pituitary– adrenal axis and increased glucocorticoid exposure.

leptin association to CNS
Creative commons
https://www.researchgate.net/publication/303707219_Rare_Genetic_Forms_of_Obesity_Clinical_Approach_and_Current_Treatments_in_2016/figures?lo=1

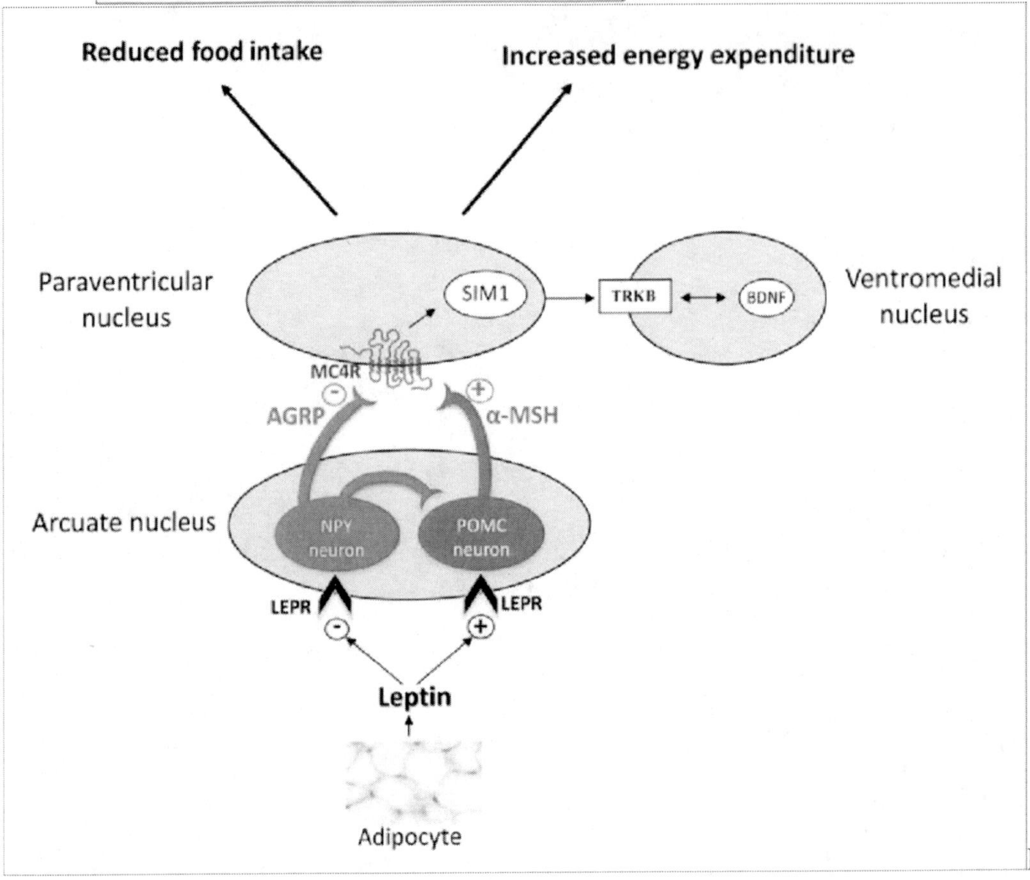

Leptin, ghrelin, and natriuretic peptide roles in the brain are reviewed. Leptin plays a role in reward and motivation. It does this by acting on dopaminergic neurons in the ventral tegmental area (a region of the brain involved in reward and motivation) to influence eating behavior. In obesity the ability of leptin to decrease food intake is impaired due to a central leptin resistance.

The arcuate nucleus in the hypothalamus uses neuropeptides to control energy balance. This balance is central and peripheral. Patients with obesity have lower levels of natriuretic peptides. The natriuretic peptides mediate endocrine and behavioral response to stress.

Ghrelin crosses the blood brain barrier and impacts the arcuate nucleus in the hypothalamus as well as the hippocampus, dorsal nucleus of the raphe, ventral tegmental area, nucleus accumbens, amygdala, prefrontal cortex nucleus and the olfactory bulb impacting the control of feeding.

This review of pathophysiology provides an overview of the biological basis of obesity – far from the myth of willpower.

Physical Assessment

Subjective Data

Weight history

- History of weight gain and loss overtime (see weight history figure)
- Details of previous weight loss attempts including previous anti

Obesity medications or over the counter substances

- Current eating habits – ask about any food sensitivities or allergies
- Current physical activity
- Current medications to identify any obesogenic medications that may need changed or medications that would interact with anti-obesity medications
- Current medical problems – evaluating for obesity related complications or comorbidities (for staging of disease as well as assistance with medication selection) that treating obesity could impact
- Alcohol and illicit drug use – alcohol use can impact medication choices

- Smoking history – recent cessation can add to weight gain

Past Medical History (PMH)

- History of stroke, cardiovascular disease, arteriosclerosis, valvular heart disease, uncontrolled hypertension, glaucoma, hyperthyroidism, seizures, renal disease, pulmonary hypertension, and/or pancreatitis. Each of these can assist in choosing medication management if that becomes part of the treatment plan (which it does in 80-90% of my patients).

Family History

- Overweight or obesity
- Family history of medullary thyroid cancer

Objective Data

- Vital Signs
    - Patient is identified as being at risk for obesity based on BMI $\geq$25kg/m^2/Asian $\geq$ 23 kg/m^2 (assure height was measure in stocking feet – not stated)

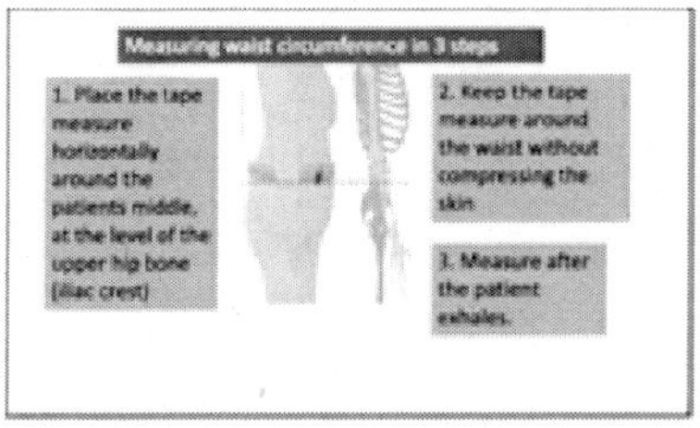

Measure waist circumference for patients with BMI 25- 35 kg/m^2 to help identify visceral adiposity (known to carry the highest risk of cardiometabolic disease)

- High-risk for cardiometabolic abnormalities: >88 cm/35 inches in women and >102 cm/40 inches in men (Asian females, waist circumference >80 cm (31.5 inches) and in Asian males a value >90 cm (35.4 inches)

Table 15.3: Physical Findings in Obesity

Physical exam specific to obesity	Finding	Indicates possibility of:
Skin	rashes in skin folds	Possible fungal infections
	hirsutism in women	Excess testosterone or possible PCOS
	Acanthosis nigricans	Insulin resistance
Cardiovascular	Irregular heart rate	Arrhythmias like a fib
	PMI shifted	Cardiomegaly
	Peripheral edema or varicosities	
Respiratory	Decreased diaphragmatic excursion	Respiratory insufficiency
Abdomen	Enlarged liver measurement	NALFD possibility
	Striae	Excess cortisol
Extremities	Peripheral edema or varicosities	CHF, PVD
	Joint deformities	Pressure alterations, arthritis
General	Lipodystrophic fat distribution	Insulin resistant

Screening tools

- PHQ9 – evaluate for depression since many AOMs can have an impact and is a comorbidity – presence of either worsens the other
- BED-7 – evaluations for binge eating, 30% of patients with obesity have BED as well and will require treatment for this psychiatric disorder with obesity

treatment. At this time assess for eating disorders screening for purging behaviors

- STOP BANG – screening for sleep apnea a comorbidity with obesity, they each worsen the other, and PARQ.

Table 15.4: Laboratory and Diagnostic Tests to Assess for Obesity

Laboratory	Assessing
Complete blood cell count	R/O anemia, complications of bariatric surgery, etc.
Comprehensive metabolic panel (electrolytes, renal and liver function tests, glucose)	important to have baseline values and evaluate kidneys and liver with obesity
Thyroid function tests	Hypothyroidism
Fasting lipid profile	dyslipidemia or metabolic syndrome may be present
Urinalysis	evaluate for obesity related glomerulopathy
Uric acid	underlying hyperuricemia may be present (hyperinsulinemia and diuretics increase risk for increased uric acid and gout)
Vitamin D	Frequently occurs with obesity due to Vitamin D in adipose tissue
Other vitamin and minerals levels	If bariatric surgery to look for deficiency
hemoglobin A1c, glucose tolerance test, serum insulin, c-peptide, urine for microalbumin	further testing for metabolic dysfunction (insulin resistance, prediabetes, diabetes)
cortisol testing	If suspect Cushing's syndrome
hormonal testing	if hypogonadism is suspected

Diagnostics (majority based on evaluating for obesity related complications)

- Body Composition
- Electrocardiogram
- Sleep study
- Imaging studies of the liver
- Coronary calcium score
- Echocardiogram, cardiac stress test
- Ankle-brachial index
- Brain MRI: If a structural lesion of the pituitary/hypothalamus is suspected (e.g., craniopharyngioma, pituitary tumor, etc.)

Management

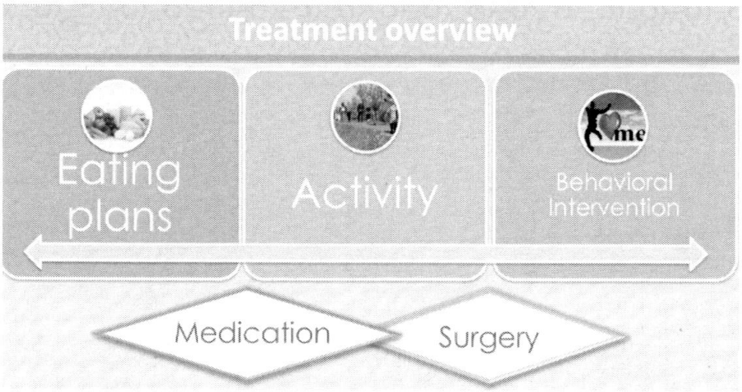

Food is a primary treatment modality. Most obesity experts consider it the first component or pillar of treatment. One thing to keep in mind is that the vast majority of our patients have "dieted" so many times in their lives and they don't want to diet again. That is good and you can use that to your advantage as you talk about long term treatment for long term success.

Eating Plans

No observable differences among the four diets Atkins, Ornish, Weight Watchers, and Zone diets. Studies have found that some patients gained, and some patients lost on each of the eating plans.

Assessment

Prior to starting changes or decisions on eating an assessment needs to be completed. There are several ways to do an assessment of eating habits. A 24-hour diet recall, 3-day diary, or tracking in an app.

Guiding principles for starting nutrition as therapy in the management of obesity:

- Minimize intake of highly processed foods
- Encourage consumption of whole foods
- Encourage consumption of high-fiber, complex, carbohydrates
- Emphasize reading labels
- Beware marketing claims

Table 15.5: Eating Plan

Eating plan overview		
Plan	Requirements	Benefits
Low Fat	15-20% fat intake	Weight loss Improved metabolic markers Improved BP Reduce all cause premature mortality
Low Carbohydrate	20-60 g of carbohydrates depending on plan Protein between 1.2-1.6g/kg/day	Weight loss Improved metabolic markers Improved insulin sensitivity Decreased triglycerides
Mediterranean	Whole food Point program over a week based on none specific dietary components	Improvement in existing heart disease Anti-inflammatory Protection against neurocognitive decline Decrease in all cause of death
Whole Food Plant Based	Plant-Based foods with minimal processing, high in fiber Avoid animal products Avoid highly refined grains, processed foods, added sugars and oils	Improved metabolic markers Improved BP Reduction in all-cause mortality Decrease in visceral adipose tissue
Fasting	Varies from concentrated timed feeding (8 hours eating, 16 hours fasting) up to 72 hours of fasting. May also be 25% of	Decreased inflammation Decreased visceral adipose tissue Improved BP and metabolic and lipid profile

	caloric needs on several days a week	
LCD/VLCD	Primarily meal replacement plans Calories vary from 800-1600 calories a day	Helpful for patients with difficulty in making food choices by removing those choices Assist in learning serving and portion control Short term weight loss

PRACTICE PEARLS FOR EATING:

- Determine patients current eating to assess patterns
- DON'T assume a patient with obesity is eating substantial number of calories
- Used shared decision making to make modifiable changes or an eating plan
- Patient ability to adhere to a plan long term is the most critical

Physical Activity

The second foundational component is physical activity. Activity alone is unlikely to treat obesity, however it has significant impact on the maintenance of successful long-term treatment. It is started early in treatment to make it an underpinning of the patient's treatment plan for life.

Moving into the activity component it is important to understand that although physical activity may not be integral to the active phase of obesity treatment it has been shown to have many benefits. It increases metabolic health, supports maintenance of weight loss, improves body composition, and improves insulin sensitivity to name just a few of the benefits.

Assessment:

Before recommending any activity there needs to be an assessment completed. Starting with the patient's current physical activity. This is done by taking a history of work and leisure activity (see table activity level examples).

Table 15.6: Activity Levels

Activity level examples		
Activity level	Leisure	Work
Very light	Watching TV, reading books	sitting at a computer or desk most of the day
Light activity	walking or non-strenuous cycling or gardening once a week	sales or office work that comprises light activities – minimal walking or lifting
Moderate activity is,	walking, bicycling, or gardening more than once a week like	Cleaning, kitchen staff, delivering mail on foot or by bicycle.
Heavy or active activity	intense walking, bicycling or sports several times a week	heavy industrial work, construction work or farming

Before prescribing an activity plan consider the screening tool PARQ-7 (http://eparmedx.com/wpcontent/uploads/2013/03/PARQPlus2019ImageVersion2.pdf) to see if the patient needs further evaluations like from cardiology or orthopedics before any prescription for activity. The PARQ7 screening tool is looking for symptoms of heart disease or musculoskeletal issues that would impact the patient's ability to safely increase activity from the baseline. A yes answer to any question may lead to further evaluation. A no to all seven PARQ7 questions likely tells you that your patient is cleared for low to moderate physical activity such as walking.

It's also important to assess mobility, balance, and gait. People with preobesity/overweight or obesity could have compromised mobility, and this could create an increase in the risk of injury.

Patients with diminished mobility may benefit from physical therapy evaluation as part of the treatment team. This professional can then guide activity options such as chair-based activities, pool-based exercises or classes designed for people with arthritis. [Author's note: Be sure that person understands obesity as a disease so that the patient is not going into a practice that could be biased or shaming in any way.]

Table 15.7: F.I.T.T.E. Exercise Prescription

F.I.T.T.E exercise prescription (ACSM)	
Frequency	number of activity sessions for a given time – the idea is to work up to 3-5 times a week
Intensity	Level the activity places on the body – this is often done through HR or ability to speak - moderate intensity is preferred – increased HR but without breathlessness
Time	Number or minutes engaged in activity – first goal is to work up to 30 minutes a day: This could be 6-5-minute engagement, 3-10 minutes engagement, or 2 - 15 minutes engagements.
Type	mode or activity used – any activity can be used – stairs versus elevators, parking further from a door, dancing, gardening
Enjoyment	Deriving pleasure from the activity

Practice Pearls

- Assessing patient's physical ability and safety is the 1st step
- Next assess baseline of activity, increase slowly with the goal of long term being 200-300 minutes a week.

- Write the physical activity as a prescription for the patient using F.I.T.T.E.
- In my clinical practice I generally start with simple step counting. Most everyone can afford a pedometer, or their phone can track steps. If they don't have a safe place or they have inclement weather many malls allow walkers and often there are places at their work sites they can walk.
- Increase physical activity through shared decision making so that it is ENJOYABLE, and the patient will have a greater chance of sticking with the plan. Listening to a book may make a walk enjoyable for someone that doesn't like walking – local libraries have online audible books so there would be no cost.

Behavior Intervention

This component of obesity treatment links with eating and activity. It is really the cornerstone of treatment where we are making the difference in long term effective treatment. This is critical to helping patients recognize roadblocks and how to go around, over or under them to keep them moving towards their goals.

What is Behavioral Intervention?

It is education, goal setting, evaluation of successes and any difficulties. The primary goal is to do problem solving for any setbacks or struggles since the last visit. It is often referred to as Intensive Behavior Therapy (IBT) or Intensive Lifestyle Intervention (ILI). Three programs that provide evidence this can be accomplished in primary care are the Look Ahead trial,

Diabetes Prevention Program and Canadian Obesity Network. All three of these demonstrate frequent follow up for the IBT using the 5As: Ask, Assess, Advise, Agree, Assist (Arrange FU). SMART goals are an easy way to assist patients in being accountable. SMART goals are specific, measurable, attainable, realistic, and timely.

Table 15.8: Behavioral Interventions

Common Components to begin	
1	Education about obesity and overview of EB plan
2	Self- monitoring
3	Eating plan selection
4	Activity prescription
5	Goals of treatment and Why patient is getting treating 5-10% weight loss to start Quality of life indicator of success

Pharmacologic management

First line treatment:

Table 15.9: FDA-Approved Short-Term (Anti) Obesity Therapies

Generic Drug*	Dose	Contraindications	Side Effects
phentermine	8mg-37.5mg	Anxiety disorder, CVD, hypertension,	Insomnia, palpitations,

diethylpropion	25 mg or 75 mg, SR	MAO inhibitors, glaucoma, hyperthyroidism, seizures, pregnancy/ breastfeeding, drug abuse history	tachycardia, dry mouth, taste alterations, dizziness, tremors, headache, diarrhea, constipation, vomiting, gastrointestinal distress, anxiety, restlessness, increased blood pressure
phendimetrazine	17.5-70 mg or 105 mg, SR		
benzphetamine	25-50 mg		

Table 15.10: FDA-Approved (Anti) Obesity Therapies

Generic Drug (alphabetically)	Mechanism of Action	Dosage	Side Effects/Cautions
liraglutide (subcutaneous injection)	GLP-1 receptor agonist	Initiate at 0.6 mg/day SQ for 1 week; increase in weekly intervals until 3-mg dose is reached	**Drug interactions:** delays gastric emptying so may impact concurrent oral medications **Adverse effects:** nausea, hypoglycemia, diarrhea, constipation, vomiting, headache, decreased appetite, dyspepsia, fatigue, dizziness, abdominal pain, increased lipase **Contraindications:** personal or family history of medullary thyroid carcinoma, multiple endocrine neoplasia syndrome type 2 (MENS 2), pregnancy, gastroparesis
naltrexone/bupropion ER (oral)	Opioid receptor antagonist; dopamine and noradrenaline reuptake inhibitor	8 mg/90 mg, 1 tab PO once daily am; titrating to max of 2 tabs PO once daily am and 1 tab PO	**Monitoring:** Cr at baseline, BP, HR, depression/suicide risk **Drug interactions:** opioid analgesics, interaction with CYP2D6 metabolized medications; beware drugs

		once daily pm	that lower seizure threshold **Adverse effects:** nausea, constipation, headache, vomiting, dizziness, insomnia, dry mouth, and diarrhea **Contraindications:** within 14 days of MAO inhibitor dose, uncontrolled hypertension, seizure disorders, eating disorders, chronic opioid use, pregnancy
orlistat (oral)	Pancreatic lipase inhibitor—impairs gastrointestinal energy absorption, causing excretion of approximately 30% of ingested triglycerides in stool	Prescription: 120 mg PO TID OTC: 60 mg PO daily	**Drug interactions:** may decrease absorption of fat-soluble vitamins **Adverse effects:** oily and frequent bowel movements; bowel urgency; fecal incontinence; flatus; increased risk for cholelithiasis and urinary oxalate (rare); post marketing reports of liver injury
phentermine/ topiramate-ER (oral) DEA Schedule IV	Noradrenergic + GABA-receptor activator, kainite/AMPA glutamate receptor inhibitor causing appetite suppression	3.75 mg/23 mg PO starting dose; titrate to 7.5 mg/46 mg, 11.25 mg/69 mg; maximum dose 15 mg/92 mg	**Monitoring:** depression, hypokalemia, CV evaluation at baseline; consider ECHO **Drug interactions:** may potentiate CNS depressants and hypokalemia of non-potassium-sparing diuretics **Adverse effects:** paresthesias, constipation, dysgeusia, insomnia, dizziness, HA, nausea, back pain, fatigue, diarrhea, blurred vision, anxiety, alopecia,

			hypesthesia, irritability, attention disturbance, GERD, tachycardia, metabolic acidosis, nephrolithiasis

NOTE: February 13, 2020 the FDA requested Eisai withdraw lorcaserin from the market due to a concern related to possible cancer increase. The CAMILLA-TIMI study had 12,000 patients and was a cardiovascular outcome trial, not a cancer risk study. The study demonstrated no increase in cardiovascular risk and a reduction in risk of diabetes. The New England Journal of Medicine article reported no difference in cancer risk. The three years of data demonstrated lorcaserin with a 3.59% cancer incidence and 3.50% cancer incidence in placebo. The FDA reported a 7.7% increase in individuals receiving lorcaserin and 7.1% with placebo. There was no hearing and no publication from the FDA. *https://www.fda.gov/drugs/drug-safety-and-availability/fda-requests-withdrawal-weight-loss-drug-belviq-belviq-xr-lorcaserin-market*

Table 15.11: Long-Term Efficacy for Anti-Obesity Medications

Therapy (alphabetically)	Length of Trial	Total Weight Loss	Mean Weight Loss
liraglutide*	≥1 year	-8.4kg	-8.0%
naltrexone/bupropion	≥1 year	-6.1 kg	-5.4%
orlistat	≥1 year	-5.3 kg	-6.1%
phentermine/topiramate	≥1 year	-10.2 kg	- 9.8%

SURGERY and Devices

The guidelines for the use of surgery or devices are in the following patients

- BMI < 40 kg/m2
    - If any case, providing surgical risk acceptable
- BMI < 35 kg/m2
    - If there is > 1 obesity-related disease
- BMI between 30 and 34.9 kg/m2
    - For Type 2 diabetes and/or Metabolic syndrome
- Inability to achieve a healthy weight loss sustained for a period of time with prior weight loss efforts

Bariatric surgery works though a change in microbiomes, as well as changing the hunger and satiety hormones. These surgeries are not merely restriction or malabsorption. Bariatric surgery has shown resolution or improvement of many ORCs including, T2DM, sleep apnea, HTN, PCOS, GERD, and NALFD.

Contraindications to surgery are active substance abuse, active psychiatric disease, active binging/bulimia, noncompliance, and poor competence.

Maintaining weight loss through treatment

Weight regain typically occurs when medication/treatment is stopped. This is not any different than someone with hypertension. The medications are not stopped when they reach goal, they are continued. Obesity is a chronic disease that will require lifetime treatment.

- Successful weight maintenance includes:
  - Self-monitoring
  - Self-belief that weight can be controlled
  - Activity at 250-400 minutes per week
  - Continued treatment
- Maintaining weight loss is made difficult by the reduction in energy expenditure that weight loss induces

Special considerations

- Obesity is unique in the bias and stigma that are associated with the disease process for patients. For this reason, the disease requires a different approach. Patients need to be asked for permission to talk and about their weight. The Stop Obesity Alliance has many recommendations for starting this conversation with patients. http://whyweightguide.org
- Pregnancy: no current medications to treat obesity can be used in pregnancy
- Pediatrics: requires a family approach to changing eating and physical activity
- Geriatrics: sarcopenic obesity is often found in elders. This is a form of obesity that may not be found with BMI as it is based on decreased muscle mass

and increased fat mass. Waist circumference is most beneficial for this diagnosis.

Complications/comorbidities:

There are 236 known obesity associated disorders. Complications (obesity causes these disorders) include these examples; Type 2 Diabetes, Hypertension, Hyperlipidemia, NALFD, PCOS, infertility, pain syndromes, osteoarthritis, 14 cancers (including breast, lung, liver, pancreas, multiple melanoma, thyroid, kidney, ovaries and more). Comorbidities (items that occur concurrently and impact each other) are obstructive sleep apnea, depression (and other psychiatric disorders)

Referrals:

Obesity Specialist: https://obesitymedicine.org/find-obesity-treatment/

NPs and PAs: OMA NP/PA Certificate of Advanced Education

Physician, NPs, and PAs: CSOWM Commission on Dietetic Registration Interdisciplinary Specialist Certification in Obesity and Weight Management credential), SCOPE certification.

Physicians Board Certification in Obesity (American Board of Obesity Medicine)

Bariatric Surgery Programs: https://asmbs.org/patients/find-a-provider

References

Chapter 1

Centers for Disease Control and Prevention. (2019, January 4). *Conjunctivitis in newborns*. Retrieved from Centers for Disease Control and Prevention: https://www.cdc.gov/conjunctivitis/newborns.html

Hubert, R. & VanMeter, K. (2018). *Gould's pathophysiology for the health professions* (6th ed.). St. Louis, MO: Elsevier.

American Academy of Pediatrics (2021). *Acute Otitis Media* pediatriccare.solutions.aap.org

American Academy of Ophthalmology (2021). *Quick Home Remedies for Pink Eye* https://www.aao.org/eye-health/diseases/ pink-eye-quick-home-remedies

Chapter 2

Achar, S., & Yamanaka, J. (2020). Back pain in children and adolescents. *American Family Physician. 102*(1):19-28.

Ali, A., Arif, A.W., Bhan, C., Kumar, D., Malik, B., Sayyed, Z., Akhtar, K.H., & Ahmad, M.Q. (2018). Managing chronic pain in the elderly: An overview of the recent therapeutic advancements. *Cureus.10*(9): e3293. doi: 10.7759/cureus.3293

American Academy of Orthopedic Surgeons (2020). *Diseases and conditions: Fractures.* Retrieved from American Academy of Orthopedic Surgeons: https://orthoinfo.aaos.org/en/diseases--conditions/fractures-broken-bones/

American Pregnancy Association (2017). Back pain during pregnancy. https://americanpregnancy.org/healthy-pregnancy/pregnancy-health-wellness/back-pain- during-pregnancy-943/

Domino, F.J., Baldor, R.A., Golding, J. & Stephens, M.B. (2019). *5-Minute clinical consult 2020.* Philadelphia: Lippincott Williams and Wilkins.

Epocrates. (2021a). *Acetaminophen.* Epocrates.com

Epocrates. (2021b). *Nonsteroidal anti-inflammatory.* Epocrates.com

Epocrates. (2021c). *Cyclobenzaprine.* Epocrates.com

Fitzgerald, P. A. (2020). Osteoporosis. In S. McPhee, M. Rabow, & M. Papadakis (Eds.), *Current medical diagnosis and treatment.* New York: McGraw-Hill.

Johnson, B. (2015). Arthritis: osteoarthritis, gout, & rheumatoid arthritis, In J. South-Paul, S. Matheny, ad E. Lewis (Eds.), *Current Diagnosis & Treatment in Family Medicine.* New York, NY: Lange

Kim, H.S.; Wu, P.H.; Jang, I.-T. (2020). Lumbar Degenerative Disease Part 1: Anatomy and pathophysiology of intervertebral discogenic pain and radiofrequency ablation of basivertebral and sinuvertebral nerve treatment for chronic discogenic back pain: A prospective case series and review of literature. International Journal of Molecular Science, 21, 1483. https://doi.org/10.3390/ijms21041483

National Institutes of Health. (2018, December). *Pregnancy, breastfeeding and bone health.* Retrieved from National Institutes of Health: https://www.bones.nih.gov/health-info/bone/bone-health/pregnancy

National Institute of Neurological Disorders and Stroke. (2020). Low back pain fact sheet. Low Back Pain Fact Sheet | National Institute of Neurological Disorders and Stroke (nih.gov)

Sehmbi, H, D'Souza, R., & Bhatia, A. (2017). Low back pain in pregnancy: Investigation, management, and role of neuraxial analgesia and anaesthesia: A systemic review. *Gynecologic and Obstetric Investigation. 82*:417-436. https://doi.org/10.59/000471764

Will. J.S., Bury, D.C. & Miller, J.A. (2018) Mechanical low back pain. *American Family Physician. 98*(7):421-428.

Chapter 3

Barthel, A., Willenberg, H. S., Gruber, M., Bornstein, S. R. (2019). Adrenal insufficiency. In Jameson, L.J., de Kretser, D.M., Grossman, A.B., Potts, J.T., De Groot, L.J., Guidice, L.C., Melmed, S., Weir, G.C. (Eds.), *Endocrinology: Adult and pediatric* (pp. 1763-1774). Philadelphia: Elsevier Saunders. https://doi.org/10.1016/B978-0-323-18907-1.00102-5

Biggers, A., Macon, B. L., Yu, W. (2019). *Addison's disease.* Healthline. Retrieved from https://www.healthline.com/health/addisons-disease

Bishop, P. M. F. (1950). *The history of the discovery of Addison's disease.* National Institutes of Health. https://www.ncbi.nlm.nih.gov/pmc/articles/PMC2081266/pdf/procrsmed00600-0036.pdf

Bornstein, S. R., Allolio, B., Arlt, W., Barthel, A., Don-Wauchope, A., Hammer, G. D., . . . Torpy, D. J. (2016). Diagnosis and treatment of primary adrenal insufficiency: An endocrine society clinical practice guideline. *Journal of Clinical Endocrinology & Metabolism, 101*(2), 364-389. doi:10.1210/jc.2015-1710

Domino, F.J., Baldor, R.A., Golding, J. & Stephens, M.B. (2019). *5-Minute clinical consult 2020.* Philadelphia: Lippincott Williams and Wilkins.

Fitzgerald, P. (2019). Cushing syndrome (Hypercortisolism). In Papadakis M.A., McPhee S.J., Rabow M.W. (Eds). *Current medical diagnosis and treatment.* New York: McGraw-Hill.

Fitzgerald, P.A. (2019). Hyperthyroidism. In S. McPhee, M. Rabow, & M. Papadakis (Eds.), *Current medical diagnosis and treatment.* New York: McGraw-Hill

Fitzgerald, P. A. (2020). Diabetes mellitus. In S. McPhee, M. Rabow, & M. Papadakis (Eds), *Current medical diagnosis and treatment.* New York: McGraw-Hill.

Garber, J. (2018). T*hyroid disease: Understanding hypothyroidism & hyperthyroidism.* Harvard Health Publishing.

Hossein G., Enrico P., Jeffrey G., Daniel D, R. Mack H., Laszlo H., Ralf P., Roberto V., & Paolo V. (*2016*). American Association of Clinical Endocrinologists, American College of Endocrinology, and Associzaone Medici Endocrinologi Medical Guidelines for Clinical Practice for the diagnosis and management of thyroid nodules- 2016 Update. *Endocrine Practice*. 22(1), 1-60. https://doi.org/10.4158/EP161208.GL

Jameson, L.J., Mandel, & Weetman, A.P. (2018). Hypothyroidism. In L. Jamesons., A. Fauci., S. Kaspter, S.D. Hause, & J. Longo (Eds.), *Harrison's principles of internal medicine* (20ed.). New York: McGraw-Hill.

Munir, S.,Quintanilla Rodriguez BS, Waseem M. (2021). *Addison Disease*. In: StatPearls [Internet]. Treasure Island (FL): StatPearls Publishing. https://www.ncbi.nlm.nih.gov/books/NBK441994/

National Organization for Rare Disorders. (2018). *Addison's disease.* https://rarediseases.org/rare-diseases/addisons-disease/

Nieman, L. K., Biller, B. M., Findling, J. W., Murad, M. H., Newell-Price, J., Savage, M. O., & Tabarin, A. (2015, August). Treatment of Cushing's syndrome: An Endocrine Society clinical practice guideline. *Journal of Clinical Endocrinology and Metabolism, 100*(8), 2807-2831. doi:10.1210/jc.2015-1818

Nieman, L., Lacroix, A., & Martin, K. (2019). *Treatment of adrenal insufficiency in adults.* UpToDate. https://www.uptodate.com/contents/treatment-of-adrenal-insufficiency-in adults?search=addisons%20disease%20adult%20treatment&source=search_result&selectedTitle=1~150&usage_type=default&display_rank=1

Papadakis M.A., McPhee S.J., Bernstein J. (2020). Goiter, endemic. *Quick medical diagnosis & treatment 2020.* New York: McGraw-Hill.

Ropper A.H., Samuels M.A., Klein J.P., Prasad S. (2019). The hypothalamus and neuroendocrine disorders. *Adams and Victor's Principles of Neurology (11th ed).* New York: McGraw-Hill.

Slovik, D. (2014) Evaluation of thyroid nodules. In Goroll, A., Mulley, A. (Eds.). *Office evaluation and management of the adult patient* (7th Ed). Philadelphia: Wolters Kluwer Health.

Chapter 4

American Headache Society. (2019). The American Headache Society position statement on integrating new migraine treatments into clinical practice. *The Journal of Head and Face Pain, 59*(1), 1-18. https://doi.org/10.1111/head.13456

American Stroke Association. (2020). *Ischemic stroke treatment.* Retrieved from https://www.stroke.org/en/about-stroke/treatment/ischemic-stroke-treatment

Boling, B., & Keinath, K. (2018). Acute ischemic stroke. *AACN Advanced Critical Care, 29*(2), 152-162. doi:10.4037/aacnacc2018483

Buttaro, T. M., Trybulski, J., Polgar-Bailey, P., & Sandberg-Cook, J. (2017). *Primary care: A collaborative practice* (5th ed.). Elsevier.

Clinch C. (2020). Evaluation & management of headache. In South-Paul J.E., Matheny S.C., Lewis E.L. (Eds). *Current diagnosis & treatment: Family medicine* (4th ed., pp.293-297). McGraw-Hill.

Coutts, S. B. (2017). Diagnosis and management of transient ischemic attack. *Continuum, 23*, 82-92. doi:10.1212/CON.0000000000000424

Douglas V.C. & Aminoff, M.J. (2020). Headache. In Papadakis M.A., McPhee S.J. & Rabow M.W. (Eds). *Current medical diagnosis and treatment 2020* (24-01 headache). McGraw-Hill.

Epilepsy Foundation. (2020). *Epilepsy terminologies.* https://www.epilepsy.com/living-epilepsy/toolbox/glossary

Evans, R.W., Burch, R.C., Frishberg, B.M., Marmura, M.J., Mechtler, L.L., Silberstein, S.D. &Turner, D.P. (2020), Neuroimaging for migraine: The American Headache Society systematic review and evidence-based guideline. *Headache: The Journal of Head and Face Pain, 60,* 318-336. https://doi.org/10.1111/head.13720

Falk, N., Cole, A. & Meredith, T.J. (2018). Evaluation of suspected dementia. *American Family Physician, 97*(6), 398-405.

Fisher, R.S., Cross, J.H., French, J.A., Higurashi, N., Hirsch, E., Jansen, F.E., Lagae, L., Moshé, S.L., Peltola, J., Roulet Perez, E., Scheffer, I.E., & Zuberi, S.M. (2017). Operational classification of seizure types by the International League Against Epilepsy: Position paper of the ILAE commission for classification and terminology. *Epilepsia, 58*(4), 522-530. doi:10.1111/epi.13670

Goadsby P.J. (2018). Migraine and other primary headache disorders. In Jameson J., Fauci A.S., Kasper D.L., Hauser S.L., Longo D.L., Loscalzo J. (Eds). *Harrison's principles of internal medicine* (20th ed., pp2-15-222). McGraw-Hill.

Golde, T. E., DeKosky, S. T., & Galasko, D. (2018). Alzheimer's disease: The right drug, the right time. *Science, 362*(6420), 1250-1251. https://doi.org/10.1126/science.aau0437

Goldenberg M. M. (2010). Overview of drugs used for epilepsy and seizures: Etiology, diagnosis, and treatment. *P & T: A Peer-reviewed Journal for Formulary Management,*

35(7), 392–415.

Hubert, R. J., & VanMeter, K. C. (2018). *Gould's pathophysiology for the health professions*. Saunders.

International Headache Society (2018). The international classification of headache disorder (3rd ed.). *Cephalalgia,38(*1), 1-211. https://doi.org/10.1177/0333102417738202

LeBlond R. F., Brown D.D., Suneja M., & Szot J.F. (2015). Recurrent headache syndromes. In *DeGowin's Diagnostic Examination* (10th ed.) McGraw-Hill.

Leone, M. A., Brathen, G., Chick, J., Faggiano, F., Hillbom, M., McIntosh, C., & Leone, M. A. (2016). Pharmacotherapy for preventing and treating alcohol withdrawal seizures. *Cochrane Database of Systematic Reviews*, *5*. DOI:10.1002/14651858.CD005223.pub2

Luzio, C. & Langond, F. (2019) *Multiple sclerosis.* Medscape. https://emedicine.medscape.com/article/1146199-overview

Powers, W. J., Rabinstein, A. A., Ackerson, T., Adeoye, O. M., Bambakidis, N. C., Becker, K., . . . Tirschwell, D. L. (2018). 2018 Guidelines for the early management of patients with acute ischemic stroke: A guideline for healthcare professionals from the American Heart Association/American Stroke Association. *Stroke, 49*(3), e46-e99. https://doi.org/10.1161/STR.0000000000000158

Pruitt, A. (2017). Migraine headache. In Goroll, A. H., Mulley, A. (Eds.) *Primary care medicine.* (7th ed, pp.1190-1197). Wolters Kluwer Health.

Roodhooft, J. M. (2009) Ocular problems in early stages of multiple sclerosis. *Bulletin de la Societe Belge d'Ophtamologie*, 313, 65-8.

Stafstrom, C. E., & Carmant, L. (2015). Seizures and epilepsy: An overview for neuroscientists. *Cold Spring Harbor Perspectives in Medicine*, *5*(6), a022426. https://doi.org/10.1101/cshperspect.a022426

Trapp, B. D., Peterson, J., Ransohoff, R. M., Rudick, R., Mörk, S., Bö, L. (1998). Axonal transection in the lesions of multiple sclerosis. *New England Journal of Medicine, 338*(5), 278-85. doi:10.1056/NEJM199801293380502

Trapp, B. D., Vignos, M., Dudman, J., Chang, A., Fisher, E., Staugaitis, S. M., . . . Rudick, R. A. (2018). Cortical neuronal densities and cerebral white matter demylelination in multiple sclerosis: A retrospective study. *Lancet Neurology, 17*(10), 870-884. doi:10.1016/S1474-422(18)30245-X

Vallerand, A., & Sanoski, C. (2019). *Davis' drug guide for nurses* (16th ed.) F.A. Davis.

Wu, G., & Alvarez, E. (2011.) The immuno-pathophysiology of multiple sclerosis. *Neurology Clinics. 29*(2), 252-278. doi:10.1016/j.ncl.2010.12.009

American Academy of Allergy and Immunology. (n.d.) *Asthma overview.* https://www.aaaai.org/conditions-and-treatments/asthma

Baldor, R. (2015). Sleep apnea, obstructive. In Domino, F.J. (Ed.). *The 5-minute clinical consult* (23rd ed.) Lippincott Williams & Wilkins.

Douglass, J., & Holgate, S.T. (2010) *Fast facts: Asthma.* Health Press Limited, Oxford.

Eekholm, S., Ahlström, G., Kristensson, J., & Lindhardt, T. (2020). Gaps between current clinical practice and evidence-based guidelines for treatment and care of older patients with community-acquired pneumonia: A descriptive cross-sectional study. *BMC Infectious Disease, 20*(73). doi:10.1186/s12879-019-4742-4

Eckert, D. J., & Malhotra, A. (2008). Pathophysiology of adult obstructive sleep apnea. *Proceedings of the American Thoracic Society, 5*(2), 144–153. https://doi.org/10.1513/pats.200707-114MG

Goolsby, M., & Jones, C. *Advanced assessment: Interpreting findings and formulating differential diagnoses* (4 ed.) F.A Davis.

Holgate, S., Casale, T., Wenzel, S., Bousquet, J., Deniz Y., & Reisner C. (2005). The anti-inflammatory effects of omalizumab confirm the central role of IgE in allergic inflammation. *Journal of Clinical and Allergy Immunology. 115*(3), 459–65. doi:10.1016/j.jaci.2004.11.053

Kline, J.A. (2020). Venous thromboembolism in pulmonary embolism. In Tintinalli J.E., Ma, O., Yealy, D.M., Meckler G.D., Stapczynski J., Cline D.M., & Thomas S.H. (Eds). *Tintinalli's emergency medicine: A comprehensive study guide* (9th ed.) McGraw-Hill.

Landis, S.H., Muellerova, H., Mannion, D.M., Meneze, A.M., Han, M.K., van der Molen, T., Ichinose, M., Aisanov, Z., Oh, Y.M., & Davis, M.K. (2014). Continuing to confront COPD international patient survey: Methods, COPD prevalence, and disease burden in 2012-2013. *International Journal of Chronic Obstructive Pulmonary Disease. 6*(9), 414-420. doi:10.2147/COPD.S61854

National Heart, Lung, and Blood Institute. (2007). *Expert panel report 3: Guidelines for the diagnosis and management of asthma.* https://www.nhlbi.nih.gov/health-topics/guidelines-for-diagnosis-management-of-asthma

Papadakis, M. & McPhee, S. (2020). *Current medical diagnosis & treatment.* McGraw Hill.

Parth, R., Rali, M., & Sockrider, M. (2018). ATS patient education series. *American Journal of Respiratory Critical Care Medicine*, 197, 15-16.

Rance, K.S. (2011). Helping patients attain and maintain asthma control: Reviewing the role of the nurse practitioner. *Journal of Multidisciplinary Healthcare*, 4, 299–309. doi:10.2147/JMDH.S2296

Singh, D., Agusti, A., Anzueto, A., Barnes, P. J., Bourbeau, J., Celli, B. R., . . . Vogelmeier, C. (2019). Global strategy for the diagnosis, managment, and prevention of chronic obstructive lung disease: The GOLD science committee report 2019. *European Respiratory Society, 18*(53), 1900164. doi:10.1183/13993003.00164-2019

Stewart, J.G. (Ed.) (2010). Atlas of pathophysiology. Wolters Kluwer Health/Lippincott Williams & Wilkins.

Tarbox, A. K., & Swaroop, M. (2013). Pulmonary embolism. *International Journal of Critical Illness and Injury Science, 3*(1), 69–72. https://doi.org/10.4103/2229-5151.109427

van Deursen, A. M., van Houten, M. A., Webber, C., Patton, M., Scott, D. A., Patterson, S., . . . Sanders, E. A. (2017). Immunogenicity of the 13-valent pneumococcal conjugate vaccine in older adults with and without comorbidities in the community-acquired pneumonia immunization trial in adults (CAPiTA). *Clinical Infectious Disease, 65*(1), 787-795. doi:10.1093/cid/cix419

Wellman A., & Redline, S. (2021). Sleep apnea. In Jameson, J. Fauci A.S., Kasper D.L., Hauser S.L., Longo D.L., & Loscalzo J. (Eds). *Harrison's principles of internal medicine* (20th ed.) McGraw-Hill.

White, D.P. (2005). Pathogenesis of obstructive and central sleep apnea. *American Journal of Respiratory Critical Care Medicine*, 172, 1363–1370. https://doi.org/10.1164/rccm.200412-1631SO

Whyte, A., & Gibson, D. (2020). Adult obstructive sleep apnea: Pathogenesis, importance, diagnosis and imaging. *Journal of Medical Imaging and Radiation Oncology*, 64 (1), 52-66. https://doi.org/10.1111/1754-9485.12978

Whyte, A., Gibson, D. (2018). Imaging of adult obstructive sleep apnoea. *European Journal of Radiology, 102, 176-187.* doi:10.1016/j.ejrad.2018.03.010

Chapter 6

Ahn, J. M., Lee, K. H., Yoo, S. Y., Cho, Y. R., Suh, J., Shin, E., Park, S. J. (2016). Prognosis of variant angina manifesting as aborted sudden cardiac death. *Journal of The American College of Cardiology, 68*(2), 137-145. doi:10.1016/j.jacc.2016.04.050

Agarwala, A., Mehta, A., Yand, E., and Parapid, B. (2020). Older adults and hypertension: beyond the 2017 guideline for prevention, detection, evaluation, and management of high blood pressure in adults. www.acc.org/latest-in-cardiology/articles/2020/02/26/06/24/older-adults-and-hypertension

American Family Physician Practice Guidelines (2018). High blood pressure: ACC/AHA releases updated guideline. *American Family Physician, 97*(6):413-415.

Benetos, A., Petrovic, M., Strandberg, T. (2019). Hypertension management in older and frail older patients. *Circulation Research, 124*:1045–1060https://doi.org/10.1161/CIRCRESAHA.118.313236

Bickley, L. (2013). *Bates' guide to physical examination and history taking.* (2013). Lippincott Williams & Wilkins.

Chapman, J. (2007). Statins and antiplatelet agents: Complementary mechanisms of action at the coronary artery level. *American Journal of Cardiovascular Drugs,* 7, 5–8. doi:10.1007/BF03262466

Croke, L. (2019). Practice guidelines: Managing chronic hypertension in pregnant women: ACOG releases updated practice bulletin. *American Family Physician, 100*(12):782-783.

Dunphy, L. M. (2015). Primary care: The art and science of advanced practice nursing (4th ed.). F.A. Davis.

Epocrates Medical Resources. (2020). *Epocrates plus* (Version 20.2) [Mobile application software]. https://online.epocrates.com/

Ferri, F. F. (2019). *Ferri's clinical advisor 2019: 5 books in 1.* Elsevier.

Flynn J.T, Kaelber, D. C., Baker-Smith, C.M., Blowey, D., Carroll, A.E., Daniels, J.M., Ferranti, S.D., Dionne, J.M., Falkner, B., Flinn, S.K., et al. (2017). Clinical practice guideline for screening and management of high blood pressure in children and adolescents. *Pediatrics, 140*(3):e20171904

Hubert, R. & VanMeter, K. (2018). *Gould's pathophysiology for the health professions* (6th ed.). Elsevier.

Jameson, L.J., Mandel, & Weetman, A.P. (2018). Hypothyroidism. In L. Jamesons., A. Fauci., S. Kaspter, S.D. Hause, & J. Longo (Eds.), *Harrison's principles of internal medicine* (20ed.). New York: McGraw-Hill.

Jarvis, C. (2020). *Physical examination and health assessment, 8th edition.* Evolve.

Juarez, M., Johnson, K., & Ali, F. (2018). Acute coronary syndromes: STEMI. In F. J. Domino (Ed.). *The 5-minute clinical consult standard 2018* (26th ed., pp. 14-17). Wolters Kluwer.

Katzung, B.G. (2018). Drugs used in heart failure. In Katzung, B.G. (Ed.), *Basic & Clinical Pharmacology, 14e.* McGraw-Hill

Kornusky, J. & Oji, O. (2018). Angina: Coronary artery vasospasm (Prinzmetal's or Variant Angina). *CINAHL Nursing Guide*, EBSCO Publishing, Ipswich, MA

Kossmann, C.E. (1964). *Diseases of the heart and blood vessels: Nomenclature and criteria for diagnosis 6th ed.* New York Heart Association.

Kwong, J. C., Schwartz, K. L., Campitelli, M. A., Chung, H., Crowcroft, N. S., Karnauchow, T., & Gubbay, J. B. (2018). Acute myocardial infarction after laboratory-confirmed influenza infection. *New England Journal of Medicine, 378*(4), 345-353. doi:10.1056/NEJMoa1702090

Mann, D.L., & Chakinala, M. (2018). Heart failure: Pathophysiology and diagnosis. In L. Jamesons., A. Fauci., S. Kaspter, S.D. Hause, & J. Longo (Eds.), *Harrison's principles of internal medicine* (20ed.). McGraw-Hill.

Mekaj, Y.H., Daci, F.T., & Mekaj. A.Y. (2015). New insights into the mechanisms of action of aspirin and its use in the prevention and treatment of arterial and venous thromboembolism. *Therapeutics and Clinical Risk Management, 24*(11), 1449-1456. doi:10.2147/TCRM.S92222

Papadakis, M. & McPhee, S. (2020). *Current medical diagnosis & treatment.* McGraw Hill.

Riley, M., Hernandez, A.K., and Kuznia, A.L. (2018). High blood pressure in children and adolescents. *American Family Physician, 98*(8):486-494.

Schub, T. B. (2018). *Acute myocardial infarction in older adults. CINAHL Nursing Guide*, EBSCO Publishing, Ipswich, MA

Spears, D., & Elkayam, U. (2019). Cardiac arrhythmias and pregnancy. In Elkayam, U. (Ed.), *Cardiac Problems in Pregnancy*, 220-251. https://doi.org/10.1002/9781119409861.ch15

Swartz, M.H. (2021). *Textbook of physical diagnosis: History and examination.* Elsevier.

Yancy, C. W., Jessup, M., Bozkurt, B., Bulter, J., Casey Jr., D. E., Colvin, M. M., . . . Westlake, C. (2017). 2017 ACC/AHA/HFSA focused update of the 2013 ACCF/AHA guideline for the management of heart failure: A report of the American College of Cardiology/American Heart Association task force on clinical practice guidelines. *Circulation,* 136, 137-161. https://doi.org/10.1161/CIR.0000000000000509

Yang, I. H., Hwang, H. J., Jeon, H. K., Sohn, I. S., Park, C. B., Jin, E. S., . . . Lee, T. G. (2019). Slow heart rate recovery is associated with increase exercise-indcued arterial stiffness in normotensive patients without

Woo, T.M., & Robinson, M. V. (2016). *Pharmacotherapeutics for advance practice nurse prescribers* (4th ed.). F. A. Davis Company.

Ziegler, T., Rahman, F. A., Jurisch, V., & Kupatt, C. (2020). Atherosclerosis and the capillary network; Pathophysiology and potential therapeutic strategies. *Cells, 9*(1), 1–13. doi:10.3390/cells9010050

Chapter 7

Ahn, I. E., Sun, C., & Wiestner, A. (2019). Chronic lymphocytic leukemia. In Rodgers, G. P. & Young, N. S. (Eds.), *The Bethesda handbook of clinical hematology*. (4th Ed.). Wolters Kluwer.

American Academy of Pediatrics. (2020). *Periodicity schedule*. Retrieved from Engaging Patients and Families: www.aap.org/en-us/professional-resources/practice-support/Pages/PeriodicitySchedule.aspx

Auerbach, M., & Adamson, J. W. (2016). How we diagnose and treat iron deficiency anemia. *American Journal of Hematology*, *91*(1), 31–38. https://doi.org/10.1002/ajh.24201

Bizzaro, N., & Antico, A. (2014). Diagnosis and classification of pernicious anemia. *Autoimmunity Reviews*, *13*(4–5), 565–568. https://doi.org/10.1016/J.AUTREV.2014.01.042

Blackburn, L. M., Bender, S. Brown, S. (2019). Acute leukemia: Diagnosis and treatment. *Seminars in Oncology Nursing, 35,* 1-7. https://doi.org/10.1016/j.soncn.2019.150950

Bristol-Myers Squibb Company. (2019). *Hydrea package insert.* https://packageinserts.bms.com/pi/pi_hydrea.pdf

Camaschella, C. (2019). Iron deficiency. *Blood*, *133*(1), 30–39. https://doi.org/10.1182/blood-2018-05-815944

Chan, C. Q. H., Low, L. L., & Lee, K. H. (2016). Oral Vitamin B12 Replacement for the Treatment of Pernicious Anemia. *Frontiers in Medicine, 3*(38). doi:10.3389/fmed.2016.00038

Ciesla, B. (2012). *Hematology in practice.* (2nd ed.). F. A. Davis Company.

deHaas, V., Ismaila, N., & Zhang, L. (2018). Initial diagnosis workup of acute leukemia: ASCO clinical practice guidelines endorsement summary of the CAP and ASH guideline. *Journal of Oncology Practice, 15*(2), 101-106. https://doi.org/10.1200/JOP.18.00613

DeVita, V. T., Lawrence, T. S., & Rosenberg, S. A. (2016). *Lymphomas and leukemias. Cancer: principles & practices of oncology.* (10th ed). Wolters Kluwer.

Djulbegovix, M., Dugdale, L. S., & Lee, A. I. (2018). Evaluation of Polycythemia: A teachable moment. *JAMA Internal Medicine, 178*(1), 128-130. doi:10.1001/jamainternmed.2017.6213

Dufour, C., Samarasinghe, S., & Miano, M. (2017). Management of acquired aplastic anemia in children. Congenital and Acquired Bone Marrow Failure. In Aljurk, M. D., Gluckman, E., & Dufour, C. (Eds.), *Congenital and acquired bone marrow dailure.* P127-139. Elsevier. https://doi.org/10.1016/B978-0-12-804152-9.00011-7

Harmening, D. M. (2009). *Clinical hematology and fundamentals of hemostasis.* (5th ed.). F. A. Davis Company.

Hillman, R. (2011). *Hematology in clinical practice* (5th ed). The McGraw-Hill Companies, Inc.

Hourigan C. S. & Malkovska, V. (2019) Acute myeloid leukemia. In Rodgers, G. P. & Young, N. S. (Eds.), *The Bethesda handbook of clinical hematology.* (4th Ed.). Wolters Kluwer.

Hsieh, M. M., Tisdale, J. F., & Rodgers, G. P. (2019). Sickle cell anemia and thalassemia. In Rodgers, G. P. & Young, N. S. (Eds.), *The Bethesda handbook of clinical hematology.* (4th Ed.). Wolters Kluwer.

Jacob, E., Childress, C., & Nathanson, J. D. (2016). Barriers to care and quality of primary care services in children with sickle cell disease. *Journal of Advanced Nursing, 72*(6), 1417-1439. doi:10.1111/jan.12756

Jain, P., Kantarjian, H, & Cortes, J. (2013). Chronic myeloid leukemia: Overview of new agents and comparative analysis. *Current Treatment Options in Oncology,* 14, 127-143. doi:10.1007/s11864-013-0234-8

Keohane, E. M., Otto, C. N., & Walenga, J. M. (2020). *Rodak's hematology clinical principles and applications.* (6th ed.). Elsevier.

Kimrey, S. & Saving, K. L. (2020). Sickle cell disease: A primer for primary care providers. *Pediatric Annuals, 49*(1), e43-e49. doi:10.3928/19382359-20191210-01

Lo, C., Glader, B., Sakamoto, K. (2020). Bone marrow failure. In Keohane, E. M., Otto, C. N., & Walenga, J. M. (Eds.), *Rodak's hematology clinical principles and applications.* (5th Ed.). Elsevier.

Olnes, M. J. (2019). The Myeloproliferative neoplasms: Polycythemia vera, essential thrombocythemia, primary myelofibrosis, and chronic myelomonocytic leukemia. In Rodgers, G. P. & Young, N. S. (Eds.), *The Bethesda handbook of clinical hematology.* (4th Ed.). Wolters Kluwer.

Parkin, P. C., Koroshegyi, C., Mamak, E., Borkhoff, C. M., Birken, C. S., Maguire, J. L., … Mason, D. (2020). Association between serum ferritin and cognitive function in early childhood. *Journal of Pediatrics*, *217*, 189-191.e2. https://doi.org/10.1016/j.jpeds.2019.09.051

Perkins, S. L. (2009). Aplastic anemia including pure red cell aplasia, congenital dyserythopoietic anemia, and paroxysmal nocturnal hemoglobinuria. In Harmenin, D. M. (Ed.), *Clinical hematology and fundamentals of hemostasis* (5th ed.). F. A. Davis Company.

Peslak, S. A., Olson, T., & Babushok, D. V. (2017). Diagnosis and treatment of aplastic anemia. *Current Treatment Options in Oncology,* 18, 70. https://doi.org/10.1007/s11864-017-0511-z

Prchal, J.T. (2019). Diagnosing or ruling out polycythemia vera in patients with erythrocytosis. *Clinical Advances in Hematology & Oncology, 17*(1), 24-27.

Scheinber, P., Young, N. S. & Liu. J. M. (2019). Bone marrow failure syndromes: Aplastic Anemia, Acquired and constitutional; Paroxysmal nocturnal hemoglobinuria; Pure red blood cell aplasia; and agranulocytosis. In Rodgers, G. P & Young, N. S. (Eds.), *The Bethesda handbook of clinical hematology* (4th ed., pp. 66-89). Wolters Kluwer.

Shephard, E. A., Neal, R. D., Rose, P. W., Walter, F. M., & Hamilton, W. (2016). Symptoms of adult chronic and acute leukaemia before diagnosis: Large primary care case-control studies using electronic records. *British Journal of General Practice,* e182-e. 188. doi:10.3399/bjgp16X683989

Toh, B. H. (2017). Pathophysiology and laboratory diagnosis of pernicious anemia. *Immunologic Research*, *65*(1), 326–330. https://doi.org/10.1007/s12026-016-8841-7

Yawn, B. P. & John-Sowah, J. (2015). Management of Sickle cell disease: Recommendation from the 2014 expert panel report. *American Family Physician, 92*(12), 1069-1077.

Yong, A. S. & Barrett, A. J. (2019). Chronic myelogenous leukemia. In Rodgers, G. P. & Young, N. S. (Eds.), *The Bethesda handbook of clinical hematology*. (4th Ed.). Wolters Kluwer.

Young, N. S. (2018). Aplastic anemia. *New England Journal of Medicine,* 379, 1643-56. doi:10.1056/NEJMra1413485.

Chapter 8

Abraham, S.; Rivero, G.; Erlikh, I.; Griffith, L.; Kondamudi, V. (2014). Surgical and nonsurgical management of gallstones, *American Family Physician*, *89*(10).795-802.

Aggarwal, R. (2011). Hepatitis E: Historical, contemporary and future perspectives. *Journal of Gastroenterology and Hepatology*, *26*, 72-82. https://doi.org/10.1111/j.1440-1746.2010.06540.x

Aggarwal, R. (2012). Diagnosis of chronic hepatitis E. *Nature Reviews Gastroenterology & Hepatology, 10*(2), 124-124. https://doi.org/10.1038/nrgastro.2012.187-c2

Al-Hawary, M. (2016). Role of imaging in diagnosing and staging pancreatic cancer. *Journal of the National Comprehensive Cancer Network, 14*(5S), 678-680. doi:10.6004/jnccn.2016.0191

Alonso, S., Pera, M., Parés, D., Pascual, M., Gil, M. J., Courtier, R., & Grande, L. (2010). Outpatient treatment of patients with uncomplicated acute diverticulitis. *Colorectal Disease, 12*(10Online), e278-e282. doi:10.1111/j.1463-1318.2009.02122.x

Ajani, J. A., D'Amico, T. A., Almhanna, K., Bentrem, D. J., Chao, J., Das, P., ... & Gerdes, H. (2016). Gastric cancer, version 3.2016, NCCN clinical practice guidelines in oncology. *Journal of the National Comprehensive Cancer Network, 14*(10), 1286-1312. doi:10.6004/jnccn.2016.0137

Barry, K. (2018). Chronic pancreatitis: Diagnosis and treatment. *American Family Physician, 97(*6), 385-393.

Boyce, T. G. (2019). *Gastroenteritis.* Retrieved from Merck Manual Professional Version: https://www.merckmanuals.com/professional/gastrointestinal-disorders/gastroenteritis/gastroenteritis

Centers for Disease Control and Prevention. (2016). *Viral Hepatitis surveillance: United States, 2013.* https://www.cdc.gov/hepatitis/statistics/2014surveillance/pdfs/2014HepSurveillanceRpt_Rev2016-09-26.pdf

Centers for Disease Control and Prevention. (2020). *Hepatitis A questions and answers for health professionals.* Retrieved from Viral Hepatitis: http://www.cdc.gov/hepatitis/hav/havfaq.htm#general

Crockett, S., Wani, S., Gardner, T., Falck-Ytter, Y. & Barkun, A. (2018). American Gastroenterological Association Institute guideline on initial management of acute pancreatitis. *Gastroenterology, 154*, 1096 – 1101. doi:10.1053/j.gastro.2018.01.032

Dunphy, L.M., Winland-Brown, J.E., Porter, B.O., & Thomas, D.J. (2019) Primary care: Art and science of advanced practice nursing – An interprofessional approach. F.A. Davis.

Fashner, J., & Gitu, A.C. (2019). Diagnosis and treatment of peptic ulcer disease and H. pylori infection. *American Family Physician,91*(4), 236-42.

Feuerstein, J. D., & Falchuk, K. R. (2016, August). Diverticulosis and diverticulitis. In *Mayo Clinic Proceedings* (Vol. 91, No. 8, pp. 1094-1104). Elsevier.

Ghany, M. G., & Morgan, T. R. (2020). Hepatitis C guidance 2019 update: American association for the study of liver diseases–Infectious Diseases Society of America recommendations for testing, managing, and treating Hepatitis C virus infection. *Hepatology, 71*(2), 686-721. https://doi.org/10.1002/hep.31060

Granlund, J., Svensson, T., Olén, O., Hjern, F., Pedersen, N. L., Magnusson, P.K.E., & Thelin Schmidt, P. (2012). The genetic influence on diverticular disease--a twin study. *Alimentary Pharmacology & Therapeutics*, *35*(9), 1103-1107. doi:10.1111/j.1365-2036.2012.05069.x

Greenberger, N., Blumberg, R., & Burakoff, R. (2009). Current diagnosis & treatment *Gastroenterology, hepatology, & endoscopy* (3rd ed.). McGraw Hill Professional.

Hart, P. A., Stanich, P. P., & Hampel, H. (2018). Screening for pancreatic cancer: Who to screen and how-to follow-Up? In *Current and Emerging Therapies in Pancreatic Cancer* (pp. 97-108). Springer.

Hepatitis C guidance: AASLD-IDSA recommendations for testing, managing, and treating adults infected with hepatitis C virus. (2015). *Hepatology*, *62*(3), 932-954. https://doi.org/10.1002/hep.27950

Hubert, R. & VanMeter, K. (2018). *Gould's pathophysiology for the health professions (6th ed.)*. Elsevier.

Kamisawa, T., Wood, L. D., Itoi, T., & Takaori, K. (2016). Pancreatic cancer. *The Lancet*, *388*(10039), 73-85. https://doi.org/10.1016.S0140-6736(16)00141-0

Kasper, D. L., Hauser, S. L., Loscalzo, J., Longo, D. L., Jameson, J. L., & Fauci, A. S. (2018). *Harrison's principles of internal medicine.* McGraw-Hill.

Katz, P., Gerson, L., & Vela, M. (2013). Guidelines for the diagnosis and management of gastroesophageal reflux disease. *American Journal of Gastroenterology*,*108* (3), 308-328; doi:10.1038/ajg.2012.444

Kornusky, J. & Caple, C. (2018). Quick lesson: Pancreatitis, acute. *CINAHL Nursing Guide*, EBSCO Publishing, Ipswich, MA

King, D., Dosanjh, A., Patel, P., Leeds, J., Nayar, M., Oppong, K., & Trudgill, N. (2019). PTU-113 How commonly is pancreatic cancer diagnosed following an endoscopic ultrasound that did not diagnose cancer? *Gut*, 68, A50-A51. http://dx.doi.org/10.1136/gutjnl-2019-BSGAbstracts.102

Kleef, J., Korc, M., Apte, M., La Vecchia, C., Johnson, C. D., Biankin, A. V., . . . Neoptolemos, J. P. (2016, April 21). Pancreatic cancer. *Nature Reviews Disease Primers*, 16022. doi:10.1038/nrdp.2016.22

Laméris, W., van Randen, A., Bipat, S., Bossuyt, P. M., Boermeester, M. A., & Stoker, J. (2008). Graded compression ultrasonography and computed tomography in acute colonic diverticulitis: Meta-analysis of test accuracy. *European Radiology*, *18*(11), 2498. doi:10.1007/s00330-008-1018-6

Lin, B., & Win, G.Y. (2018). *Viral gastroenteritis*. Retrieved from Medscape:https://emedicine.medscape.com/article/176515-treatment#d7

Lindenmeyer, C.C. (2020). Acute cholecystitis. Retrieved from: Merck Manual Professional Version. https://www.merckmanuals.com/professional/hepatic-and-biliary-%20%20disorders/gallbladder-and-bile-duct-disorders/acute-cholecystitis

Linder, K. A., & Malani, P. N. (2017). Hepatitis A. *Journal of the American Medical Association, 318*(23), 2393. https://doi.org/10.1001/jama.2017.17244

Lok, A. S., McMahon, B. J., Brown, R. S., Wong, J. B., Ahmed, A. T., Farah, W., Almasri, J., Alahdab, F., Benkhadra, K., Mouchli, M. A., Singh, S., Mohamed, E. A., Abu Dabrh, A. M., Prokop, L. J., Wang, Z., Murad, M. H., & Mohammed, K. (2015). Antiviral therapy for chronic hepatitis B viral infection in adults: A systematic review and meta-analysis. *Hepatology, 63*(1), 284-306. https://doi.org/10.1002/hep.28280

Mali, P. (2016). Pancreatitis in pregnancy: Etiology, diagnosis, treatment, and outcomes. *Hepatobiliary & Pancreatic Diseases International, 15*(4), 434-438. doi:10.1016/s1499-3872(16)60075-9

Phillip, V., Steiner, J., & Algul, H. (2014). Early phase of acute pancreatitis: Assessment and management. *World Journal of Gastrointestinal Pathophysiology, 5*(3), 158-168. doi:10.4291/wjgp.v5.i3.158

Provenzale, D., Gupta, S., Ahnen, D. J., Bray, T., Cannon, J. A., Cooper, G., ... & Giardiello, F. M. (2016). Genetic/familial high-risk assessment: colorectal version 1.2016, NCCN clinical practice guidelines in oncology. *Journal of the National Comprehensive Cancer Network, 14*(8), 1010-1030. doi:10.6004/jnccn.2016.0108

Puchades Renau, L., & Berenguer, M. (2018). Introduction to hepatitis C virus infection: Overview and history of hepatitis C virus therapies. *Hemodialysis International*, 22, S8-S21. https://doi.org/10.1111/hdi.12647

Quinlan, J.D. (2014). Acute pancreatitis. *American Family Physician, 90*(9), 632-639.

Rehermann, B. (2016). Advances in hepatitis C research and treatment. *Nature Reviews Gastroenterology & Hepatology, 13*(2), 70-72. https://doi.org/10.1038/nrgastro.2015.227

Rezapour, M., Ali, S., & Stollman, N. (2018). Diverticular disease: An update on pathogenesis and management. *Gut and Liver, 12*(2), 125. doi:10.5009/gnl16552

Strate, L. L., Modi, R., Cohen, E., & Spiegel, B. M. (2012). Diverticular disease as a chronic illness: Evolving epidemiologic and clinical insights. *American Journal of Gastroenterology, 107*(10), 1486-1493. doi:10.1038/ajg.2012.194

Sureau, C., & Negro, F. (2016). The hepatitis delta virus: Replication and pathogenesis. *Journal of Hepatology, 64*(1), S102-S116. https://doi.org/10.1016/j.jhep.2016.02.013

Tavakolpour, S., Darvishi, M., & Sali, S. (2019). Tenofovir alafenamide: A new drug with various ambiguous aspects in treatment of chronic Hepatitis B infection. *Archives of Clinical Infectious Diseases, 14*(1). https://doi.org/10.5812/archcid.65343

Tempero, M. A., Malafa, M. P., Al-Hawary, M., Asbun, H., Bain, A., Behrman, S. W., ... & Chiorean, E. G. (2017). Pancreatic adenocarcinoma, version 2.2017, NCCN clinical practice guidelines in oncology. *Journal of the National Comprehensive Cancer Network*, *15*(8), 1028-1061. doi:10.6004/jnccn.2017.0131

Terrault, N. A., Lok, A. S., McMahon, B. J., Chang, K., Hwang, J. P., Jonas, M. M., Brown, R. S., Bzowej, N. H., & Wong, J. B. (2018). Update on prevention, diagnosis, and treatment of chronic hepatitis B: AASLD 2018 hepatitis B guidance. *Hepatology*, *67*(4), 1560-1599. https://doi.org/10.1002/hep.29800

Tursi, A., Brandimarte, G., Elisei, W., Giorgetti, G. M., Inchingolo, C. D., Danese, S., & Aiello, F. (2008). Assessment and grading of mucosal inflammation in colonic diverticular disease. *Journal of Clinical Gastroenterology*, *42*(6), 699-703. doi:10.1097/MCG.0b013e3180653ca2

Yapali, S., Talaat, N., & Lok, A. S. (2014). Management of Hepatitis B: Our practice and how it relates to the guidelines. *Clinical Gastroenterology and Hepatology*, *12*(1), 16-26. https://doi.org/10.1016/j.cgh.2013.04.036

You, H., Sweeny, A., Cooper, M. L., Von Papen, M., & Innes, J. (2019). The management of diverticulitis: A review of the guidelines. *Medical Journal of Australia*, *211*(9), 421-427. doi:10.5694/mja2.50276

Wheat, C. L., & Strate, L. L. (2016). Trends in hospitalization for diverticulitis and diverticular bleeding in the United States from 2000 to 2010. *Clinical Gastroenterology and Hepatology*, *14*(1), 96-103. doi:10.1016/j.cgh.2015.03.030

World Health Organization. (2020, July 27). *Hepatitis E*. Retrieved from World Health Organization: http://www.who.int/mediacentre/factsheets/fs280/en/

Zaman, K., Goyal, K., & P Singh, M. (2016). Hepatitis E vaccines – Current scenario. *Gastroenterology, Hepatology and Endoscopy*, *1*(3), 69-72. https://doi.org/10.15761/ghe.1000117

American Gastroenterological Associaiton (AGA), (2019). Hepatitis C Care Pathway. https://gastro.org/guidelines/liver-diseases/

Chapter 9

American Cancer Society. (2020). *Key statistics for prostate cancer.* Accessed from American Cancer Society: https://www.cancer.org/cancer/prostate-cancer/about/key-statistics.html

American College of Surgeons. (2017). *AJCC cancer staging manual* (8th ed.). Springer International Publishing.

American Kidney Fund. (2020). *Kidney failure (ESRD) causes, symptoms, and treatments*. Retrieved from American Kidney Fund: https://www.kidneyfund.org/kidney-disease/kidney-failure/

American Kidney Fund. (2020). *Glomerulonephritis: Symptoms, causes and treatment.* Retrieved from American Kidney Fund: www.kidneyfund.org/kidney-disease/other- kidney-conditions/rare-diseases/glomerulonephritis/

American Urological Association. (2018). *Early detection of prostate cancer.* Retrieved from American Urological Association: https://www.auanet.org/guidelines/prostate-cancer-early-detection-guideline

American Urological Association. (2019). *Benign prostatic hyperplasia: Surgical management of benign prostatic hyperplasia/lower urinary tract symptoms.* Retrieved from American Urological Association: https://www.auanet.org/guidelines/benign-prostatic-hyperplasia-(bph)-guideline

Bachmann, L.H. (2020). *Urethritis in adult men.* Retrieved from UpToDate: https://www.uptodate.com/contents/urethritis-in-adult-men?search=urethritis&source=search_result&selectedTitle=1~84&usage_type=default&display_rank=1

Ball, J. W., Dains, J. E., Flynn, J. A., Solomon, B. S., & Stewart, R. W. (2014). Se*idel's guide to physical examination.* Elsevier Health Sciences.

Barratt, J., Harris, K. P. G., & Topham, P. (2009). *Oxford desk reference: Nephrology.* Oxford University Press.

Bomback, A. S., Gilbert, S. J., Perazella, M. A., Tonelli, M., & Weiner, D. E. (2018). *National kidney foundation's primer on kidney diseases (7th ed).* Elsevier.

Bonkat, G., Pickard, R., Bartoletti, R., Cai, T., Bruyere, F., Geerlings, S.E., & Wagenlehner, F. (2018). *EAU guidelines on urological infections.* Retrieved from Urology Web: https://uroweb.org/wp-content/uploads/EAU-Guidelines-on-Urological-Infections-2018-large-text.pdf

Capriotti, T. (2020). *Pathophysiology introductory concepts and clinical perspectives.* F.A. Davis Company.

Floege, J., Barbour, S.J., Cattran, D.C., Hogan, J.J., Nachman, P.H., Tang, S.C., . . . Rovin, B.H. (2020). Management and treatment of glomerular diseases (part 1): Conclusions from a kidney DISEASE: Improving global outcomes (KDIGO) controversies conference. *Nephrology, 24*(2), 22-41. doi:10.36485/1561-6274-2020-24-2-22-41

Gilbert, S. & Weiner, D. (2013). *Primer on kidney diseases* (6th ed.). Elsevier.

Hobbs, A.L., Shea, K.M., Daley, M..J., Huth, R.G., Jaso, T.C., Bissett, J., & Hemmige, V. (2016). Are first-generation cephalosporins obsolete? A retrospective, non-inferiority, cohort study comparing empirical therapy with cefazolin versus ceftriaxone for acute pyelonephritis in hospitalized patients. *Journal of Antimicrobial Chemotherapy*, *71*(6), 1665-71. doi:10.1093/jac/dkw03

Johnson, J. R., & Russo, T. A. (2018). Acute pyelonephritis in adults. *New England Journal of Medicine*, *378*(1), 48-59. https://doi.org/10.1056/nejmcp1702758

Kasper, D.L., Longo, D.L., Fauci, A.S., Hauser, S.L., Jameson, J.L., & Loscazo, J. (2015). *Harrison's principle of internal medicine.* (19th ed.). McGraw-Hill Medical.

LeBlond, R., Brown, D., & DeGowin, R. (2020). *DeGowin's diagnostic examination* (11th ed.). McGraw Hill Professional.

Lotti, T., & Porena, M. (Eds.). (2004). *Physiopathology, medical therapy and prevention of urinary lithiasis.* Club of Urinary Lithiasis, Florence. https://doi.org/10.1159/isbn.978-3-318-01079-4

Maier, R. & Katsufrakis, P.J. (2015). Sexually transmitted diseases. In South-Paul, J.E., Matheny, S.C. & Lewis E.L. (Eds.), *Current diagnosis & treatment: Family medicine (4th ed.).* McGraw-Hill

Marshall, K. & Hale, D. (2017). Urinary tract infections. *Home Healthcare Now, 35*(8), 448–449. doi:10.1097/NHH.0000000000000597.

Michels, T.C., & Sands, J.E. (2015). Dysuria: Evaluation and differential diagnosis in adults. *American Family Physicians*, *92*(9), 778-86.

Moe, O. W. (2006). Kidney stones: pathophysiology and medical management. T*he Lancet, 367*(9507), 333-344. doi:10.1016/s0140-6736(06)68071-9

National Kidney Foundation. (2020). *Chronic kidney disease (CKD) symptoms and causes.* Retrieved from National Kidney Foundation: https://www.kidney.org/atoz/content/about-chronic-kidney-disease

Papadakis, M.A., McPhee, S.J., & Bernstein, J. (2019). Cystitis, acute (urinary tract infection). *Quick medical diagnosis & treatment, 2020.* McGraw Hill.

Papadakis, M.A., & McPhee, S.J. (2019). *Current medical diagnosis & treatment. 58th Edition.* McGraw Hill Education.

Pearle, M. S., & Lotan, Y. (2012). Urinary lithiasis. *Campbell-Walsh Urology*, 1257-1286.e9. https://doi.org/10.1016/b978-1-4160-6911-9.00045-1

Pearson, R. & Williams, P. (2014). Common questions about the diagnosis and management of benign prostatic hyperplasia. *American Family Physician, 90*(11), 769-774.

Sayammagaru, S. (2017). *Pyelonephritis.* Retrieved from Med India: https://www.medindia.net/patientinfo/pyelonephritis.htm

Schaeffer, E. M. (2018). Re: Acute pyelonephritis in adults. *Journal of Urology*, *200*(2), 226-226. https://doi.org/10.1016/j.juro.2018.05.029

Stone, C. K., & Humphries, R. L. (2017). *Current diagnosis and treatment emergency medicine (8th ed.).* McGraw Hill Professional.

Ceftriaxone: Drug Information. In: Up to Date, Post W (Ed), *UpToDate*, Waltham, MA. Accessed May 26, 2021

Vallerand, A., & Sanoski, C. (2019). *Davis' drug guide for nurses* (16th ed.). F.A. Davis.

Wang, S., Zhang, Y., Zhang, X., Tang, Y., & Li, J. (2020). Upper urinary tract stone compositions: The role of age and gender. *International Brazilian Journal of Urology, 46*(1), 70-80. https://doi.org/10.1590/s1677-5538.ibju.2019.0278

Whitaker, D.L., Hatcher, P.A., Talavera, F., & Kim, E.D. (2020). *Urethritis.* Retrieved from Medscape: https://emedicine.medscape.com/article/438091-overview

Xiang, H., Han, J., Ridley, W. E., & Ridley, L. J. (2018). Bear paw sign: Xanthogranulomatous pyelonephritis. *Journal of Medical Imaging and Radiation Oncology*, 62, 56-56. https://doi.org/10.1111/1754-9485.04_12784

Chapter 10

Becker, J.D. (2018). *Pediatric allergic rhinitis*. Retrieved from Medscape: https://emedicine.medscape.com/article/889259-overview

Bermas, B.L., & Smith, N.A. (2018). *Pregnancy in women with systemic lupus erythematosus*. Retrieved from UpToDate: https://www.uptodate.com/contents/pregnancy-in-women-with-systemic-lupus-erythematosus

Centers for Disease Control and Prevention. (2019). *Welcome to the HIV risk reduction tool.* Retrieved from Centers for Disease Control and Prevention: https://wwwn.cdc.gov/hivrisk/what_is/stages_hiv_infection.html

Cho, C., Covar, R. A., Fleischer, D. M., & Boguniewicz, M. (2016). Allergic disorders. In R. R. Deterding, R.R., Hay, W.W., Levin, M.J., & Abzug, M.J. (Eds.), *Current diagnosis & treatment: Pediatrics* (23rd ed., pp. 1147-1149). McGraw-Hill Education.

Dailey, A.F., Hoots, B.E., Hall, I., Song, R., Hays, D., Fulton, P., ...Valleroy, L.A. (2017). Vital signs: Human immunodeficiency virus testing and diagnosis delays - United States. *Morbidity and Mortality Weekly Report, 66*(47), 1300-1306.

Greer, F.R., Sicherer, S.H. & Burks, A.W. (2019) The effects of early nutritional interventions on the development of atopic disease in infants and children: The role of maternal dietary restriction, breastfeeding, hydrolyzed formulas, and timing of introduction of allergenic complementary foods. *American Academy of Pediatrics, 143*(4), e20190281. https://doi.org/10.1542/peds.2019-0281

Gupta, R.S., Warren, C.M., Smith, B.M., Blumenstock, J.A., Jiang, J., Davis, M.M., & Nadeau, K.C. (2018). The public health impact of parent-reported childhood food allergies in the United States. *Pediatrics, 142*(6), e20181235. doi:10.1542/peds.2018-1235

Marcel, C. (2019).Food allergies. *CINAHL Nursing Guide*, EBSCO Publishing, Ipswich, MA

March,P. & Holle, M. (2018). HIV Infection during pregnancy. *CINAHL Nursing Guide,* EBSCO Publishing, Ipswich, MA

Pravikoff D, (2018). Systemic Lupus Erythematosus and Pregnancy Complications. *CINAHL Nursing Guide*, EBSCO Publishing, Ipswich, MA

2020.United States Census Bureau. (2019). *Quick facts (2015 and 2016 estimates).* Retrieved from United States Census Bureau: https://www.census.gov/quickfacts/fact/table/US/RHI225218

United States Department of Health and Human Services. (2019). *What are HIV and AIDS?* Retrieved from HIV.gov: https://www.hiv.gov/hiv-basics/overview/about-hiv-and-aids/what-are-hiv-and-aids

United States Preventive Services Task Force. (2019). Screening for HIV Infection: US preventive services task force recommendation statement. *Journal of the American Medical Association, 321*(23), 2326–2336. doi:10.1001/jama.2019.6587

Al Abound, A.M. & Nigam, P.K. (2020). Wart. *StatPearls [Internet].* StatPearls Publishing. Retrieved from National Center for Biotechnology Information: https://www.ncbi.nlm.nih.gov/books/NBK431047/

American Cancer Society (2020). *Survival rates for melanoma skin cancer.* Retrieved from American Cancer Society: https://www.cancer.org/cancer/melanoma-skin-cancer/detection-diagnosis-staging/survival-rates-for-melanoma-skin-cancer-by-stage.html

Blumberg, G., Long, B., & Koyfman, A. (2017). Clinical mimics: An emergency medicine-focused review of cellulitis mimics. *The Journal of Emergency Medicine*, *53*(4), 475-484. https://doi.org/10.1016/j.jemermed.2017.06.002

Bobonich, M. A., & Nolen, M. E. (2015). *Dermatology for advanced practice clinicians.* Wolters Kluwer.

Brown, B.D., & Hood Watson, K.L. (2019). Cellulitis. *StatPearls.* StatPearls Publishing. Retrieved from National Center for Biotechnology Information: https://www.ncbi.nlm.nih.gov/books/NBK549770/

Bruun, T., Oppegaard, O., Kittang, B.R., Mylvaganam, H., Langeland, N., & Skrede, S. (2016). Etiology of cellulitis and clinical prediction of streptococcal disease: A prospective study. *Open Forum Infectious Diseases, 3*(1), 181. https://doi.org/10.1093/ofid/ofv181

Centers for Disease Control and Prevention. (2015). Human papillomavirus (HPV) infection. Retrieved from Centers for Disease Control and Prevention: https://www.cdc.gov/std/tg2015/hpv.htm

Cranendonk, D.R., Lavrijsen, A.P.M., Prins, J.M., & Wiersinga, W.J. (2017). Cellulitis: Current insights into pathophysiology and clinical management. *The Netherlands Journal of Medicine*, *75*(9), 366-378. http://www.njmonline.nl/getpdf.php?id=1907

Ferri, F.F. (2016). *Ferri's clinical advisor: Warts.* Elsevier.

Focht, D.R., Spicer, C., & Fairchok, M.P. (2002, Oct15). The efficacy of duct tape vs cryotherapy in the treatment of verruca vulgaris (the common wart). *Archives of Pediatric and Adolescent Medicine, 156(10)*, 971-974. doi:10.1001/archpedi.156.10.971

Gilboy, J. (2012, January 3). Updated information on MRSA infections. *The Clinical Advisor*, 43-52. https://issuu.com/clinicaladvisor/docs/december2011

Gutzmer, R., Wiegand, S., Kölbl, O., Wermker, K., Hepp, M., & Berking, C. (2019). Actinic keratosis and cutaneous squamous cell carcinoma: Treatment options. *Deutsches Aerzteblatt International, 116*(37), 616–626. doi:10.3238/arztebl.2019.0616

Habif, T. P. (2016). *Clinical dermatology: A color guide to diagnosis and therapy.* (6th ed.) Mosby.

Herman Reinehr, C.P., & Bakos R.M., (2019). Actinic keratosis: Review of clinical, dermoscopic, and therapeutic aspects. *Anais Brasileiros de Dermatologia. 94*(6), 637-657. doi:10.1016/j.abd.2019.10.004

Hosking, A., Elsensohn, A., Makdisi, J., Grando, S., de Feraudy, S. (2018). Keratosis pilaris rubra with mucin deposition. *Journal of Cutaneous Pathology, 45*(12), 958-961. doi:10.1111/cup.13365

Kanani, A., Betschel, S., & Warrington, R. (2018). Urticaria and angiodema. *Allergy, Asthma & Clinical Immunology,* 14, 115-127. doi:10.1186/s13223-018-0288-z

Kemnic, T. R., & Coleman, M. (2019). Trimethoprim sulfamethoxazole. *StatPearls*. StatPearls Publishing. Retrieved from National Center for Biotechnology Information: https://www.ncbi.nlm.nih.gov/books/NBK513232/

May, D.B., Hooper, D.C., & Mitty, J. (2020). *Trimethoprim-sulfamethoxazole: An overview.* Retrieved from UpToDate: https://www.uptodate.com/contents/trimethoprim-sulfamethoxazole-an-overview

McPhee, S. J. & Papadakis, M.A. , R.A. (2019). *Current medical diagnosis & treatment. 58th Edition*. McGraw Hill Education.

Nardi, N., & Schaefer, T. (2019) Impetigo. *Stat Pearls [Internet].* StatPearls Publishing. Retrieved from National Center for Biotechnology Information: https://www.ncbi.nlm.nih.gov/books/NBK430974/

Pfizer. (2020). *CLEOCIN® HCL* capsules (clindamycin). Retrieved from Pfizer: https://www.pfizermedicalinformation.com/en-us/cleocin-hcl-capsules

Raff, A.B., & Kroshinsky, D. (2016). Cellulitis: A review. *Journal of the American Medical Association, 316*(3), 325-337. https://doi.org/10.1001/jama.2016.8825

Raff, A.B., Weng, Q.Y., Cohen, J.M., Gunasekera, N., Okhovat, J.P., Vedak, P., Joyce, C., Kroshinsky, D., & Mostaghimi, A. (2017). A predictive model for diagnosis of lower extremity cellulitis: a cross-sectional study. *Journal of the American Academy of Dermatology, 76*(4), 618-625. https://doi.org/10.1016/j.jaad.2016.12.044

Rendon, A., & Schakel, K. (2019). Psoriasis pathogenesis and treatment. *International Journal of Molecular Sciences, 20*(6), 1475. doi:10.3390/ijms2006147

Richmond, J. M., & Harris, J. E. (2014). Immunology and skin in health and disease. *Cold Spring Harbor Perspectives in Medicine, 4*(12), a015339. https://doi.org/10.1101/cshperspect.a015339

Roberts, M.C. (1996). Tetracycline resistance determinants: Mechanisms of action, regulation of expression, genetic mobility, and distribution. *FEMS Microbiology Reviews, 19*(1), 1-24. https://doi.org/10.1111/j.1574-6976.1996.tb00251.x

Schaefer, P. (2017). Acute and chronic urticaria: Evaluation and treatment. *American Family Physician, 95*(11), 717-724.

Stevens, D.L., Bisno, A.L., Chambers, H.F., Dellinger, E.P., Goldstein, E.J., Gorbach, S.L., Hirschmann, J.V., Kaplan, S.L., Montoya, J.G., & Wade, J.C. (2014). Practice guidelines for the diagnosis and management of skin and soft tissue infections: 2014 update by the Infectious Diseases Society of America. *Clinical Infectious Diseases, 59*(2), e10-e52. https://doi.org/10.1093/cid/ciu296

Sullivan, T., & de Barra, E. (2018). Diagnosis and management of cellulitis. *Clinical Medicine*, *18*(2), 160. https://doi.org/10.7861/clinmedicine.18-2-160

Summers, J.B., & Kaminski, J. (2003, November 15). Is duct tape occlusion therapy an effective treatment of warts? *American Family Physicians, 68*(10), 1912-1916.

Weber, D.J., Tolkoff-Rubin, N.E., & Rubin, R.H. (1984). Amoxicillin and potassium clavulanate: An antibiotic combination mechanism of action, pharmacokinetics, antimicrobial spectrum, clinical efficacy and adverse effects. *Pharmacotherapy: The Journal of Human Pharmacology and Drug Therapy*, *4*(3), 122-133. https://doi.org/10.1002/j.1875-9114.1984.tb03333.x

Weng, Q.Y., Raff, A.B., Cohen, J.M., Gunasekera, N., Okhovat, J.P., Vedak, P., Joyce, C., Kroshinsky, D., & Mostaghimi, A. (2017). Costs and consequences associated with misdiagnosed lower extremity cellulitis. *JAMA Dermatology*, *153*(2), 141-146. https://doi.org/10.1001/jamadermatol.2016.3816

Wolff, K., Fitzpatrick, T.B., Johnson, R.A., Roh, E., & Saavedra, A.P. (2017). *Fitzpatrick's color atlas and synopsis of clinical dermatology*. (8th ed.) McGraw Hill Education.

Zimmerman, E.E., & Crawford, J. (2012, December 15). Cutaneous cryosurgery. *American Family Physicians*, *86*(12), 1118-24.

Chapter 12

Access Medicine (2020). *Drug monographs*. Retrieved from Access Medicine: https://accessmedicine.mhmedical.com/drugs.aspx#letter=R&groupId=320&resourceIndexType=0&tab=tab0

Access Medicine. (2020). *Penicillin G benzathine*. Wolthers Kluwer.

Ader, D.N., South-Paul, J., Adera, T., & Deuster, P.A. (2001). Cyclical mastalgia: Prevalence and associated health and behavioral factors. *Journal of Psychosomatic Obstetrics & Gynecology*, *22*(2), 71-76. https://doi.org/10.3109/01674820109049956

Ameen, F., Reda, S.A., El-Shatoury, S.A., Riad, E.M., Enany, M.E., & Alarfaj, A.A. (2019). Prevalence of antibiotic resistant mastitis pathogens in dairy cows in Egypt and potential biological control agents produced from plant endophytic actinobacteria. *Saudi Journal of Biological Sciences*, *26*(7), 1492-1498. https://doi.org/10.1016/j.sjbs.2019.09.008

American Cancer Society. (2019). Cancer facts & figures 2019. Retrieved from American Cancer Society: https://www.cancer.org/research/cancer-facts-statistics/all-cancer-facts-figures/cancer-facts-figures-2019.html

American Cancer Society. (2020). *Hormone therapy for prostate cancer*. Retrieved from American Cancer Society:

https://www.cancer.org/cancer/prostate-cancer/treating/hormone-therapy.html

American College of Obstetricians and Gynecologists. (2015). Practice bulletin no 149: Endometrial cancer. (2015). *Obstetrics & Gynecology, 125*(4), 1006-1026. doi:10.1097/01.AOG.0000462977.61229.de

American College of Surgeons. (2017). *AJCC Cancer staging manual* (8th ed.). Springer International Publishing.

American Psychiatric Association. (2013). *Diagnostic and statistical manual of mental disorders* (5th ed.). American Psychiatric Publishing.

American Urological Association. (2019). Diagnostic and treatment of early stage testicular cancer: AUA Guideline (2019). Accessed from American Urological Association: https://www.auanet.org/guidelines/testicular-cancer-guideline#x14301

Bell, K.J., Del Mar, C., Wright, G., Dickinson, J., & Glasziou, P. (2015). Prevalence of incidental prostate cancer: A systematic review of autopsy studies. *International Journal of Cancer, 137*(7), 1749-1757. doi:10.1002/ijc.29538

Bermudez, A., Bhatla, N., & Leung, E. (2015). Cancer of the cervix uteri. *International Journal of Gynecology & Obstetrics, 131*(S2), S88-S95. https://doi.org/10.1016/j.ijgo.2015.06.004

Bernaldi, M., Lazzeri, L., Perelli, F., Reis, F.M., & Petraglia, F. (2017). Dysmenorrhea and related disorders. *F1000 Research, 28*(5), 24-28. doi:10.12688/f1000research.11682.1

Brkic, M., Vujovic, S., Ivanisevic, M.F., Ivovic, M., Gajic, M.T., Marina, L., Barac, M., Barac, B., Djogo, A., Malesevic, G., & Franic, D. (2016). The influence of progesterone gel therapy in the treatment of fibrocystic breast disease. *Open Journal of Obstetrics and Gynecology, 6*(5), 334-341. https://doi.org/10.4236/ojog.2016.65042

Buggio, L., Somigliana, E., Borghi, A., & Vercellini, P. (2019). Probiotics and vaginal microecology: Fact or fancy? *BMC Women's Health,* 19, 25. doi:10.1186/s12905-019-0723

Burnett, M., & Lemyre, M., (2017). Primary dysmenorrhea consensus guideline. *Journal of Obstetrics and Gynaecology Canada, 39*(7), 585-595. doi:10.1016/j.jogc.2016.12.023

Burney, R. O., & Giudice, L. C. (2012). Pathogenesis and pathophysiology of endometriosis. *Fertility and Sterility, 98*(3), 1-19. http://dx.doi.org/doi:10.1016/j.fertnstert.2012.06.029

Capriotti, T.M., & Frizzell, J.P. (2016). *Pathophysiology: Introductory concepts and clinical perspectives.* F.A. Davis.

Carter, H.B., Albertsen, P.C., & Barry, M.J. (2018). *Early detection of prostate cancer (2018).* Retrieved from American Urological Association: https://www.auanet.org/guidelines/prostate-cancer-early-detection-guideline

Centers for Disease Control and Prevention. (2015). *Pelvic inflammatory disease (PID).* Retrieved from Centers for Disease Control and Prevention: https://www.cdc.gov/std/tg2015/pid.htm

Centers for Disease Control and Prevention. (2015). *Trichomoniasis.* Retrieved from Centers for Disease Control and Prevention: https://www.cdc.gov/std/tg2015/trichomoniasis.htm

Centers for Disease Control and Prevention. (2016). *Chlamydia treatment and care.* Retrieved from Centers for Disease Control and Prevention: https://www.cdc.gov/std/chlamydia/treatment.htm

Centers for Disease Control and Prevention. (2020). *Candidiasis*. Retrieved from Centers for Disease Control and Prevention: http://www.cdc.gov/fungal/diseases/candidiasis/index.html/

Centers for Disease Control and Prevention. (2021). *Genital herpes - CDC factsheet (Detailed)*. Retrieved from Centers for Disease Control and Prevention: https://www.cdc.gov/std/herpes/stdfact-herpes-detailed.htm

Chien, J., & Poole, E. M. (2017). Ovarian cancer prevention, screening, and early detection: Report from the 11th biennial Ovarian Cancer Research Symposium. *International Journal of Gynecological Cancer: official journal of the International Gynecological Cancer Society*, *27*(S5), S20–S22. https://doi.org/10.1097/IGC.0000000000001118

Danino, M.A., El Khatib, A.M., Doucet, O., Dao, L., Efanov, J.I., Bou-Merhi, J.S., & Iliescu-Nelea, M. (2019). Preliminary results supporting the bacterial hypothesis in red breast syndrome following postmastectomy acellular dermal matrix–and implant-based reconstructions. *Plastic and Reconstructive Surgery*, *144*(6), 988e-992e. https://doi.org/10.1097/PRS.0000000000006227

Davila, G.W., Kapoor, D., Alderman, E., Hiraoka, M.K.Y., Ghoniem, G.M., & Peskin, B.D. (2018). Endometriosis clinical presentation. *Medscape Obstetric and Gynecology,* 1-27. http://emedicine.medscape.com/article/271899-overview#a1

DermNet NZ. (2009). *Fungal skin infections*. Retrieved from DermNet NZ: https://www.dermnetnz.org/cme/fungal-infections/candida-infection/

De Sanctis, V., Soliman, A., Bernasconi, S., Bianchin, L., Bona, G., Bozzola, M., …. Perissinotto, E. (2015). Primary dysmenorrhea in adolescents: Prevalence, impact and recent knowledge. *Pediatric Endocrinology Reviews,* 13(2), 465-471.

Diallo A.C., Tendeng J.N., Ndong, A., Diao, M.L., Thiam, O., Thiam, J.A., …Konate, I. (2019). Peritonitis by spontaneous rupture of ovarian dermoid cyst: A case report. *Open Scientific Journal of Surgery*. 1-3, 60-62. doi:10.36811/osjs.2019.110009

Domino, F.J., Baldor, R.A., Golding, J., & Stephens, M.B. (2019). *The 5-Minute Clinical Consult (27th ed.).* Lippincott Williams & Wilkins.

Ferri, F.F. (2019). *Ferri's clinical advisor 2019: 5 books in 1*. Elsevier.

Flobbe, K., Bosch, A.M., Kessels, A.G., Beets, G.L., Nelemans, P.J., von Meyenfeldt, M.F., & van Engelshoven, J.M. (2003). The additional diagnostic value of ultrasonography in the diagnosis of breast cancer. *Archives of Internal Medicine*, *163*(10), 1194-1199. https://doi.org/10.1001/archinte.163.10.1194

Fox, H., Walker, L.G., Heys, S.D., Ah-See, A.K., & Eremin, O. (1997). Are patients with mastalgia anxious, and does relaxation therapy help? *The Breast*, *6*(3), 138-142. https://doi.org/10.1016/S0960-9776(97)90554-3

Garcia, A.C., Viñas, M.T., Guitart, J., Cabiscol, A.A., Pareses, E.C., & Barragan, F.B. (2018, February 28). *Could contrast ultrasound replace contrast pelvic MRI in the follow-up of patients with symptomatic fibroids treated with uterine artery embolization (UAE)?* [Scientific Exhibit]. European Congress of Radiology, Vienna, Austria. http://dx.doi.org/10.1594/ecr2018/C-2750

Giuliani, E., Sawsan, A.S., & Marsh, E.E. (2020). Epidemiology and management of uterine fibroids. *International Journal of Gynecology & Obstetrics, 149*(1), 3-9. http://dx.doi.org/10.1002/ijgo.13102

Goeminne, A., Maggen, C., Timmermna, D., & Neven, P. (2019). P03 management of ovarian cysts in premenopausal women with tamoxifen. *International Journal of Gynecological Cancer, 29*(4), 1. http://dx.doi.org/10.1136/ijgc-2019-ESGO.68

Goldberg, A.E. (2018). *Benign lesions of the ovaries.* Retrieved from Medscape: https://emedicine.medscape.com/article/265548-overview#a6

Grabosch, S. (2018). *Ovarian cysts.* Retrieved from Medscape: **https://emedicine.medscape.com/article/255865-** overview#a1

Gradison, M. (2012). Pelvic inflammatory disease. *American Family Physician, 85*(8), 791-796.

Groves, M.J. (2016). Genital herpes: A review. *American Family Physician, 93*(11), 928-934.

Habibi, N., Huang, M.S., Gan, W.Y., Zulida, R., & Safavi, S.M., (2015). Prevalence of primary dysmenorrhea and factors associated with its intensity among undergraduate students: A cross-sectional study. *Pain Management Nursing, 16*(6), 855-861. doi:10.1016/j.pmn.2015.07.001

Hantsoo, L., Epperson, C.N. (2015). Premenstrual dysphoric disorder: Epidemiology and treatment. *Current Psychiatry Reports, 17*(85). https://doi.org/10.1007/s11920-015-0628-3

Harp, D. F. & Chowdhury, I. (2011). Trichomoniasis: Evaluation to execution. *European Journal of Obstetrics & Gynecology and Reproductive Biology, 157*(1), 3-9. doi:10.1016/j.ejogrb.2011.02.024

Hawkins, J.W., Roberto-Nichols, D.M., & Stanley-Haney, J.L. (2015). *Guidelines for nurse practitioners in gynecologic settings.* Springer Publishing Company.

Holland, A.C., Hodges, A., Catron., Bevis, K.S. Berman, N.R., & Meneses, K. (2016). Endometrial cancer: Using evidence to impact practice and policy. *The Journal of Nurse Practitioners, 12*(6), 395-402. https://doi.org/10.1016/j.nurpra.2016.04.006

Horner, N.K., & Lampe, J.W. (2000). Potential mechanisms of diet therapy for fibrocystic breast conditions show inadequate evidence of effectiveness. *Journal of the American Dietetic Association, 100*(11), 1368-1380. https://doi.org/10.1016/S0002-8223(00)00383-7

Hubert, R.J., & VanMeter, K.C. (2018). *Gould's pathophysiology for the health professions.* Saunders.

Iacovides, S., Avidon, I., & Baker, F.C., (2015). What we know about primary dysmenorrhea today: A critical review. *Human Reproduction Review, 21*(6), 762-778. doi:10.1093/humupd/dmv039

Jahdi, F., Tolouei, R., Samani, L. N., Hashemian, M., Haghani, H., Mojab, F., & Memarzadeh, M. (2018). Effect of evening primrose oil and vitamin B6 on pain control of cyclic mastalgia associated with fibrocystic breast changes: A triple-blind randomized controlled trial. *Shiraz E-Medical Journal*, *20*(5), e81243. https://doi.org/10.5812/semj.81243

Jeanmonod, R., & Jeanmonod, D. (2020). Vaginal candidiasis (Vulvovaginal candidiasis). In *StatPearls* [Internet]. Stat Pearls Publishing.

Jo, J., & Lee, S.H., (2018). Heat therapy for primary dysmenorrhea: A systematic review and meta-analysis of its effects on pain relief and quality of life. *Scientific Reports,* 8, 1-8. doi:10.1038/s41598-018-34303-z

Johnson, N.P., Hummelshoi, L., Adamson, G.D., Keckstein, J., Taylor, H.S., Abrao, M.S... Giudice, L.C. (2016). World endometriosis society consensus on the classification of endometriosis. *Gynecology, 32*(2), 315–324. http://dx.doi.org/10.1093/humrep/dew293

Kaganov, H., & Ades, A. (2016). Uterine fibroids: Investigation and current management trends. *Australian Family Physician, 45*(10), 722–725.

Kasper, D.L., Longo, D.L., Fauci, A.S., Hauser, S.L., Jameson, J.L., Loscazo, J. (2015). *Harrison's principle of internal medicine*. McGraw-Hill Medical.

Kuchenbaecker, K.B., Hopper, J.L., Barnes, D.R., Phillips, K.A., Mooij, T.M., Roos-Blom, M.J., …Antoniou, A.C. (2017). Risks of breast, ovarian, and contralateral breast cancer for BRCA1 and BRCA2 mutation carries. *Journal of the American Medical Association, 317*(23), 2402-2416. doi:10.1001/jama.2017.7112

Lucidi, R.S., (2019). *Polycystic ovarian syndrome.* Retrieved from Medscape: https://emedicine.medscape.com/article/256806-overview#a4

Malherbe, K., & Fatima, S. (2019). Fibrocystic Breast Disease. In *StatPearls [Internet].* StatPearls Publishing. https://www.ncbi.nlm.nih.gov/books/NBK551609/

March, P. (2018). Candidiasis, Oral (Thrush). *CINAHL Nursing Guide*, EBSCO Publishing, Ipswich, MA

Mark Lu, C., McPhee, S.J. & Nicoll, D. (2017). *Algorithms*. In Nicoll, D., Mark Lu, C., & McPhee, S.J. (Eds). *Guide to diagnostic tests (7th ed.)* McGraw-Hill.

Mattei, P.L., Beachkofsky, T.M., Gilson, R.T. & Wisco, O.J. (2012). Syphilis: A reemerging infection. *American Family Physician*, *86*(5), 433-440.

Mayor, M.T., Roett, M.A., & Uduhiri,K.A. (2012). Diagnosis and management of gonococcal infections. *American Family Physician*, *86*(10), 931-938.

McMullen, E.R., Zoumberos, N.A., & Kleer, C.G. (2019). Metaplastic breast carcinoma: Update on histopathology and molecular alterations. *Archives of Pathology & Laboratory Medicine*, *143*(12), 1492-1496. https://doi.org/10.5858/arpa.2019-0396-RA

McNamara, M. & Walsh, J. (2020). Mastalgia. In Papadakis, M.A., McPhee, S.J. & Rabow, M.W. (Eds.). *Current medical diagnoses and treatment 2020.* McGraw-Hill.

Meattini, I., Poortmans, P., Kirova, Y., Saieva, C., Visani, L., Salvestrini, V., Kim, J., Jung, W., Olmetto, E., Mariotti, M., Desideri, I., Fourquet, A., Livi, L., & Kim, K. (2019). Hypofractionated whole breast irradiation after conservative surgery for patients aged less than 60 years: A multi-centre comparative study. *Acta Oncologica*, *59*(2), 1-8. https://doi.org/10.1080/0284186X.2019.1695061

Meier, K. (2018). Male infertility differential diagnoses. Retrieved from Medscape: https://emedicine.medscape.com/article/436829-differential#1

Moy, L., Slanetz, P.J., Moore, R., Satija, S., Yeh, E.D., McCarthy, K.A., Hall, D., Staffa, M., Rafferty, E.A., Halpern, E., & Kopans, D.B. (2002). Specificity of mammography and US in the evaluation of a palpable abnormality: Retrospective review. *Radiology*, *225*(1), 176-181. https://doi.org/10.1148/radiol.2251010999

Murshid, K.R. (2011). A review of mastalgia in patients with fibrocystic breast changes and the non-surgical treatment options. *Journal of Taibah University Medical Sciences*, *6*(1), 1-18. https://doi.org/10.1016/S1658-3612(11)70151-2

National Cancer Institute SEER Program (n.d.). *Cancer stat facts: Testicular cancer.* Accessed from National Cancer Institute: https://seer.cancer.gov/statfacts/html/testis.html

National Cancer Institute SEER Program. (n.d.). *Cancer stat fact sheets: Uterine cancer.* Retrieved from National Cancer Institute: https://seer.cancer.gov/statfacts/html/corp.html

Oehninger, S., & Ombelet, W. (2019). Limits of current male infertility testing. *Fertility and Sterility, 111*(5). https://doi.org/10.1016/j.fertnstert.2019.03.005

Osafo, N., Agyare, C., Obiri, D.D., & Antwi, A.O. (2017). Mechanism of action of nonsteroidal anti-inflammatory drugs. In A. Al-Kaf (Ed.) *Nonsteroidal anti-inflammatory drugs.* http://dx.doi.org/10.5772/68090

Pappas, P.G., Kauffman, C.A., Andes, D.R., Clancy, C.J., Marr, K.A., Ostrosky-Zeichner, L., ...Sobel, J.D. (2016). Clinical practice guideline for the management of candidiasis: 2016 update by the Infectious Disease Society of America. *Clinical Infectious Diseases*, *62*(4), e1-e50. https://doi.org/10.1093/cid/civ933

Pavone, D., Turrini, I., Sorbi, F., Vannuccini, S., Capezzuoli, T., Fambrini, M., & Petraglia, F. (2019). Hormones and inflammation: An update on endometriosis. *Menstrual Cycle Related Disorders,* 177–192. http://dx.doi.org/10.1007/978-3-030-14358-9_14

Puscheck, E.E. (2020). Infertility. Retrieved from Medscape: https://emedicine.medscape.com/article/274143-overview#a1

Read, J.R., Perz, J., & Ussher, J.M. (2014). Ways of coping with premenstrual change: Development and validation of a premenstrual coping measure. *BMC Women's Health, 14*(1). doi:10.1186/1472-6874-14-1

Reed, B.G., & Carr, B.R. (2018). The normal menstrual cycle and the control of ovulation. In Feingold, K.R., Anawalt, B., Boyce, A., et al. (Eds.). *Endotext [Internet].* Medtext.com, Inc.

RelayHealth (2020) Eye conjunctivitis: chlamydial infection. https://www.summitmedicalgroup.com/library/adult_health/oph_chlamydial_conjunctivitis/

Reid, R.L. (2017). Premenstrual dysphoric disorder (Formerly Premenstrual Syndrome). In Feingold K.R.,Anawalt, B., Boyce, A, et al. (Eds). *Endotext* [Internet]. MDText.com, Inc. https://www.ncbi.nlm.nih.gov/books/NBK279045/

Rosolowich, V., Saettler, E., & Szuck, B. (2006). Mastalgia. *Journal of Obstetrics and Gynaecology Canada, 28*(1), 49-57. https://doi.org/10.1016/S1701-2163(16)32027-8

Salzman, B., Collins, E. & Hersh, L. (2019). Common breast problems. *American Family Physician, 99(8),* 505-514.

Santen, R.J. (2018). Benign breast disease in women. In Feingold, K.R., Anwalt, B., Boyce, A., et al. (Eds). *Endotext [Internet].* MDText.com, Inc. https://www.ncbi.nlm.nih.gov/books/NBK278994/

Schuiling, K.D., & Likis, F E. (2016). *Women's gynecologic health*. Jones & Bartlett Learning.

Schünemann, H.J., Lerda, D., Quinn, C., Follmann, M., Alonso-Coello, P., Rossi, P.G., Lebeau, A., Nyström, L., Broeders, M., Ioannidou-Mouzaka, L., Duffy, S.W., Borisch, B., Fitzpatrick, P., Hofvind, S., Castells, X., Giordano, L., Canelo-Aybar, C., Warman, S., Mansel, R., …Saz-Parkinson, Z. (2019). Breast cancer screening and diagnosis: A synopsis of the European breast guidelines. *Annals of Internal Medicine*, *172*(1), 46-56. https://doi.org/10.7326/M19-2125

Shetty, M.K., Shah, Y.P., & Sharman, R.S. (2003). Prospective evaluation of the value of combined mammographic and sonographic assessment in patients with palpable abnormalities of the breast. *Journal of Ultrasound in Medicine*, *22*(3), 263-268. https://doi.org/10.7863/jum.2003.22.3.263

Siegel, R.L., Miller, K.D., & Jemal, A. (2020). Cancer statistics, 2020. *A Cancer Journal for Clinicians, 70*(1),7-30. https://doi.org/10.3322/caac.21590

Simans, S.M. & Pate, K.A. (2014). Epidemiology, diagnosis, and management of polycystic ovary syndrome. *Clinical Epidemiology,* 1-30. https://www.ncbi.nlm.nih.gov/pmc/articles/PMC3872139/

Simon, A., Chang, W.Y., DeCherney, A.H. (2019). Amenorrhea. In DeCherney, A.H., Nathan, L., Laufer, N., Roman, A.S. (Eds.). *Current diagnosis & treatment: Obstetrics & gynecology (*12th ed.). McGraw-Hill.

Smith, D.S., Holderman, J.C., & Bugayong, K.T. (2020). *Trichomoniasis*. Retrieved from Medscape: https://emedicine.medscape.com/article/230617-overview#a3

Smith, G.E.C., & Burrows, P. (2008). Ultrasound diagnosis of fibroadenoma - is biopsy always necessary? *Clinical Radiology*, *63*(5), 511-515. https://doi.org/10.1016/j.crad.2007.10.015

Soo, M.S., Rosen, E.L., Baker, J.A., Vo, T.T., & Boyd, B.A. (2001). Negative predictive value of sonography with mammography in patients with palpable breast lesions. *American Journal of Roentgenology*, *177*(5), 1167-1170. https://doi.org/10.2214/ajr.177.5.1771167

Speroff, L., & Darney, P.D. (2019). *A clinical guide for contraception*. Lippincott Williams & Wilkins.

Stachs, A., Stubert, J., Reimer, T., & Hartmann, S. (2019). Benign breast disease in women. *Deutsches Ärzteblatt International, 116*(33-34), 565. https://doi.org/10.3238/arztebl.2019.0565

Stahl, S.M. (2013). *Stahl's essential psychopharmacology: Neuroscientific basis and practical applications* (4th ed.). Cambridge University Press.

Steele, G.S., Richie, J.P., Oh, W.K., & Michaelson, M.D. (2020). Clinical manifestation, diagnosis, and staging of testicular germ cell tumors. Retrieved from UpToDate: https://www.uptodate.com/contents/clinical-manifestations-diagnosis-and-staging-of-testicular-germ-cell-tumors

Stewart, C., Ralyea, C. & Lockwood, S. (2019). Ovarian Cancer: An integrated review. *Seminars in Oncology Nursing, 35*(2),151-156. doi:10.1016/j.soncn.2019.02.001

Stewart, E.A., Cookson, C.L., Gandolfo, R.A., & Schulze-Rath, R. (2017). Epidemiology of uterine fibroids: A systematic review. *British Journal of Obstetrics and Gynaecology, 124*(10), 1501–1512. doi:10.1111/1471-0528.14640

Tu, C., Ren, X., He, J., Zhang, C., Chen, R., Wang, W., & Li, Z. (2019). The value of LncRNA BCAR4 as a prognostic biomarker on clinical outcomes in human cancers. *Journal of Cancer, 10*(24), 5992. https://doi.org/10.7150/jca.35113

Unnikrishnan, A.G., Kalra, S., Purandare, V., & Vasnawala, H. (2018). Genital infections with sodium glucose cotransporter-2 inhibitors: Occurrence and management in patients with type 2 diabetes mellitus. *Indian Journal of Endocrinology and Metabolism, 22*(6), 837–842. https://doi.org/10.4103/ijem.IJEM_159_17

Vallerand, A., & Sanoski, C. (2019). *Davis' drug guide for nurses* (16th ed.). F.A. Davis.

Vane, J.R., & Botting, R.M. (1998). Mechanism of action of nonsteroidal anti-inflammatory drugs. *The American Journal of Medicine, 104*(3S1), 2S-8S. https://doi.org/10.1016/S0002-9343(97)00203-9

Vercellini, P., Somigliana, E., Vigano, P., Abbiati, A., Barbara, G., & Fedele, L. (2009). Chronic pelvic pain in women: Etiology, pathogenesis, and diagnostic approach. *Gynecological Endocrinology, 25*(3), 149–158. http://10.1080/09513590802549858

Winkler, U.H., Schindler, A.E., Brinkmann, U.S., Ebert, C., & Oberhoff, C. (2001). Cyclic progestin therapy for the management of mastopathy and mastodynia. *Gynecological Endocrinology, 15*(6), 37-43. https://doi.org/10.1080/gye.15.s6.37.43

Witchel, S., Burghard, A.C. , Tao, R.H., & Oberfield, S.E. (2019). The diagnosis and treatment of PCOS in adolescents an update. *Endocrinology and metabolism, 31*(4), 562-569. doi:10.1097/MOP.0000000000000778

World Health Organization (2019). Human papillomavirus (HPV) and cervical cancer. Retrieved from World Health Organization: https://www.who.int/news-room/fact-sheets/detail/human-papillomavirus-(hpv)-and-cervical-cancer

Youlden, D.R., Baade, P.D., Walker, R., Pyke, C.M., Roder, D.M., & Aitken, J. F. (2019). Breast cancer incidence and survival among young females in Queensland, Australia. *Journal of Adolescent and Young Adult Oncology*. Advance online publication. https://doi.org/10.1089/jayao.2019.0119

Zagouri, F., Sergentanis, T.N., Chrysikos, D., & Bartsch, R. (2013). Platinum derivatives during pregnancy in cervical cancer: A systematic review and meta-analysis. *Obstetrics & Gynecology*, 121, 337-343. doi:10.1097/aog.ob013a31827.5822

Zeiger Roni, F. (2014) *Diagnosaurus 4.0.* McGraw-Hill.

Chapter 13

AAP Committee on Fetus and Newborn and ACOG Committee on Obstetric Practice (2017). *Guidelines for perinatal care* (8th ed.). American Academy of Pediatrics and American College of Obstetrics and Gynecology.

Abramowitz, A., Miller, E.S., & Wisner, K.L. (2017). Treatment options for hyperemesis gravidarum. *Archives of Women's Mental Health*, *20*(3), 363–372. https://doi.org/10.1007/s00737-016-0707-4

Access Medicine. (2020). *Drug monographs.* Retrieved from Access Medicine: https://accessmedicine.mhmedical.com/drugs.aspx#letter=A&groupId=320&resourceIndexType=0&tab=tab0

Afreen, N., Sultana, H., & Affreen, R. (2017). Role of transvaginal sonography in the objective diagnosis of incompetent cervix. *International Archives of Integrated Medicine 4*(11), 61-75.

Al-Dughaishi, T., Al-Jabri, M.M., Al-Haddabi, A H., & Gowri, V. (2019). Trends of patients' preferences in the management of first and early second trimester pregnancy loss towards the choice of medical or surgical termination of pregnancy in a tertiary care center in Oman. *Journal of Reproduction & Infertility, 20*(1), 52-56.

Amaral, L.M., Wallace, K., Owens, M., & LaMarca, B. (2017). Pathophysiology and current clinical management of preeclampsia. *Current Hypertension Reports*, *19*(8), 61. doi:10.1007/s11906-017-0757-7

American College of Obstetricians and Gynecologists. (2018). *ACOG Practice Bulletin.* Retrieved from The American College of Obstetricians and Gynecologists: https://www.acog.org/-/media/project/acog/acogorg/clinical/files/practice-bulletin/articles/2018/11/early-pregnancy-loss.pdf

Buttaro, T. & Trybulski, J., Polgar-Bailey, P., & Sandberg-Cook, J. (2017). *Primary Care* (5th ed.). Elsevier Health Sciences.

Cunningham F., Leveno K.J., Bloom S.L., Dashe, J.S., Hoffman B.L., Casey, B.M., & Spong C.Y. (Eds.). (2018). *Williams Obstetrics (25th ed.).* McGraw-Hill.

Davis, M., & Sanders, B. (2019). Preeclampsia and future stroke risk in women: What NPs need to know. *Nurse Practitioner, 44,* 50-54. https://doi.org/10.1097/01.NPR.0000554088.97825.ad

Doyle, J., & Silber, A. (2015). Preterm labor: Role of the nurse practitioner. *Nurse Practitioner, 40*(3), 49-54. doi:10.1097/01.NPR.0000445957.28669.51

Fisher, A.L., & Nemeth, E. (2017). Iron homeostasis during pregnancy. *The American Journal of Clinical Nutrition, 106*(6), 1567S–1574S. doi:10.3945/ajcn.117.155812

Fitzpatrick, J.E., High, W.A., & Kyle, W.L. (Eds.). (2018). Urticarial and Indurated Eruptions. *Urgent Care Dermatology: Symptom-Based Diagnosis* (pp. 63-82). Elsevier.

Gatzke, N., & Johnson, L. (2014). Ectopic pregnancy: A red flag diagnosis. *The Nurse Practitioner, 39*(12), 42-47. doi:10.1097/01.NPR.0000456394.77661.8e

HER Foundation. (2019). *About hyperemesis gravidarum.* (2019). Retrieved from HER Foundation: https://helpher.org/hyperemesis-gravidarum/

Hobbins, J. (2011). Special feature: Preterm birth - A synopsis of current methods of prediction and prevention. *OB GYN Clinical Alert.* doi:10.29309/TPMJ/2019.26.05.3487

Hurst, H., & Lemoine, J. (2016). Diagnosing dermatologic conditions of pregnancy. *The Journal for Nurse Practitioners, 12*(2), e57-e58. doi:10.1016/j.nurpra.2015.08.008

Khuu, G. & Dika, C. (2017). Iron deficiency anemia in pregnant women. *Nurse Practitioner,* 42, 42-47. https://doi.org/10.1097/01.NPR.0000516124.22868.08

Klauser, C.K., & Saltzman, D. H. (2019). Gastrointestinal disorders in pregnancy. In DeCherney A.H., Nathan. L., Laufer, N., & Roma, A.S. (Eds.), *Current diagnosis & treatment: Obstetrics & Gynecology* (12th ed.) McGraw-Hill.

McParlin, C., O'Donnell, A., Robson, S.C., Beyer, F., Moloney, E., Bryant, A., … Vale, L. (2016). Treatments for hyperemesis gravidarum and nausea and vomiting in pregnancy: A systematic review. *Journal of the American Medical Association, 316*(13), 1392–1401. doi:10.1001/jama.2016.14337

Plows, J.S., Stanley, J.L., Baker, P.N., Reynolds, C.M. & Vickers, M.H. (2017). The pathophysiology of gestational diabetes. *International Journal of Molecular Sciences, 19*(11), 3342. doi:10.3390/ijms19113342

Schub, T., & Parks-Chapman, J. (2018). *Diabetes mellitus, gestational.* Retrieved from CINAHL Information Systems: https://www.ebscohost.com/assets-sample-content/Diabetes_Mellitus_Type_2.pdf

Seehusen, D.A., & Grogan, S.P. (2015). Magnesium sulfate for prevention of preterm birth. *American Family Physician, 91*(7), 444-445.

Shuiling, K.D. & Likis, F.E. (2017). *Women's gynecologic health* (3rd ed). Jones & Bartlett.

Siu, A.L. (2015). Screening for iron deficiency anemia and iron supplementation in pregnant women to improve maternal health and birth outcomes: U.S. Preventive Services Task Force recommendation statement. *Annals of Internal Medicine, 163*(7), 529–536. doi:10.7326/M15-1707

Tufail, N., Bano, N., Asif, U., & Asif, M. (2019). Cervical incompetence; Role of cervical cerclage in cervical incompetence. *Professional Medical Journal, 26*(5), 831-835. doi:10.29309/TPMJ/2019.26.05.3487

United States Preventative Services Task Force (2018). Screening for preeclampsia: Recommendation statement. *American Family Physician, 97*(2).

Chapter 14

American Psychiatric Association (2013). *Diagnostic and statistical manual of mental disorders (5th ed.).* American Psychiatric Publishing.

Capriotti, T., & Frizell, J.P. (2016). *Pathophysiology: Introductory concepts and clinical perspectives.* F.A. Davis.

Flint, A.J., & Gagnon, N. (2012). Diagnosis and management of panic disorder in older patients. *Drugs & Aging,* 20, 881–891. https://doi.org/10.2165/00002512-200320120-00002

Hirotsu, C., Tufik, S., & Andersen, M.L. (2015). Interactions between sleep, stress, and metabolism: From physiological to pathological conditions. *Sleep Science, 8*(3), 143-152. doi:10.1016/j.slsci.2015.09.002

Holt, S.R., Segar, N., Cavallo, D.A., & Tetrault, J.M. (2017). The addiction recovery clinic. *Academic Medicine, 92*(5), 680-683. doi:10.1097/acm.0000000000001480

Jacobson, S. A. (2014). *Clinical manual of geriatric psychopharmacology* (2nd ed.). American Psychiatric Publishing.

Johnson, K., & Phoenix, B. (2017). Integrative management of anxiety-related conditions. In K.R. Tusaie & J.J. Fitzpatrick (Eds.), *Advanced practice psychiatric nursing: integrating psychotherapy, psychopharmacology, and complementary alternative approaches across the lifespan.* Springer.

Kalmbach, D.A., Anderson, J.R., & Drake, C.L. (2018). The impact of stress on sleep: Pathogenic sleep reactivity as a vulnerability to insomnia and circadian disorders. *Journal of Sleep Research, 27*(6), e12710. doi:10.1111/jsr.12710

Matheson, E., & Hainer, B.L. (2017). Insomnia: Pharmacologic therapy. *American Family Physician, 96*(1), 29-35.

Miller, S. (2018). *The ASAM principles of addiction medicine.* Lippincott Williams & Wilkins.

Muza, R.T. (2015). Central sleep apnoea: A clinical review. *Journal of Thoracic Disease, 7*(5), 930-937. doi:10.3978/j.issn.2072-1439.2015.04.45

Obesity Medicine Association. (2020). *Obesity algorithm eBook presented by the Obesity Medicine Association.* Retrieved from the Obesity Medicine Association: https://obesitymedicine.org/obesity-algorithm/

Preston, J.D., Talaga, M.C., & O'Neal, J.H. (2015). *Child and adolescent clinical psychopharmacology made simple* (3rd ed.). New Harbinger Publications.

Rastegar, D.D., & Fingerhood, D.M. (2015). *The American Society of Addiction Medicine handbook of addiction medicine.* Oxford University Press.

Rhoads, J., & Murphy, P.J.M. (2015). *Clinical consult to psychiatric nursing for advanced practice.* Springer.

Shelgikar, A.V., & Chervin, R. (2013). Approach to and evaluation of sleep disorders. *Continuum: Lifelong Learning in Neurology, 19*(1), 32-49. Doi:10.1212/01.CON.0000427214.00092.0f

Stahl, S.M. (2013). *Stahl's essential psychopharmacology: Neuroscientific basis and practical applications* (4th ed.). Cambridge University Press.

Stahl, S.M. (2017). *Prescriber's guide: Stahl's essential psychopharmacology* (6th ed.) Cambridge University Press.

Takahashi, L. (2019) Neurobiology of schizophrenia, mood disorders, anxiety disorders, and obsessive-compulsive disorder. In McCance, K.L., Huether, S.E., Brashers, V.L., & Rote, N.S. (Eds.), *Pathophysiology: The biological basis for disease in adults and children* (8th ed., pp. 611-613). Elsevier.

Chapter 15

Apovian, C.M., Aronne, L.J., Bessesen, D.H., McDonnell, M.E., Murad, M.H., Pagotto, U., …Still, C.D. (2015). Pharmacological management of obesity: An Endocrine Society clinical practice guideline. *The Journal of Clinical Endocrinology & Metabolism, 100*(2), 342-362. https://doi.org/10.1210/jc.2014-3415

Armstrong, M.J., Mottershead, T.A., Ronksley, P.E., Sigal, R.J., Campbell, T.S., & Hemmelgarn, B.R. (2011). Motivational interviewing to improve weight loss in overweight and/or obese patients: A systematic review and meta-analysis of randomized controlled trials. *Obesity Reviews,* 12, 709–723. doi:10.1111/j.1467-789X.2011.00892.x

Bays, H.E., McCarthy. W., Christensen. S., Tondt, J., Karjoo, S., Davisson, L., Ng, J., Golden A. et al. (2020). Obesity Algorithm eBook, presented by the Obesity Medicine Association. www.obesityalgorithm.org. https://obesitymedicine.org/obesity-algorithm/

Blackstone, R.P. (2017). *Bariatric surgery complications: The medical practitioners essential guide.* Springer International Publishing. doi:10.1007/978-3-319-43968-6

Fruh, S. (2017). Obesity: Risk factors, complications, and strategies for sustainable long-term weight management. *Journal of the American Association of Nurse Practitioners, 29*(S1), S3-S14. doi:10.1002/2327-6924.12510

Garvey, J.F., Pengo, M.F., Drakatos,P., & Kent B.D. (2015). Epidemiological aspects of obstructive sleep apnea. *Journal of Thoracic Disease, 7*(5),920-929. doi:10.3978/j.issn.207-1439.2015.04.52

Garvey, W.T., Mechanick, J.I., Brett, E.M., Garber, A.J., Hurley, D.L., Jastreboff, A.M., …Plodkowski, R. (2016). American Association of Clinical Endocrinologists and American College of Endocrinology comprehensive clinical practice guidelines for medical care of patients with obesity. *Endocrine Practice,* 22, Suppl 3:1-203. doi:10.4158/EP161365.GL

Golden, A. (2017). Current pharmacotherapies for obesity: A practical perspective. *Journal of the American Association of Nurse Practitioners, 29*(S1), S43-S52. doi:10.1002/2327-6924.12519

Rogge, M., & Gautam, B. (2017). Biology of obesity and weight regain: Implications for clinical practice. *Journal of the American Association of Nurse Practitioners, 29*(S1):S15-S29. doi:10.1002/2327-6924.12504

Sumithran, P., Prendergast, L.A., Delbridge, E., Purcell, K., Shulkes, A., Kriketos, A., & Proietto, J. (2011). Long-term persistence of hormonal adaptations to weight loss. *New England Journal of Medicine, 365*(17), 1597-1604. doi:10.1056/NEJMoa1105816

Vallis, M., Piccinini–Vallis, H., Sharma, A.M., & Freedhoff, Y. (2013). Modified 5 As: Minimal intervention for obesity counseling in primary care. *Canadian Family Physician*, *59*(1), 27-31.

Made in United States
Cleveland, OH
06 November 2026

47762403R00262